Introduction to Crowd Management

Claudio Feliciani · Kenichiro Shimura ·
Katsuhiro Nishinari

Introduction to Crowd Management

Managing Crowds in the Digital Era: Theory
and Practice

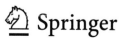 Springer

Claudio Feliciani 🆔
Research Center for Advanced Science
and Technology
The University of Tokyo
Meguro, Tokyo, Japan

Kenichiro Shimura 🆔
Industrial Research Institute for Japan Ltd.
Chiyoda, Tokyo, Japan

Katsuhiro Nishinari 🆔
Research Center for Advanced Science
and Technology
The University of Tokyo
Meguro, Tokyo, Japan

ISBN 978-3-030-90014-4   ISBN 978-3-030-90012-0   (eBook)
https://doi.org/10.1007/978-3-030-90012-0

This Springer imprint is published by the registered company Springer Nature Switzerland AG
The registered company address is: Gewerbestrasse 11, 6330 Cham, Switzerland

This book is dedicated to our parents who, despite being different in culture and customs, all helped us growing up and choose the right path unconsciously leading to the publication of this book.

Foreword

All of us participate in traffic, every day. It has become so natural that we usually do not even think about it. Therefore, one would expect that we know very well how traffic works. While this is (arguably) true for vehicular traffic, the situation is rather different for pedestrian and crowd dynamics.

So why—despite its relevance for everyday life—are several aspects of pedestrian dynamics not yet fully understood, especially on a quantitative level (compared to vehicular traffic)? And what could be done to change this?

Of course there are good reasons behind the gaps in our understanding. In contrast to vehicular traffic, pedestrian motion is truly two-dimensional with people moving in arbitrary directions. It is also much less restricted by legal rules whereas cars have to use streets, in a given direction, stay in lanes, and obey regulations, e.g., at intersections. There is also an important difference from a physics point of view. The motion of cars is very much restricted by inertia which plays little role in pedestrian motion. Pedestrians are able to accelerate, change the direction of motion, etc. almost instantaneously. Therefore, their motion is less controlled by physics, but more by psychological effects. Depending on their goals, desires, emotions, etc., pedestrians can change their state of motion very quickly, e.g., to follow the quickest path to their destination. Pedestrians are able to learn and their behavior will be influenced by previous experiences in similar situations. This makes their movement much less predictable than the motion of cars which well described by rather simple physical theories due to limited acceleration capability and the legal rules that restrict the motion.

Despite these difficulties, new techniques and approaches have allowed to make substantial progress in our understanding of pedestrian motion and crowd dynamics in recent years. Using laboratory experiments, the behavior of pedestrians could be studied in some detail, at least in relatively simple, but well-defined scenarios. Sophisticated modeling approaches, like multi-agent models, allow to incorporate much more details that are relevant for crowd motion. Last but not least, the ever-increasing capabilities of computers have made it possible to perform simulations of large crowds faster than real time thus making predictions (forecasts) possible, at least in principle.

There are other potential differences between different modes of traffic related to safety. Usually, we are aware about its risks, e.g., in cars and planes. But what about the risks in large crowds? Usually we feel rather safe, although sometimes uncomfortable. Nevertheless, we more and more hear of crowd disasters on the news, often with many injuries and even casualties. To address the problems associated, e.g., with large-scale public events, crowd control and risk management have become increasingly important. Using modern techniques both in planning and surveillance of crowd events, it has become possible to reduce the risk for participants in large crowd gatherings.

What exactly is "crowd management"? It is not just "tell people what to do, where to go", etc. Instead, it is a scientific discipline that requires an ingenious combination of very different fields in a truly interdisciplinary way. Crowds are different from pure physical systems which are similar in certain aspects as e.g. granular media. Crowds involve different persons who have their own will, goals, etc. Thus, understanding its dynamics requires the inclusion of social and psychological aspects.

In this book, the authors give a comprehensive review of the state of the art of every aspect of pedestrian dynamics and crowd motion, starting from empirical techniques for data acquisition to sophisticated modeling approaches. They put the latest scientific insights into perspective of applications, thus reducing the gap between scientists and stakeholders. Practitioners are interested in the identification and analysis of risks and methods to make crowd dynamics safer and more comfortable. They will find valuable introductions to information management, methods of crowd control and risk management which are essential tools in the planning of large events and mass gatherings.

The authors are renowned experts and have made seminal contributions to the field, ranging from theory to experiments and practical applications. Through the "Crowd Management Research Center" founded by Prof. Nishinari, they are engaged in close collaborations with practitioners in the context of crowd management. Their expertise has made them sought after advisors, e.g., for the 2020 Tokyo Olympic and Paralympic Games. Their track record makes them perfectly suited to write an insightful and wide-ranging overview of all relevant aspects of crowd dynamics and crowd management. I have learned a lot from this book, and I am sure other readers will as well!

Cologne, Germany   Andreas Schadschneider
August 2021

Preface

On May 2017, Prof. Katsuhiro Nishinari founded the "Crowd Management Research Center" with the aim to reinforce collaboration between academics and stakeholders involved in crowd management. In the three-year project, a number of meetings, workshops, site visits, and symposiums have been hold with our partner private companies. From our side, we tried to teach them the theory behind crowd dynamics and allow them to discover the latest technological trends in the discipline. At the same time, we took the opportunity to understand what are the most common problematics in the frame of crowd management and what are the solutions most typically used on a daily basis from people dealing with pedestrian traffic and crowds on-site.

This book is the result of this three-year project. On one side, we tried to summarize the theoretical knowledge accumulated in over 20 years of research on crowd dynamics based on research performed by researchers throughout the world while also including the contributions of the authors themselves. On the other side, we tried to relate this theoretical background with practical aspects involved in the daily activity of crowd management to allow readers understanding how theory can be used for practical applications. The result is a book that we hope can be of interest for people working in the field of crowd management, but also a good starting point for researchers or students approaching the field of crowd dynamics and wishing to get an overall view on this complex, interdisciplinary, and fascinating topic.

As such, this book addresses methods and technologies used in managing and controlling crowds in busy places (train stations, airports, shopping malls, exhibition halls, etc.) and during events like concerts and sport competitions by addressing fundamental aspects related to crowd management using simple concepts requiring little or no knowledge of mathematics or engineering. A large number of images and tables have been used to clearly illustrate the most important points. In addition, we structured the book in way in which theoretical notions are presented first and practical advices are given at the end to allow understanding the link between both parts.

Although this book has been conceived over this three-year project by continuous discussions between the authors, each of us took different roles in writing it. Below, the contributions of each author are listed along with a short description on their background.

Claudio Feliciani received his Ph.D. from The University of Tokyo in 2017, and he is currently working in the same institution as Project Associate Professor. Although having a background in engineering, he has always had a profound interest on social sciences. As a consequence, his research path has naturally drawn him to pedestrian traffic and crowd management where he made use of his knowledge on physics and mathematics to create new methods to assess crowd condition and develop new models for simulation. He has authored or co-authored numerous works mostly relating to crowd dynamics and traffic, but also covering animal behavior and social issues. In 2021, he shared the Ig Nobel Prize in kinetics (with Katsuhiro Nishinari among others) for having helped in the discovery that distracted pedestrians are more likely to bump into others. Beside academic research, he has also been active as a volunteer firefighter in his hometown in Switzerland for several years. In the frame of this book, he has been the main responsible in composing Chaps. 2, 4, 5 and 6. In addition, he has also been working to unify the writing style and presentation throughout the book, has helped extending the accidents accounted in the Appendix, and has prepared most of the final figures of this book.

Kenichiro Shimura is the Representative Director of Industrial Research Institute for Japan, Ltd. and is the Visiting Research Fellow at The University of Tokyo since April 2021, followed by being the Project Lecturer from 2017. He has extensive research experience in the field of crowd dynamics and safety management of crowd control for over a decade. He specializes in crowd control, simulation and safety analysis. He received a bachelor's degree (Aerospace) from The University of Glasgow, UK in 1995 and a master's degree (Automatic Control and Systems Engineering) from The University of Sheffield, UK in 1998. He then received his Ph.D. in Quantum Engineering and Systems Science from The University of Tokyo in 2003. He has been involved in various areas such as, nuclear engineering, materials science and hydrogen energy, researching the modelling and simulation by the use of Cellular Automata since then. In this book he introduces the analytical methods to assess crowd accidents, developed by him in order to help readers design appropriate planning and control of crowds to prevent crowd accident in the future. The details can be found in the academic papers published by Shimura. Chapter 3 is written by Shimura, with reflection of comments by Claudio Feliciani, who has contributed to increase the statistical samples of past accidents.

Katsuhiro Nishinari received his Ph.D. from The University of Tokyo in 1995, and he has been holding a Full Professor position in the same institution since 2009. His research interests include "jamology", which is an interdisciplinary field related to transportation and jamming phenomena including vehicular traffic, pedestrian motion, queuing networks, and supply chain by means of applied mathematics, fluid dynamics, and statistical physics. He has authored over 150 scientific publications and written several books on a variety of subjects. He his also active in cooperating with private institutions and has been a consultant for over 100 companies while also being an external advisor for the 2020 Tokyo Olympic and Paralympic Games organizing committee. For this book, he has written the original texts for Chaps. 1, 7, 8 and 9. In addition, he found the financial means to support this project and has overseen the whole work.

To summarize in a simpler form, the contributions of the single authors within this book can be listed as follows:

Chapter 1 Katsuhiro Nishinari
Chapter 2 Claudio Feliciani
Chapter 3 Kenichiro Shimura
(with contributions from Claudio Feliciani and Katsuhiro Nishinari)
Chapter 4 Claudio Feliciani
Chapter 5 Claudio Feliciani
Chapter 6 Claudio Feliciani
(with contributions from Katsuhiro Nishinari)
Chapter 7 Katsuhiro Nishinari
(with contributions from Claudio Feliciani and Kenichiro Shimura)
Chapter 8 Katsuhiro Nishinari
(with contributions from Claudio Feliciani)
Chapter 9 Katsuhiro Nishinari

Tokyo, Japan   Claudio Feliciani
August 2021

Acknowledgements

This book has been written in the frame of a project involving a close cooperation between the authors and industrial/private partners. The authors are therefore grateful to the nine companies involved in the project and would like to thank them for the precious discussions, which helped us to understand the crowd management problem from the point of view of institutions having to deal with it on a daily basis and thus allowing us to create a book combining theoretical and practical expertise. The companies taking part in the "Crowd Management Research Center" (active between 2017 and 2020) are listed as follows (in alphabetical order): ANA Holdings Inc., East Japan Railway Company, Goodfellows Co., Ltd, Kajima Corporation, Mitsubishi Electric Corporation, Narita International Airport Corporation, SECOM Co., Ltd, Tokyo Dome Corporation, and Tokyo Metro Co., Ltd.

In addition to the companies listed above, part of the research behind some contents presented in this book was also founded by the JST-Mirai Program Grant Number JPMJMI17D4 and JPMJMI20D1 and the JSPS KAKENHI Grant Number 20K14992. The authors wish to express their gratitude to the institutions that founded us and allowed us to perform the research need to better grasp important aspects of crowd motion making this publication not only possible but also more complete and accurate.

The authors would also like to acknowledge the help from the members of the Nishinari laboratory, who helped to better shape minor, but still relevant, parts of this book. In particular we would like to thank Hisashi Murakami, Xiaolu Jia, Sakurako Tanida, Daichi Yanagisawa, Takahiro Ezaki, and Satori Tsuzuki, who constantly provided feedback, support, and encouragement to the authors, allowing us to stay focused on this book. Among them a special thanks to Hisashi Murakami, who, by winning the Ig Nobel Prize (shared with Yuta Nishiyama and two authors of this book) helped spreading the awareness on crowd research to a wider audience.

We are also very grateful to our secretaries: Yuko Tsumori, En Fujimoto, Isako Tanaka, Yuriko Yokoyama, and Erika Shihara, who, not only provided administrative support, but also kept us in good spirits. In addition, we would like to thank all the students who have been part of the Nishinari laboratory during the three-years period in which the book was written for having helped organizing a number of experiments that are used as content in this book. Among them a special thanks to Akihiro Fujita and Fumitaka Sumiyama who often instructed participants to our experiments, allowing us to focus on the observation of crowd behavior. The acknowledgment is also extended to previous students, whose research topics have been of inspiration in the writing of this book, and to Enago (www.enago.jp) for the English language review of parts of this book.

Finally, we would like to thank colleagues throughout the world that helped us finding the right point of view through discussions and joint research. In particular, we are grateful to Andrea Gorrini, Andreas Schadschneider, Francesco Zanlungo, Zeynep Yücel, Luca Crociani, Akihito Nagahama, Masahiro Furukawa, Shuqi Xue, Xiaomeng Shi, Iker Zuriguel, Angel Garcimartin, Maik Boltes, Alessandro Corbetta, Jasmin Thurau, Giuseppe Vizzari, Stefania Bandini, Bastien Chopard, Leonel Aguilar, Armin Seyfried, Mohcine Chraibi, Milad Haghani, Ruggiero Lovreglio, Yu-Li Tsai, Dražen Brščic, Agnes Grisoglio, Catherine Henot, and Heinrich Marti (while also, obviously, including the people we forgot).

Contents

1   **What Is Crowd Management?**   1
    1.1   Introduction   1
    1.2   Objectives of This Chapter   3
    1.3   Definitions and Fundamental Principles of This Book   3
    1.4   Stakeholders and Crowd Information   6
    1.5   The Crowd Manager   9
    1.6   Structure of This Book   10
    References   12

2   **Crowd Properties and Characteristics**   13
    2.1   Introduction   13
    2.2   Objectives of This Chapter   15
    2.3   Qualitative Crowd Characteristics   15
        2.3.1   Types of Crowds and Classification   16
        2.3.2   Crowd Behavior Under Normal Conditions   23
        2.3.3   Crowd Behavior in Emergencies   32
    2.4   Quantitative Crowd Characteristics   36
        2.4.1   Speed, Density, and Flow   36
        2.4.2   Fundamental Diagram of Pedestrian Traffic: Theory
                 and Limitations   43
        2.4.3   Level of Service (LOS)   46
    References   48

3   **Analysis of Past Crowd Accidents**   51
    3.1   Introduction   51
    3.2   Objectives of This Chapter   52
    3.3   Crowd Incident Mechanisms   52
        3.3.1   Crowd Domino   53
        3.3.2   Crowd Avalanche   54
    3.4   Classification and Analysis of Crowd Incidents   56
        3.4.1   Causality of Crowd Incidents   56
        3.4.2   External Factors (Environmental)   58

3.4.3   Internal Factors (Crowd Intrinsic)   63
3.5   Role of Crowd Management   71
References   73

4   Pedestrian and Crowd Sensing Principles and Technologies   75
4.1   Introduction   75
4.2   Objectives of This Chapter   78
4.3   Computer Vision   79
       4.3.1   Detection and Tracking   80
       4.3.2   Optical Flow   84
       4.3.3   Density Estimation   85
       4.3.4   Advantages/Disadvantages   86
4.4   Distance Sensors   89
       4.4.1   Advantages/Disadvantages   92
4.5   Localization Technologies (GPS, Indoor Positioning, Etc.)   93
       4.5.1   Direct and Indirect User Involvement   94
       4.5.2   Advantages/Disadvantages   95
4.6   Instrumented Detection   96
       4.6.1   Mobile Network Antennas   97
       4.6.2   Bluetooth, WiFi, and RFID Tags   97
       4.6.3   Advantages/Disadvantages   99
4.7   Alternative Methods   100
       4.7.1   Gate/Transit Counting   100
       4.7.2   Manual Counting   101
       4.7.3   Estimation by Total Mass   101
       4.7.4   Thermocamera   102
       4.7.5   Inertial Sensors   103
       4.7.6   Chemosensors   104
       4.7.7   Pressure Sensors   104
4.8   Sensing Method Selection and Comparison   105
       4.8.1   Sensing Accuracy   110
4.9   Future and Emerging Trends in Sensing Technology   111
       4.9.1   Detection of Complex Patterns by Machine-Learning
               Algorithms   111
       4.9.2   Sensor Fusion   112
       4.9.3   Emotional State and Mood Detection   113
References   113

**5   Crowd Simulators: Computational Methods, Product
     Selection, and Visualization**   119
5.1   Introduction   119
5.2   Objectives of This Chapter   120
5.3   Types of Crowd Simulators and Space Representation   121
       5.3.1   Macroscopic Models   121
       5.3.2   Network Models   123
       5.3.3   Microscopic Models   124

5.4   State-of-the-Art Modeling Approaches 125
    5.4.1   The Behavioral Levels and Multiscale Simulation 125
    5.4.2   Procedural Steps in Setting up a Simulation Scenario 127
    5.4.3   Concluding Remarks 131
5.5   Typical Models Employed in Crowd Simulation 132
    5.5.1   Cellular Automata 132
    5.5.2   Social Force Model 136
    5.5.3   Network Models 139
    5.5.4   Alternative Approaches 143
5.6   Simulator Selection and Comparison 146
    5.6.1   Selection Criteria and Relevance 146
    5.6.2   Commercial Software, Code Development,
           or Outsourcing? 148
    5.6.3   Choosing a Commercial Software 150
5.7   Evaluation and Improvement of Simulation Results 150
    5.7.1   Evaluation of Simulated Motion 152
    5.7.2   Improving Simulation Results 154
5.8   Result Visualization 156
References 162

6   **Crowd Control Methods: Established and Future Practices** 167
6.1   Introduction 167
6.2   Objectives of This Chapter 171
6.3   Information Management—Laying the Fundamentals
    for an Effective Crowd Control 173
    6.3.1   Static Information Provision: Wayfinding and Its Role
           in Crowd Control 175
    6.3.2   Dynamic Information Provision: Adding the Time
           Variable to Wayfinding 189
    6.3.3   Communicating with the Crowd: Efficiently Adapting
           Style and Content 198
6.4   Physical Methods to Safely Steer Crowds—Potentials
    and Limitations 202
    6.4.1   Crowd Control Barriers (Barricades) 204
    6.4.2   Waiting Lines/Queuing Systems 205
    6.4.3   Access Gates and Ticket Control 207
    6.4.4   Flow Control and Bottleneck Effect 208
    6.4.5   Dynamic Routing and Guidance Staff 211
6.5   The "Nudge" Approach in Crowd Control 212
6.6   The "Self-Regulation" Approach 213
References 215

7 Risk Management: From Situational Awareness to Crowd Control 217
  7.1 Introduction 217
  7.2 Objectives of This Chapter 218
  7.3 Risk Definition and Approach 218
  7.4 A Framework for Risk Management in Crowds 220
       7.4.1 Off-Site Risk Management 221
       7.4.2 On-Site Risk Management 221
  7.5 Risk Assessment 222
       7.5.1 General Principles 223
       7.5.2 Risk Identification 224
       7.5.3 Risk Analysis 225
       7.5.4 Risk Evaluation 228
  7.6 Limitations and Best Practices in Risk Assessment 229
       7.6.1 Risk Assessment in Case of Sporadic Information 229
       7.6.2 Risk Assessment Using Multiple Quantities 230
       7.6.3 Choice of Numerical Values 231
       7.6.4 Best Practices and Future Trends 231
       7.6.5 Taking Special Conditions into Account 232
       7.6.6 Risk Assessment Diversification 233
       7.6.7 Risk Assessment Accounting for Secondary Elements 233
  7.7 From Risk Assessment to Crowd Control 235
  References 236

8 Planning of Mass Gatherings and Large Events 237
  8.1 Introduction 237
  8.2 Objectives of This Chapter 238
  8.3 Planning Approach 238
  8.4 Setting Conditions and Operating Modes 241
       8.4.1 Conditions 243
       8.4.2 Operating Modes 245
  8.5 Risk Assessment for Normal Operation 248
       8.5.1 Important Points to Check 252
  8.6 Risk Assessment for Abnormal Operations 253
       8.6.1 Risk Factors 255
  8.7 From Planning to On-Site Operation 258
  References 259

9 Conclusion: The Seven Knows 261

Appendix A: Historical List of Crowd Incidents 263

Glossary 297

Index 301

Acronyms

AI	Artificial intelligence
API	Application program interface
BIM	Building information modeling
BLE	Bluetooth low energy
BPM	Beat per minute
CA	Cellular automata
CAD	Computer-aided Design
CCTV	Closed circuit television
CPU	Central processing unit
DRC	Democratic Republic of the Congo
ESIM	Elaborated social identity model
GPS	Global Positioning System
HD	High definition
ISO	International Organization for Standardization
IT	Information technology
LADAR	Laser radar
LIDAR	Laser imaging detection and ranging
LOS	Level of service
LSO	Landing Signal Officer
MAC	Media access control
OD	Origin destination
RFID	Radio frequency identification
SDK	Software Development Kit
TBD	To be determined
UK	United Kingdom
USA	United States of America
USSR	Union of Soviet Socialist Republics
UUID	Universally Unique Identifier
VIP	Very important person

Chapter 1
What Is Crowd Management?

Abstract Crowds of people have been studied for more than a century, but their behavior has not been (and may possibly never be) fully understood. Nonetheless, the presence of crowds of people is becoming a dominant part of our modern civilization, and it is therefore important to find efficient ways to manage them in order to guarantee safety and comfort for people living in increasingly urbanized areas. This chapter introduces the definition of crowd management and explains the differences between managing and controlling crowds. Crowd management strategies are discussed in regard to safety and comfort, explaining how it is possible to keep a balance between both contrasting goals. In addition, the role of the stakeholders involved in crowd management is also discussed putting an emphasis on the importance of their cooperation and information sharing. In fact, success is guaranteed in crowd events or user experience maximized in large facilities (to consider some examples) only when all stakeholders work together toward a common goal. In this regard, an official responsible for crowd management, which we define as "crowd manager," should be instructed to have sufficient knowledge on crowd behavior and dynamics and act as a mediator between stakeholders to advice them on policies related to crowd management and control.

1.1 Introduction

The social nature of humans has always led to gatherings of people and crowds have been observed from the early times of civilization. In some ways, humans can be considered as social animals, which possess an individual cognition but change into a collective behavior while in group. Although understanding the collective behavior observed in animal swarms is already a difficult and challenging task, the complex social structure of humans and their abstract psychological thinking makes understanding and predicting behavior of human crowds even more difficult.

However, the need to understand crowd behavior or at least grasp some of its fundamental features has grown with the progresses of human civilization. Although crowds used to be sporadic appearances to be seen only during special occasions or in the few urbanized cities in the old times, the exploding urbanization occurring in the

© The Author(s), under exclusive license to Springer Nature Switzerland AG 2021
C. Feliciani et al., *Introduction to Crowd Management*,
https://doi.org/10.1007/978-3-030-90012-0_1

nineteenth and twentieth centuries has radically changed people's living conditions. Nowadays, crowds of people can be seen daily in train stations, airports, or other large infrastructures, and religions gatherings in densely populated areas can attract millions of people in only few days. Mobility has also seen a dramatic increase, thus adding to crowds a remarkably dynamic feature.

Research is still ongoing to understand how people behave while inside a crowd, how the crowd itself moves as a whole and which psychological state is formed by the collective bonds formed between strangers within a packed group of people. To completely understand and predict crowds, we first need to fully understand individuals, and therefore, there is still a long way to have a full understanding (and we may never have a perfect model/theory describing them). Nonetheless, human behavior in crowds has been studied for several decades (if not centuries) now and, while we do not know everything, lot has been understood through scientific research, by learning from previous tragedies and thank to a continuous feedback from people directly dealing with masses of people on a daily basis (security personnel, station staff, police, etc.). It is therefore possible to describe common phenomena and behaviors observed in crowds and, based on these, set up guidelines on how to deal with crowds and possibly control them.

This book aims at summarizing what we have learned about crowds and propose methods which can be useful to improve safety and comfort in locations experiencing congestion or related problems. Since technology increasingly plays an important role in crowd management, we gave a particular attention to technical solutions also because we believe a general understanding of technological solutions will benefit people involved with crowd management in the near future. Nonetheless, aspects related to crowd psychology and classical human intervention are also discussed, because, without neglecting the usefulness of technical solutions, crowds are unpredictable at times and, in that case, humans are usually the ones coming up with the best approaches. Also, it is very likely, that, regardless of technological improvements, at least in the near future, crowd management will be never fully automatized, thus requiring the assistance of human personnel, which, for this reason, must have an adequate understanding and preparation to be able to act in the right way.

Needless to say, this book cannot cover every aspect of crowd management since this is a multidisciplinary discipline, and there are already excellent texts considering specific aspects such as mass psychology, emergency route planning, crowd simulation, wayfinding or coping with emergencies. This book should be seen (as clearly stated in the title) as an introduction providing a sufficient and yet complete overview on all aspects involved with crowd management. People professionally involved in this area, facility managers, researchers, or interested readers may take this book as a starting point. Based on what learned here, some reader may find the need to explore more in detail one or more specific aspects discussed in this book and, in that case, specialized literature will become fundamental on the scope.

1.2 Objectives of This Chapter

This chapter aims at introducing the most fundamental principles related to crowd management, the actors involved in it, and present the general structure of this book. In particular, it is important that the reader understands how to keep a balance between safety and comfort and feels when a change in strategy is required. On that purpose, throughout the book, we will present methods to predict and control crowds' motion. While the same method may be used to achieve both the goal of safety *and* comfort, most methods are more appropriate to achieve only one goal. Thus, it is important to read this book while keeping in mind the theoretical principles introduced in this chapter on the balance between safety and comfort and understand when, how, and to which extend the focus must be gradually changed from one goal to the other.

This chapter will also outline the most relevant actors in regard to crowd management. In the same way, we will remind through the book that crowd management is never successful if conducted alone by a single person/institution and it is a team work indeed. Therefore, each of the methods presented in this book (e.g., crowd prediction/simulation and crowd control) need to be seen as a task that several actors will carry out together. In this sense, this chapter should form the foundation to construct a successful crowd management framework with the following chapters only providing the building blocks which constitute that framework. While the principles introduced in this chapter are simple and may seem even obvious, they are also easy to forget, and therefore, it is necessary to consider this chapter as the glue keeping the book (or the elements of that framework) together.

1.3 Definitions and Fundamental Principles of This Book

Let us begin by establishing the concepts behind crowd management. For the purposes of this book, crowd management is defined in the following way:

> Proactive security activities that bring safety and comfort to individuals by facilitating efficient movement of crowds

Various characteristics of crowds are discussed in the following chapters, and the term is used in the broadest possible sense of the word. Both "casual" crowds, such as those encountered when commuting, and "occasional" crowds, such as those found at events, are included in the scope of the following discussion on crowd management. In addition to moving crowds, which are more common and generally more difficult to manage, static regular crowds are often seen when people stop moving to watch sport events, during public viewing or when they line up at service counters to pass through immigration control, to check-in at airports or, again, to perform procedures at administrative offices. These types of static, accumulated gatherings are also subject to crowd management.

The topic of management being discussed regards, of course, the assembly and movement of groups of people in crowds, but this should not be considered from a simple, narrow perspective where every aspect of crowds is considered separately, but should instead be generally seen as part of a wider problem where several elements interact with each other's. Crowd management could result in deliberately restricting the movements of some groups of people in order to minimize risk and improve the overall efficiency and comfort, such as when crowds are made to leave large stadiums by seating block rather than exiting at will. To explain how this relates with the previous statement concerning the need for a wide perspective, we should note that, if each seating block is considered separately and not part of a larger structure, a simultaneous swift egress would seem as the optimal solution, but when the stadium is seen as a whole more complex and interconnected network, then benefits behind the strategy presented earlier become evident. For some people, it may take longer to leave, but congestion is reduced in the stadium, thus resulting in an overall benefit for the whole crowd.

The goal of crowd management is to ensure safety and comfort of its constituents. Avoiding stagnation and hazardous situations involving high densities of people by enabling a smooth movement of crowds helps to prevent risks. Furthermore, making movement more efficient helps to reduce wasted time, which can have great social significance. Efficient time use also increases individual comfort and enables a space to be used by more users over a single day, which is of benefit to the stakeholders involved too. Ultimately, it is important that a combination of safety and comfort is always ensured for individuals who make up a crowd, and from here on, we will examine the role of security and efficiency as necessary mechanisms for achieving this goal. Since there are many different types of crowds and because future evolution of events can be uncertain, we must be flexible in our approach.

Notoriously, a difficult problem that we face here is finding the correct balance between safety and efficiency. There is often too much emphasis placed on efficiency with the aim to improve visitors' experience, having as a result that systems that are put in place can be overwhelmed by crowds under specific conditions, which, in turn, will compromise security. Accordingly, efficiency can be considered in low-risk situations, but it is important that management systems prioritize safety when risk is high. In short, a flexible approach is necessary, in which people are able to freely move in low-risk situations, but methods and protocols are ready to be put in force when safety is under risk.

The various activities that help to achieve this flexible approach are referred to as crowd control, and this forms the core of crowd management. This topic will also be discussed in more detail in later chapters, but the key concept behind crowd control relies on accident prevention through risk management. Preventive safety measures are extremely important when trying to safeguard human lives, and obtaining a clear image on crowd's condition/state is essential when attempting to foresee and evaluate risks. If a risk is deemed to be high, it is important to use preventive crowd control in a timely manner to lower the risk level. A variety of methods of control can be

Fig. 1.1 Crowd control in response to risk and service levels

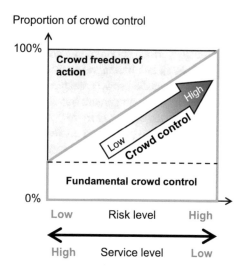

considered depending on the level of risk, from the simple information provision employing a mix of media, to compulsory guidance imposed by security staff. Furthermore, it is important to consider not only risk but also to look at the situation from the perspective of efficiency. As an example, when the number of people waiting in a line increases beyond a certain level, it is important to reduce waiting times and improve the level of service by dynamically increasing the number of service counters that are available in response. When no alternatives are available, adopting conservative measures is imperative to ensure safety, but, if enough resources are accessible, then using them straightaway in a less conservative manner is suggested since that would allow to lower risk by also ensuring an adequate level of comfort.

Figure 1.1 illustrates the general principles presented above.

In this diagram, the horizontal axis represents both risk levels and service levels, and the vertical axis represents the degree of crowd control. When risk level is low or service level is high, there is no need for special crowd control measures except, of course, for basic information provision (guidance is still required even in an almost empty building or people may get lost). This minimum and fundamental amount of crowd control is shown as the base level in the diagram. In other words, information provision should always be in place as a foundation for further crowd control, in a similar fashion to road signs (drivers could easily miss an highway exit if signs are not given and car navigation not used). When the risk level becomes elevated as the density of the crowd becomes higher, it is necessary to deploy additional crowd control measures in appropriate order. In this respect, individual freedom of behavior may need to be restricted and/or service levels reduced as necessary steps in ensuring the overall safety of the crowd.

Additionally, in emergencies such as accidents, the worst-case scenario must be assumed and consequently considered in advance. In this regard, another important part of crowd management is the prior planning that is needed to minimize damage, through such measures as ensuring that evacuation routes are secure and sufficient in number. Furthermore, during emergencies, on-site personnel need to be prepared and specifically formed to communicate with the crowd and necessary information must be provided in an efficient manner to external or third-party emergency services.

Every successful crowd management strategy should account not only for on-site, real-time crowd management but also for off-site crowd management and advance planning. In this book, we try to cover all these aspects. The concepts that we have touched upon here (including preventive flow design to identify and eliminate risks) will be described in more detail in the following chapters.

1.4   Stakeholders and Crowd Information

As already briefly stated, the key element in successful crowd management is ensuring that information is properly shared, and activities are coordinated among relevant stakeholders. There are many stakeholders when it comes to crowds; the following examples apply when organizing an event.

> Attendees, organizers, sponsors, media, firefighters, security staff, police, government officials, facility staff, transportation companies, travel agencies, local residents, etc.

From here on, we will mostly consider crowds attending an event and discuss all aspects related to their management. This choice is related to the fact that events typically involve a lot of stakeholders and attract a lot of people over a short period of time, thus representing the most complex case of crowd management. However, the concepts introduced here for the case of an event also hold true for a train station or an airport, with the exception that crowd management strategies can be improved over time by observing and analyzing crowd behavior on a daily basis (which does not eliminate the need for planning).

Coming back to the list highlighted above, we can see from this example that there are several types of stakeholder involved in crowd management. If coordination among the stakeholders does not exist, even if individual organizations are aware of their roles and come up with optimized plans, the overall plan will be only partially optimized, and it is unlikely that the individual plans will form a coherently optimized whole. If the whole plan is divided into areas of individual responsibility, it may lead to incidents involving the crowd, as we will discuss later. It is therefore important that stakeholders share information and coordinate, both during the planning stages and during the actual event. Considering the various aspects of the event as a whole allows proper decision-making about crowd management and in turn allows visitors to enjoy the event in safety and comfort.

If we look in more depth at stakeholder relationships, we can see that the general image and approach described so far is getting even more complex. For example, the primary target for crowd management at events is visitors, but local residents also have significant connections to the event since their normal routine is being affected. In this context, when scheduling an event, the traffic of visitors need to be set up so that it causes the minimum possible disruption to the daily lives of local residents. It is, however, almost impossible for an event to have no local impact at all, which means that it is necessary to establish dialog with residents and make adjustments to take their needs into account. In order to be beneficial and ensure a long-standing relationship, this communication must be a two-sided. If local residents are allowed to gain information from organizers about upcoming local events, they may be able to come up with ideas such as local festivals, flea markets or side events, adding value to the main event. However, a continuous dialogue is needed between both parties. For instance, if side events are organized by local residents without informing organizers of the main event, congestion may occur on access routes and in the worst-case emergency vehicles may not be able to enter the facility in case of accidents. To avoid such a situation and ensure that daily routine traffic, gatherings of local residents, and the flow of visitors mix in a planned, optimal, and safe way, this kind of communication and two-way information sharing is thus extremely important.

Furthermore, those who contribute financially to the organization of an event, such as investors and sponsors, are likely to have strong opinions about the planning of the event. However, single-mindedly pursuing commercial goals risks compromising crowd safety. It is of course necessary to listen to police guidance and pay attention to the law but, even if that is the case, the pursuit of profit tends to lead to underestimations of risk. If an event is held with unreasonably low margins for safety, it becomes impossible to respond to unexpected situations.

Additionally, if there are multiple organizers, the decision-making process can become unduly complicated, eventually making unclear who is responsible if something goes wrong. Accordingly, it is important for stakeholders to properly discuss the planning in advance and to establish consensus, so that each stakeholder fully understands the scope of their own responsibilities. It is essential that everyone who is involved shares the same goal, resulting in the creation of unified protocols for command and control combining all parties resources, thus eventually leading to a unified response to any expected or unexpected event. As already mentioned, it is particularly important to reach an agreement and a common vision by those stakeholders whose goal lie on both extremes in relation to safety and comfort (e.g., sponsors/investors and police/firefighters).

Next, let us look at the information that is required for proper crowd management. As shown in Table 1.1, each stakeholder has a variety of information at their disposal and will sometimes need to quickly communicate the information that they have to those who are on-site at the event. There have been many cases in which a failure to convey information to those who need it in a timely manner has led to accidents involving crowds as we will see in Chap. 3.

However, sharing this kind of information often has privacy implications, and it is important that there are rules in place for information sharing. Information that is

Table 1.1 Stakeholders and crowd information

Stakeholder	Crowd information
Visitors	Personal information (age, gender, etc.), destination, group size, scheduled arrival and travel times, etc.
Organizers	Venue information, event schedule, ticket sales, etc.
Private security companies	Location of security personnel, response protocols, CCTV locations, etc.
Police	Traffic information, data about criminal activity, etc.
Transportation companies	Timetables, transport capacity, number of vehicles, etc.
Facility operating company	Detailed facility map, venue capacity, toilet/locker locations, shop opening hours, etc.
Government	Legal regulations, data about related companies, relevant historical material, etc.
Fire and ambulance service	Evacuation sites, number of fire trucks and ambulance available, number of hospitals open, number of doctors on call, etc.
Local residents	Local events, members of residents' committees, etc.

relevant to the life and safety of those in the crowd should be shared to the maximum extent possible, but information for which prior consent for disclosure has not been obtained should be safeguarded. As it is difficult to strike a balance between security and privacy, stakeholders need to discuss the issues thoroughly and establish ground rules before a crisis occurs. At the same time, it is important to remember that it is not always possible to obtain complete information. In these instances, it is necessary to be able to manage the crowd using only the information that is available at the time and/or consider alternative methods to obtain the missing information, maybe only in part or in a summarized format.

Standardization and digitalization are needed to ensure the smooth sharing of information. Most of the times, digitization of information is particularly lacking or is available in a format that is not universally recognized and therefore not understandable by other stakeholders. Also considering that crowd control is rapidly moving toward a digitized and partially automated approach, it is therefore essential to put efforts into digital crowd information, so that communication between stakeholders is facilitated. Eventually, platforms can and should be developed to enhance crowd management in the future (possibly by also sharing part of the information with the crowd itself as we will discuss in Chap. 6).

CAD and Building Information Modeling (BIM) data are increasingly playing an important role in crowd management as they represent the starting point for simulations (as we will see in Chap. 5). Although this information is often confidential, since it reveals some vulnerable details related to venues' security, it is fundamental that at least a simplified version roughly representing the areas in which people move should be made available to organizers or related stakeholders. Such kind of data (in particularly BIM) can also help companies operating facilities to plan and schedule maintenance and identify optimal locations for security cameras and/or sensors (more in Chap. 4), thus enabling good crowd management strategies from multiple perspectives.

1.5   The Crowd Manager

Crowd management involves a variety of stakeholders who each have access to different information, and it is important that there is a central individual or organization who can make top-down adjustments in order to optimize the whole management system. Presently, this often takes the form of a person (typically in a managerial position) within the organization/company hosting the event. However, managing a crowd is a specialized job that requires extensive knowledge and experience, and it can have many implications for the lives of those who make up the crowd. Looking into the future, there is a need for certified specialists to fulfill this role. We believe that such a role should be taken by a so-called crowd manager who specializes in crowd management and makes use of her/his knowledge to act as coordinator between stakeholders to help identify lacks during planning. To some extent, this book can be taken as an effort to summarize the required knowledge for crowd managers and is intended to be used as a reference guide for the development of human resources devoted to crowd management.

It is worth noting that qualified crowd managers already exist in some countries, and their required training is substantial. In the USA, for example, any location where large numbers of people gather is required to have a crowd manager in place. As an example of this, venues such as dance halls and bars in which large crowds are common must have one crowd manager for every 250 people, and owners who violate this rule face potential jail time [1]. However, the main job for this kind of crowd manager is to guide evacuation in the event of a fire, and state fire departments provide the necessary training courses. The manager is also expected to check fire protection equipment, make sure that the venue does not exceed its capacity, and make announcements when a crisis occurs. In some countries, there are similar positions related to fire safety which partially cover these responsibilities, but it should be noted that they are slightly different to the role of crowd managers that is detailed here, and typically, only aspects related with fire prevention/extinction are covered with the "crowd" part missing in the training. In addition, venue security and police also perform many activities that are linked to the role of crowd managers although they not always possess specific knowledge on the subject (for instance police is typically trained for riots or violent scenarios, which, on the other side, are not typically within the responsibilities of crowd managers and not part of their training).

This book summarizes the knowledge that is required for successful crowd management, incorporating the latest theories and technical knowledge on the subject from academia, experience gained on-site and relevant crowd security sources from around the world.

1.6   Structure of This Book

This book covers almost all of the knowledge that is required for crowd management, and its contents and the relationship between each part are shown in Fig. 1.2. Firstly, this initial chapter defined the concept of crowd management and provided an overview of the topic.

In Chap. 2, we will learn about the characteristics of crowds and discuss various aspects of crowd psychology and crowd behavior. A deep understanding of crowds' nature forms the initial foundation for learning about crowd management.

Chapter 3 looks at historical incidents involving crowds from around the world, with particular emphasis on summarizing and classifying serious incidents that resulted in fatalities or left many people wounded. Learning about the causes of past accidents enables us to learn about common mistakes made in crowd management and helps us to consider ways to prevent the same errors being repeated.

Chapter 4 summarizes methods that can be used to detect the presence of people and thus "measure" crowds. There are many ways to do this, each with their own advantages and disadvantages. New technologies are currently being developed to help with this process and the state of the art will be reviewed as widely as possible. In doing this, we tried to explain the most important aspects avoiding details which may be difficult to understand by people without a technical background.

Chapter 5 looks at various simulation methods that have been developed in recent years as a means of attempting to predict crowd behavior. The behavior of crowds is not based on natural principles such as physics, which means that there is no unified method for predicting their actions, and various models have been proposed. These range from micro to macroapproaches, and many models are applied in real life cases around the world. It should be noted, however, that no universal almighty simulator

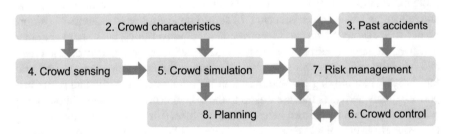

Fig. 1.2 The contents of each chapter and their relationships to each other

exists, and comparison and examination of each method/product show that they each have their own advantages and disadvantages. Also in this chapter, we tried to present the most fundamental aspects required to understand how a crowd simulator work leaving to interested readers the possibility to deepen the subject by themselves if needed.

Chapter 6 examines methods that can be used to control crowds and looks at various techniques and theories that aim to control crowd behavior according to levels of risk. When risk levels are low, techniques that range from the installation of simple, static signs to the use of dynamic signage can be implemented. Higher levels of risk require more compelling forms of crowd guidance, such as barricades. The latest research on the subject pays particular attention to using the so-called nudge theory to take a soft approach to guidance, and this chapter will summarize the various control methods that are available when aiming to minimize risk.

Chapter 7 looks at risk assessment and describes methods for assessing and classifying risk to avoid incidents when dealing with crowds. Risk assessment will be presented taking into consideration the possibilities offered by crowd simulation and sensing as described in the previous chapters.

Chapter 8 acts as a comprehensive summary of the planning topics considered so far with a particular emphasis on events that are to be planned in a short time but require a lot of attention in regard to crowd management . At the event planning stage, it is important to anticipate various sources of risk and to take steps to reduce their potential impact. It is particularly important that dangerous areas are identified and that steps are taken to plan the flow of visitors. There are also various operational constraints to consider (cost, time, safety and service level, etc.) and it is important that these factors are taken into account when designing crowd management systems.

Finally, Chap. 9 summarizes the content of this book in seven important rules (labeled the "seven knows") that should act as the fundamental principles to every crowd manager.

Depending on the location and the type of facility representing each reader's focus, one chapter may be more relevant than others. For example, when it comes to real-time, on-site crowd management, crowd sensing plays a vital role in understanding a crowd's situation, and ideally crowd behavior must be modeled in real time, using simulations that are based on this information. In such places, it is usually possible to put a certain emphasis on comfort as number of occupants is typically stable, occupants often familiar with the place and staff well acknowledged with emergency procedures. In this sense, readers interested in developing a state-of-the-art system to keep crowds under control 24-h a day all-year round may find Chaps. 4 and 5 particularly relevant on this task.

On the other side, when it comes to off-site planning (e.g., for events that takes place only for a short time, but requires extensive preparation), behavior must be predicted by using such information as the total number of expected visitors, and the estimated length of their visit. This kind of modeling can be difficult, but predictions are easier when there are a fixed number of seats available, such as stadium or ticket-based events. In this context, planning and risk assessment play the utmost important role, and flexible approaches are required in which crowd control may have to be enforced using the stricter measures. In this regard, readers who are working or focusing on such a scenario may find Chaps. 6, 7 and 8 particularly useful to them.

The above outline gives the structure of the discussion on crowd management related aspects in this book. Since each chapter is basically independent from the others, the reader may jump to the chapters that address her/his learning objectives, although following the structure of the book chapter after chapter may help to build a gradual understanding on the subject.

Reference

1. International Code Council, Inc.: International fire code (2015)

Chapter 2
Crowd Properties and Characteristics

Abstract The definition of "crowd" has been the subject of several disputes, let alone the description of its behavior and properties. Although there is no universal way to classify and describe crowds, there are some qualitative properties that can help profiling a specific crowd and manage it accordingly. In addition, there are also characteristic patterns observed when people move in large groups. Knowing them and be able to recognize them can help predicting the way people move in a given environment. Moreover, in more than a century of research on mass psychology and related fields, several theories have emerged to explain how people switch from an individual identity to a shared one when inside a crowd. Although this sort of theories had been originally developed spurred by scientific/academic interest, a number of applications have been developed and are rapidly emerging based on these theories. Understanding them can therefore help in managing crowds and the most important ones will be presented in this chapter. Nonetheless, without neglecting the importance to understand crowds qualitatively, technological development is pushing toward the need to define crowds in a numerical, quantitative way. We will therefore discuss how crowds can be measured and what are the most important quantities used in crowd management. Density, speed, and flow which represent the foundation of quantitative crowd management will be presented and discussed in detail along with the related fundamental diagram and Level of Service (LOS).

2.1 Introduction

The concept of "crowd" has always fascinated intellectuals and general public. In particular, researchers have been trying to understand how a simple, large group of people can turn into a crowd behaving with their own dynamics and when the members of a crowd "lose" their individuality in favor of a collective mindset. Crowds have also become an important topic of research after the historical events of the twentieth century, when leaders employed increasingly large crowds as a weapon to strengthen their power (with the opposite situation when crowds have challenged established leadership being also true) [1]. As research on crowds progressed, it became evident that defining a crowd and its properties is essential for a critical and structured approach. The earliest definitions of crowd were very theoretical but later definition took into account the more practical aspects.

Many crowd theories have been proposed over the years. However, no single theory can explain the phenomena observed during crowd events (and no such theory may be established in the foreseeable future). More than a hundred years of discussion and research on the topic have helped clarify the need to analyze and manage crowds and the cognitive processes transforming individuals once inside a large group of people.

The study of crowds has also been considerably influenced by historical events and technological improvements. In the '60s, when the memory of the large wars of the 20th century was still alive and globalization was an emerging phenomenon, people were mostly interested in the sociological aspects of crowds: How and why does an individual transition to a collective mindset when people gather in large groups? Why is this phenomenon particularly strong in some crowds compared to others? Moreover, with regard to tragic events, how does panic spread across escaping crowds (currently, it is believed that panic does not occur or that it occurs only in rare cases, as will be discussed later)? At the same time, more practical problematics emerged in increasingly congested cities. As mass transportation evolved with the construction of metro, tram, and bus lines, people started to move around cities in large numbers. As a consequence, more practical questions arose: How to design transportation facilities from the perspective of pedestrian users? How to define building criteria that can ensure both comfort and safety?

Because of the technological limitations and the historical context, the initial research (in the early twentieth century) on crowds mainly adopted a qualitative perspective, with some simple numerical norms appearing in the late '50s and early '60s. However, with the rapid improvements in computer technology and the decreasing costs of video components, collecting numerical data on pedestrian and crowd movements became easier. Nowadays, in the digital era where a large amount of data is available, research on crowd has taken a predominantly quantitative approach. Because of the ease of counting people, tracking their positions, and more recently, even measuring their emotional states as well as the possibility of employing machine learning approaches to analyze data, a quantitative approach is better suited.

However, the rapid development toward a quantitative approach has led to a partial neglect of crowd theories and qualitative aspects. While crowd management definitely requires quantitative data that can help performing automated tasks, crowd managers also need to be familiar with qualitative aspects to understand how the crowd theory concepts are turned into numbers. In addition, qualitative aspects related to crowd management, such as sociological theories, are an important tool to help understand crowds in new situations going beyond previous experiences or to prepare for something new.

To partially reflect the historical approach of crowd research and management and to enable a better understanding of the topics presented, this chapter will start with the discussion of the qualitative aspects of crowd behavior and then delve into the quantitative aspects.

2.2 Objectives of This Chapter

This chapter is intended to build a theoretical basis of crowd behavior and characterization/profiling. Readers may find little practical applications related to the contents of this chapter, but a sufficient understanding of the topics presented herein will help widen one's view on crowds and better contextualize the discussion of the whole book.

In particular, after reading this chapter, it should become clear that every crowd is different and should be approached in a different way. This chapter will also provide some methods and tools that can be used to schematically analyze and categorize crowds so that when preparing for a new event, crowd managers need to obtain only some information on the participants in advance and can build a profile based on that information.

Despite the increasing sophistication of crowd and group theories and their ability to explain numerous crowd phenomena, their understanding will not ensure that everything can be predicted and will not help crowd managers manage crowds at their will (as history shows some people have the gift to move crowds at their will, but most are helpless when situations get out of control). However, some knowledge of crowd theories and other theoretical aspects can surely help when planning crowd events and understand why certain approaches work while others do not.

For example, the increasingly adopted "self-policing" management approach is a direct application of a particular crowd theory (the self-categorization theory).

Another example of the use of crowd theories is the fundamental diagram of traffic flow—this diagram, which is based on a mathematical theory, is often employed in traffic management. Since the figures for pedestrian traffic used in norms and regulations are based on this diagram, learning how and why is it employed can help understand the validity and limitations of norms and can help identify situations in which it is necessary to adopt limits well below the ones set in constructional codes.

2.3 Qualitative Crowd Characteristics

As stated earlier in the introduction, the qualitative aspects of crowd behavior represent the basis for understanding several phenomena observed during crowd events and in public spaces. Crowd theories and qualitative observations cannot explain everything, and people dealing with crowds on a daily basis may have already gained an empirical knowledge enabling them to understand most aspects. However, knowledge of the theoretical and qualitative aspects of crowds can help widen one's viewpoint and build a structured way of thinking, thus also influence practical aspects related to crowd management.

In this section, we will start by defining the concept of "crowd" and various types of crowds along with their characteristics. Later, we will discuss aspects of crowd behavior by distinguishing between normal conditions and evacuations. We will learn that the latest trend in research is to disregard past theories related to crowd behavior in emergencies and assume that the behavior is not very different from that in normal situations; however, as some differences do occur between normal situations and emergencies, it is convenient to analyze both situations differently. In this regard, it is also important to remember that in normal situations, comfort can be prioritized, but safety becomes of utmost importance during emergencies.

2.3.1 Types of Crowds and Classification

Let us, now, consider the definition of the term "crowd." While a theoretical definition may not be of primary importance for management purposes, it will surely help understand the main topic of this book as well as distinguish between the group of people that we consider a crowd and the group that is simply "many people." In addition, understanding different types of crowds and their classification is of utmost importance for crowd managers. Although the accuracy of the proposed categories can be discussed, it is important to remember that every crowd is different and must be managed in a different way.

2.3.1.1 Definition of "crowd"

A large number of definitions have been provided for the concept "crowd." Providing all of them would simply create a long list of lookalike definitions. It is, therefore, better to focus on the common elements among them. In general, most scholars and researchers seem to agree that a crowd, in order to be defined as such, should contain all of the following elements [2, 3]:

- **Size**: The number of people must be sufficiently large; however, there is no agreement on what is the minimum size of a crowd. Clearly a minimum of two people is necessary, although a small number of individuals tend to be considered as groups, and only large groups are eligible to be defined as a crowd.
- **Density**: People need to be close enough to become a crowd. Generally, it can be assumed that a necessary condition is that people are face to face so that direct communication is possible. If a large number of people is spread over an immense surface, it is unlikely they will behave in a collective way.
- **Time**: The interval during which the members interact must not be very short. Literature suggest that to form a crowd, individuals should come together as a group in a specific location for a measurable amount of time. Short casual encounters are, therefore, excluded from the term "crowd."
- **Collectivity**: Individuals must share a social identity if they are to be thought of as a true "crowd." Here, collectivity is intended in terms of social identity, including goals, interests, and behaviors.

- **Novelty**: A unique aspect of a crowd is that they act in a socially coherent manner without any prior awareness, or communication, of group norms, and values. In short, in a crowd, individuals should come together in an unfamiliar or ambiguous situation and yet should be able to act as a united mass.

2.3.1.2 Types of Crowds

Each crowd is different, and therefore, it is important to distinguish different types of crowd in order to successfully prepare for, manage, and act toward it at a given time.

Both in the academic and the crowd management communities, attempts to define the types of crowd are limited. Stakeholders seem to consider only crowds typical for them (e.g., police is mostly concerned with demonstrators; music event organizers, with ravers; and building constructors, with evacuating crowds). Hence, there is a need for a universal classification of crowd types. In the following paragraphs, we will present three attempts to define types of crowds, each based on a different approach and adopting a different perspective.

Zeitz [4] defined three types of crowd by using the mood as a distinguishing element. According to Zeitz, there are fundamentally three types of crowd according to their moods (see Table 2.1): passive, active, and energetic. Passive crowds do have a collective component and present the minimal conditions to be considered a crowd. However, their degree of involvement is rather limited. Active crowds show more involvement, but their mood is expressed to a moderate extent. Energetic crowds are considerably immersed into an event, and they may exhibit violent actions if their mood is altered in a sudden and unexpected way.

Table 2.1 Crowd types based on their moods according to Zeitz [4]

Crowd type	Characteristics
Passive	• Little or no talking • Little or no physical movements • Little or no physical contact • Little or no audience participation • Cooperative
Active	• Moderate degree of talking • Moderate degree of physical movements • Moderate degree of physical contact • Moderate degree of audience participation • Cooperative
Energetic	• Considerable degree of talking • Considerable degree of physical movements • Considerable degree of physical contact • Considerable degree of audience participation • May turn into episodes of violence

In a less structured (but historically relevant) approach, Momboisse [5] distinguishes four types of crowds:

- **Casual crowds**: Crowds that are neither organized nor unified and that comprise of individuals who simply are in the same place at the same time.
- **Conventional crowds**: Crowds comprising people who have gathered for a specific purpose or to observe a specific event and where the people share common interests.
- **Expressive crowds**: Crowds the comprise people involved in some form of expressive behavior, but not disruptive behaviors; for example, crowds with dancing or singing members.
- **Aggressive hostile crowds**: Crowds that are unorganized and lack unity, but comprise members who are willing to be induced into disorder and unlawful behavior.

The most commonly used labels for crowds are the ones proposed by Berlonghi [6], who identifies crowds into 11 types as listed in Table 2.2.

Regardless of the categories used, note that many crowds are usually composed of numerous small crowds, each of which can be considered to have its own "personality" and social identity. Therefore, crowd types of the "subcrowds" should be also considered, and the differing personalities and social identities must be simultaneously managed if an event is to be effectively supervised.

2.3.1.3   Characteristics of Crowds

Given the fundamental elements required to define a crowd as such and the different types of crowds, Berlonghi proposes a list of characteristics (Table 2.3) that allow categorizing crowds from a rather theoretical perspective. Despite the theoretical nature, this approach is useful when profiling a particular crowd and preparing for an event.

More practically, the properties characterizing a specific crowd and defining its behavior may be considered from a dual perspective: internal (or intrinsic crowd) properties and external (or environmental) properties. External properties, strictly speaking, are relative to the environment surrounding a crowd and not to the crowd itself. However, the crowd and the environment are so closely related that the external properties must be considered along the internal properties of the crowd. Hence, we decided to include environmental properties in this chapter although its focus is, strictly speaking, on the crowd itself. The internal and external properties are presented separately in Tables 2.4 and 2.5 to highlight the differences. As we will see in the next chapter, this differentiation can further help when analyzing past accidents, although when accidents are concerned external properties also play a crucial role.

The combination of each of the characteristics listed in Tables 2.4 and 2.5 may contribute to characterizing crowds according to the previously presented types. For example, a large crowd composed mainly of young men who gather in a scarcely lit area at night with the purpose of watching a football game presents the most common

Table 2.2 Types of crowds according to Berlonghi [6]

Type of crowd	Description	Example
Ambulatory	A crowd entering or exiting a venue, walking to or from access points or around the venue to use its facilities	Casual crowds observed in transportation facilities or crowds moving to an event's venue
Motion limited	A crowd where people have limited or restricted mobility to some extent	Crowds comprising people with walking, visual, speaking, or hearing impairments; this may also include tourists in a foreign country
Cohesive Spectator	A crowd watching an event that they have come to see at the location or that they happen to discover once at the location	People attending public live viewing in theaters, concerts, or cinemas
Expressive Revelous	A crowd engaged in some form of emotional release	People attending an open-air music festival or fans watching a sport event
Participatory	A crowd participating in the actual activities at an event	Professional performers (such as idol groups), athletes or members of the audience invited on stage
Aggressive Hostile	A crowd which becomes abusive, threatening, boisterous, and potentially unlawful and disregards instructions from officials	Escalating crowd during a political demonstration or violent protesters during a strike
Demonstrator	A crowd, often with a recognized leader, organized for a specific reason or event, to protest, demonstrate, march, or chant	People peacefully demonstrating for political, environmental, or other reasons
Escaping Trampling	A crowd attempting to escape from real or perceived danger or life-threatening situations, including people involved in organized evacuations, or chaotic pushing and shoving by a panicking mob	People escaping a fire during an emergency, office workers taking part in an evacuation drill or people running away from a violent fight between hooligans
Dense Suffocating	A crowd in which people's physical movements rapidly decreases (eventually leading to a complete stop) due to high crowd density, resulting in serious injuries and fatalities	The crowds that form during the accidents described in the following chapter
Rushing Looting	A crowd whose main aim is to obtain, acquire, or steal something, often causing damage to property, serious injuries, or fatalities	People rushing during special sales, trying to get the best seats, or wishing to get an autograph from or a picture with a famous star
Violent	A crowd attacking, terrorizing, or rioting with no consideration for the law or the rights of other people	Organized crime groups or hooligans having little or no interest in the actual event but aiming to disrupt public order

Table 2.3 Theoretical characteristics of crowds according to Berlonghi [6]

Characteristic	Behavioral indicators
Organization *How organized is the group?*	• A demonstrator crowd is likely to be highly organized • An ambulatory crowd is likely to be unorganized • A revelous or cohesive crowd may organize themselves spontaneously
Leadership *How established is the leadership?*	• A spectator crowd will have no leadership • A demonstrator crowd will have a prespecified leader • An escaping crowd being evacuated will have clear leadership, whereas an escaping crowd being panic mobbed will not • Leadership roles for groups of rival fans at sporting events may develop spontaneously
Cohesiveness *Have members of the crowd bonded with each other?*	• Members of an expressive crowd are likely to form close bonds and may turn on rival crowds, either playfully or with harmful intent
Unity of purpose *Is the crowd united for a common purpose?*	• A participatory crowd often has a clear purpose, e.g., running a marathon
Common motive for action *Are crowd members united in their motives for action?*	• An expressive crowd chanting at a key moment in a football match has the common motive of encouraging their team and distracting the opposition
Psychological unity *Is the crowd psychologically united?*	• A participatory crowd has a strong sense of psychological unity because its members are all performing or working together • A demonstrator crowd is likely to be psychologically united • A spectator crowd at a charity concert or event to raise social awareness is likely to be psychologically united
Emotional intensity *Is the crowd emotionally intense?*	• Depends on the nature and purpose of the event, e.g., emotional intensity is likely to be high at sporting event finals or play-offs
Volatility *Has the crowd reached an explosive point?*	• Decided by whether people are acting as responsible individuals or as reckless members of a crowd, indicating the potential for disorder
Individual behavior *How much individual control and responsibility do people express?*	• A crowd is characterized by individual behavior when crowd members exercise responsibility for their own actions and for the actions of other crowd members
Group behavior *To what extent are individuals dominated by the group?*	• Individuals highly dominated by the group act with little self-awareness, low self-consciousness, and little sense of responsibility
Degree of lawlessness *How much criminal activity is taking place?*	• Throwing objects, damaging property, fighting, and pushing and shoving are all indicative of a lawless crowd
Level of violence *How violent is the crowd?*	• This can be based on both a historical assessment of previous incidents and current observations of crowd behavior
Level of property damage *How much damage to property is likely to occur?*	• The extent of likely damage can be anticipated by reviewing damage at previous events of similar nature, with a similar crowd or at the same location
Likelihood of injuries and deaths *How likely are injuries and deaths?*	• This depends on the event type and location. For instance, the age, condition and design of certain venues influence the likelihood of accidents • Escaping, rushing, dense, or violent crowds are also more likely to suffer injuries or even deaths

Table 2.4 Practical characteristics of crowds considering internal (or intrinsic crowd) properties

Characteristic	Explanation
Size *How large is the crowd?*	This is the total number of individuals comprising a crowd. Large crowds may have to be split and considered separately.
Demographic *What is the composition of the crowd?*	Age and gender are among the most relevant factors. Depending on the context, the cultural background may also be relevant.
Size of unit *How is the crowd subdivided?*	Can the crowd be considered as composed of singleton individuals or are groups a dominant part of it? Crowds where families or small groups represent a significant portion will show peculiar behaviors.
Mobility *Will mobility be limited by the presence of disabled people?*	How many of the members have limited mobility, and what kind of impairment do they have? Both physical and mental disabilities can affect mobility of the crowd.
Level of fitness / Health status *How fit are the individuals?*	Health status generally varies from individual to individual, but heat, cold, fatigue, or heavy physical activity (e.g., dancing) will affect most of the people and need to be considered.
Emotional state / Mood *What is the mood of the crowd?*	This can be also evaluated considering the criteria presented earlier while discussing crowd types.
Level of membership identification *How much do individuals recognize themselves as part of the crowd?*	Commuters will have a low level of membership identification; general public viewing a sports live event, a middle level; and organized hooligans, a high level.
Level of personal interaction *How likely is that people will interact with each other?*	For people attending an opera concert, the level of interaction will be low, whereas in the case of rock concerts, a higher level of personal interaction is likely.
Homogeneity *Can every part of the crowd be considered equivalent?*	Crowds in stadia behave differently depending on the seating location and proximity to organized fan areas. Fond fans tend to occupy places closer to the stage.
Familiarity *Are individuals familiar to the place?*	People familiar to a place will move according to precise patterns, while unfamiliar people are likely to get lost.
Luggage / Baggage *Do luggage represent an issue?*	How many people carry luggage? Do they represent a large part of the crowd? What kind of baggage is it?
Degree of intoxication *Are people under the influence of drugs?*	Alcohol, in particular, can have an adverse effect on crowd behavior. Some people may arrive already drunk, thus requiring special consideration.
Motivation / Purpose *What is the reason for people to gather?*	Highly motivated individuals gathering for a specific purpose will behave differently from casual crowd passing in a train station.
Dwell time *How long will the crowd stay in the same location?*	It may be possible to distinguish between a transit crowd (e.g., commuters), a shortly stopping crowd (e.g., a passerby looking at an event), and a staying crowd (e.g., concert fans).

Table 2.5 Practical characteristics of crowds considering external (or environmental) properties

Characteristic	Explanation
Location and boundaries *Where do individuals gather?*	Is the location delimited by a boundary, or is it an open location? Is it in a rural or an urban context? Is it a residential, business, or industrial area?
Geometry *What is the specific geometry of the location?*	Are there bottlenecks? Are there internal connections between areas? Is there a "center" or an area that is more important than others?
Time (of the day) *What part of the day is considered?*	Crowds are more difficult to manage during night or during events where there is a transition from daylight to artificial light.
Type of location / event *Which kind of event is being held?*	Presence of music or light shows and the noise generated are of particular relevance.
Media / society relevance *Do the location/event have a strong importance in media or society in general?*	The presence of an important person in an almost unknown event can change its nature. Also, some places may have particular significance to certain people because of cultural/social reasons (e.g., a religious place).
Historical meaning / significance *Is there a bond between the crowd and the location/event?*	Football fans will behave differently if they believe a stadium will bring "bad luck" to them because of previous defeats or if a match is relevant to the tournament's ranking.
Weather *How is the weather (and its forecast)?*	Both temperature and the presence of rain/snow will strongly affect crowd behavior. People may not be prepared for abrupt weather changes.
Specific operation *Are there external operations which could affect crowd dynamics?*	Transportation, parking, ticket selling, or admission control are only some of the components related to how a location is controlled and the crowd managed. Crowd behavior in a well-managed location can be affected by bad external operation (e.g., delays in connecting trains or full parking).

traits of spectator or expressive crowds, but they could turn into an aggressive or even violent crowd under particular circumstances such as alcohol intoxication and/or defeat of the team supported. A male-only idol band performing a concert in the same location, would attract a different crowd, possibly, mostly composed of young females. Even if the participating members are different from the crowd considered earlier, we may still categorize it as a spectator or expressive crowd. However, the difference in gender and purpose shifts the critical nature of that crowd, thus making a possible transition into a suffocating or a looting crowd the main concern; for example, if fans try to get as close as possible to the stage during an autograph signing session.

Finally, last but not least, it is fundamental to recognize that every crowd is characterized by a dual nature and it is composed of both a physical and a psychological component. This distinction allows considering different aspects of crowd behavior and safety, which will be presented later.

By the term "physical crowd," we simply imply a group of people in the same location. Considering crowds as physical entities is necessary for engineering purposes, when dimensions and design of pedestrian space has to be computed. However, the merging of people, each with their own personal identity but united by a common social identity as members of a particular category leads to the formation of a "psychological crowd." This dimension of crowds is relevant to understand collective behaviors and decision-making in groups of people.

Understanding the psychological dimension of crowds is important; however, collective behavior does not always occur, and in most of the cases, crowds are merely physical, in the sense that members still behave as individuals while in the presence of others. In this sense, we could state that pedestrian places need to be designed considering the physical space occupied by individuals, but crowds need to be managed taking into account their psychological dimension.

Each crowd may combine both aspects in different proportions. For example, commuters in a train station may be considered merely from their physical perspective. On the other hand, we may consider an online community as a crowd with no physical dimension. However, note that under specific circumstances, any physical crowd may rapidly turn into a psychological crowd, for example, in the case of an emergency, and it is, therefore, important to be ready to manage it appropriately.

2.3.2 Crowd Behavior Under Normal Conditions

Since early twentieth century, theories were proposed to explain different collective behaviors observed in crowds and to formulate solutions to prevent the outbreak of violence and unlawful actions. Now, there are several theories to explain different aspects of crowd and group dynamics, each with its own strengths and limitations, and listing all of them would go beyond the scope of this book.

To ensure an overall understanding of various approaches to study crowd behavior, in this section, we describe the most common behavior observed in crowds first and then present the most well-known crowd theories explaining them. Among crowd theories, we have included both the ones that had a big influence on the perception of crowds among the general public and the ones that are nowadays considered the most relevant to explain observed behaviors. Finally, we will discuss how crowds can be influenced in general terms.

2.3.2.1 Individual Behaviors of People in Crowds and Emerging Self-organization Phenomena

One of the key factors to contextualize crowd behavior and understand why crowds show peculiar characteristics is the behaviors and choices of single individuals.

Although the behavior of a crowd is not the mere sum of what observed in its individual components, by reviewing the typical behaviors of pedestrians, the connection with the wider crowd can be easily seen. In general, by studying the way in which individuals move and make decisions, the following observations can be made [2, 3]:

- Individuals typically try to minimize time required for and cost of their moves, which translates into avoiding congestion and maximize their speed.
- Individuals generally avoid moving in the opposite direction to the main flow and avoid taking detours. Typically, direct routes are preferred even if they are crowded.
- For most of the people, the fastest routes are the ones with the highest preference. If several routes with the same length are available, individuals typically prefer the one with the straightest section and the best line of sight, having the least changes in direction, for as long as possible.
- Attractiveness plays an additional role when routes with similar lengths are evaluated. Routes that are better lit, less noisy, or have an attractive environment are chosen if the overall tradeoff plays in favor of shorter routes.
- If not under stress for personal reasons, individuals prefer to walk at their desired and more comfortable speed, ultimately corresponding the most energy-efficient one.
- People always perform collision avoidance, trying to keep a certain distance from other pedestrians, walls, or obstacles. The faster people move, the more they try to stay away from potential obstacles.
- When there is congestion, to avoid collisions, people usually follow the person ahead of them, thus creating distinctive flow patterns (Fig. 2.1).
- If possible, people try to stay away from other individuals, or if in a group, from members not belonging to their group [7], thus filling spaces unevenly and forming clusters (Fig. 2.1). The tendency of people to perform short-cuts and minimize their efforts while moving (as discussed above) also leads to an uneven use of space and eventually to the so-called herding behavior (Fig. 2.1).
- Family members and groups of friends usually prefer to move together as a unit and should they be separated; they are likely to reform the same structure when conditions allow it. Also, groups with a specific hierarchy (e.g., parents and children) behave differently from groups without hierarchy (e.g., friends).
- People normally adapt to new situations by trial and error, and in already known situations, they act in an automatic way without reflecting on optimal strategies.
- Small groups are generally able perform cohesive, united decisions concerning direction and speed of motion even when only a few members have the information required to perform such decisions.

The above-described behaviors that are typical for individuals or small groups within a crowd have the capacity to create characteristic phenomena at the crowd level. In short, when a large number of people within a crowd behave in a particular way (and this occurs without the members being aware they are behaving in a coherent way), some emerging patterns are observed at the crowd level where people can be no more considered individually, but the crowd becomes a unique mass having its own

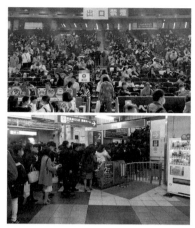
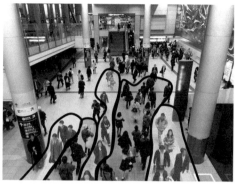

Fig. 2.1 Left: uneven space filling of crowds. In a stadium, the seats between the stairs are typically left empty as people try to minimize their effort and keep distance from the group on the other side. At the train station gate, people try to enter straight and follow people ahead of them, thus showing herding behavior and creating a large empty space next the gate. Right: typical flow patterns formed when moving in medium densities

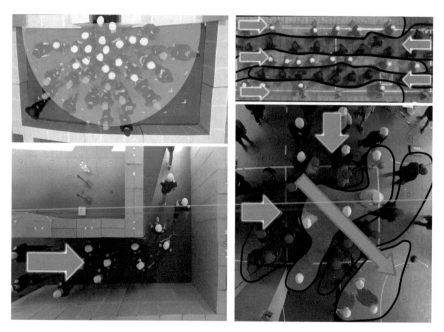

Fig. 2.2 Top-left: arch formation when people evacuate a room with a single exit. Top-right: lane formation for people walking on a sidewalk/corridor. Bottom-right: stripe formation for people walking in a two-legged crossing. Bottom-left: corner hugging for people walking in a corridor with a 90° corner

dynamics. The transition from a number of individuals behaving in an independent way from a crowd moving according to own patterns is usually defined as a self-organization phenomenon [8].

Some of the self-organization phenomena typical for collective crowd behavior are as follows:

- **"Faster is slower" effect:** This occurs when people try to pass through a bottleneck. The faster people wish to move (or the more impatient they are), the more densely the crowd is packed and the slower can individuals move.
- **Arching and clogging:** When large dense crowds push forward through a narrow exit (or bottleneck), the exit become clogged, and the crowd forms a circular shape with the exit at its center (Fig. 2.2).
- **Lane formation:** When people walk in opposite directions (e.g., in a corridor) distinct lanes are automatically formed for each direction of motion. This helps people to reduce collision with the counter-flow (Fig. 2.2). However, the stability of these lanes is hindered when the crowd density is high and people are more likely to overtake or if somebody traverses the main flow.
- **Corner hugging:** When crowds pass through a corner, people walking close to the corner will slow down to a greater extent (compared to others away from the corner), and after passing the corner, will tend to move away from it. People appear therefore to "hug" the corner (Fig. 2.2).
- **Stripe formation in two-legged crosses:** In corridors or delimited paths, when a 90° intersection is formed with two groups of people walking in perpendicular directions, stripes are formed with members of the same direction (Fig. 2.2). Stripes typically move 45° relative to each flow and do form because people attempt to minimize collisions with the other group.
- **Circular motion in four-legged crosses:** If at a given crossing, people arrive from four different directions, a circular motion is typically observed around the center as people organize themselves to reduce head-to-head collisions.
- **Jam shockwave:** When densely packed crowds attempt to move in one direction, transition is only possible by shuffle, which means that individuals can only proceed if the person in front of them proceeds. Walking is, therefore, intermittent, and a sort of shockwave (also referred as stop-and-go wave) is seen in the backward direction when observing the crowd from above.
- **Oscillations at bottlenecks:** When two large groups of people attempt to pass through a bottleneck in opposite directions, a sort of oscillation occurs between both groups. As pressure builds up in one direction, that direction will become dominant, but as pressure decreases, the opposite group will become dominant, thus reversing the direction of people passing through the bottleneck.
- **Pattern adaptation in small groups:** Self-organization phenomena are also seen in small groups within a crowd. For example, groups of two people (dyads) typically move side-by-side (defined "line abreast") at low densities but switch to a front-back (called "river-like") configuration when the densities increase. Groups of three people (triads) show a "∧" shape (with the tip oriented in the direction of

motion) when walking at low densities, but will turn into a "V" if density increases
and further change into a river-like configuration for even higher densities [9].
- **Collective intelligence:** As in the case of small groups, crowds too can efficiently
  take important decisions even if only few members have the information required
  to make those decisions. In this context, leadership plays a marginal role, but even
  when it does, it should be always considered as an emergent phenomenon. When
  an unknown situation is perceived, informed individuals are usually automatically
  recognized (or assumed) as leaders from the rest of the crowd, and the crowd will
  imitate their actions. In the crowd context, informed individuals can reach consensus regarding decisions without even knowing whether they are in the majority or
  minority, or whether the information conflicts with that of other informed members
  of the group.

2.3.2.2 Classical and Modern Crowd Theories and Their Most Important Elements

In the previous section, we explained the typical patterns formed by crowds and
showed how the behaviors of individuals in a group lead to the formation of emergent phenomena. However, the emergence of a collective identity has been not been
discussed yet. The theories presented below should help understanding this aspect.
They also represent the theoretical foundation for the sociological aspects treated in
this book. Here, only the most well known theories or the ones that are relevant for
this book are presented; for more details or less known theories readers are referred
to more specialized literature (for example the work by Challenger et al. [2, 3], which
summarizes the most relevant aspects).

Group Mind Theory

One of the earliest theories of crowd behavior was proposed by Le Bon in 1895. The
"group mind theory" of Le Bon, who was highly influential in his time, assumes that
crowd behaviors are pathological and abnormal, with savage animal instincts arising
as people gather in a group. Le Bon proposed that individuals in a crowd lose all
sense of self and responsibility and negative behaviors are transmitted as a form of
contagion.

Le Bon's theory is now widely considered inaccurate and misleading, with scientific evidence clearly showing that people are more likely to exhibit cooperative rather
than disruptive behavior when in a group. It is believed that part of the popularity of
the "group mind theory" is related to the fact that its existence legitimized repression
and allowed placing the blame on the crowd in case of accidents. In fact, according
to the theory, crowds are mindless and disruptive by nature, so people should not
gather, and if something does happen, it is the fault of the people themselves. In
short, this theory cannot be used for crowd management as it tells us nothing about
how to efficiently deal with crowds. Nonetheless, it is important to be aware of this

theory as the negative image of crowds is partly related to the lasting influence of the theory on public perception.

Deindividuation Theory

Several years later, in the 1950s, a new theory emerged to explain behavior of people when they form a part of a group: the so-called deindividuation theory. This theory still remains popular despite its demerits. The theory proposes that the normal behavioral restraints of individuals based on guilt, shame, commitment, and fear, become weakened when they are a part of a group. According to the theory, in a crowd, self-awareness and self-observation decrease, and crowd's members lose their sense of socialized individual entity. The theory further assumes that people lose their abilities to self-regulate and evaluate their own behaviors, resulting in lowered self-awareness and leading to the deindividuation of individuals (and hence, the name of the theory) as a result.

In short, partially because of arousal caused by the presence of others, the attention of group members is drawn away from themselves to focus, instead, on the group as a whole. Under such a condition, individuals are more susceptible to external cues and to the group's motives and emotions. Also, by identifying themselves as part of a group or crowd, individuals are provided with a "cloak of anonymity" that diffuses personal responsibility for actions and reduces concern for social evaluation.

As consequence, people in crowd, no longer see themselves as individuals, with proper identity and responsibility, but as an anonymous member of a collective group, they feel legitimate in behaving in a more uncivilized and antisocial manner, thus resulting in the disruptive behaviors sometimes seen in crowds.

Emergent Norm Theory

The "emergent norm theory" (proposed by Turner in the 1960s) takes a different perspective and attempts to explain how and why antisocial behaviors may emerge in crowds. This theory attempts to explain how collective action is governed by "new" norms (that is, not guided by traditional, preestablished group norms) that emerge from within the crowd.

According to this theory, when a crowd gathers, there are no clear norms indicating how to behave. The distinctive actions of the more prominent members of the crowd are attended to by the rest of the crowd and come to be seen as the characteristic of that crowd and thus act as the behavioral norms. As more crowd members follow these norms, they become more established and more influential over other members. Hence, norms typically emerge from the distinctive actions of prominent individuals within a crowd. Often, distinctive actions are the ones that are relatively rare in the lives of most individuals, for instance, antisocial behaviors. This could explain why norms which emerge are likely to be antisocial behavioral norms.

While the emergent norm theory has its own limitations (e.g., cannot explain how norms emerge in rapidly changing crowds or neglect that many people gather for specific reasons, thus already bringing a set of shared norms), it is one of the firsts assuming crowd behavior as originating from "normal" mechanisms rather than as a pathology of individuals.

Social Identity and Self-categorization Theory

From a slightly different aspect, the social identity theory (proposed by Turner in the 1970s) introduces a new concept that is still used in the analysis of crowd behaviors: the distinction between personal and social identities. According to this theory, there is a sharp distinction between the personal identity, that is, an individual's self-understanding defined in terms of one's own attributes and close relationships, and the social identity, that is, an individual's self-understanding defined in terms of one's specific group membership. Typically, every individual belongs to a variety of social groups (with associated social identities) and shifts depending on the circumstances. The same person may see himself as a football fan while watching a match in a stadium, but as a doctor when at work.

The social identity theory further proposes that as individuals, we are continually involved in three processes:

- **Categorization process:** We set a "label" categorizing ourselves and other individuals.
- **Identification process:** We associate ourselves with certain groups, known as in-groups, with whom we share a sense of identity and belonging and gain self-esteem from doing so.
- **Comparison process:** We contrast our own groups with other groups, known as out-groups, that we perceive as distinct from our in-groups.

The self-categorization theory (proposed in the 1980s) has further developed some of the concepts appearing in the social identity theory and the processes discussed above. The self-categorization theory assumes that in a group situation, individuals create a "prototype" to represent their social category, which defines and characterize the attitude, behaviors and feeling of one group (the in-group) as distinct from those of another group (the out-group). Prototypes tend to maximize the perceived differences between groups, while minimizing the perceived differences within groups. This theory assumes that when in a group, individuals behave according to the shared in-group prototype rather than their own individual characteristics.

(Elaborated) Social Identity Model of Crowd Behavior

The social identity model of crowd behavior extends the ideas of both the theories discussed above. This model was proposed by Reicher (who is called the "father" of the self-categorization theory) in the 1980s. It is one of the most modern models that explains crowd behavior and has inspired some of the latest approaches of crowd control and policing style, in particular, the so-called self-regulating (or "self-policing") approach.

As the name suggests, identity plays an important role in the identity model of crowd behavior. It argues that alongside a unique self, that is, a personal identity, each individual has a self that can be conceptualized according to his/her membership in different social groups, that is, the social identity. The social identity model, in contrast with the previous theories, proposes that when part of a crowd, individuals do not lose their identity, but simply shift from an individual to a shared social identity. Accordingly, individuals do not lose control of their behaviors, but shift from behaving in terms of their distinct, individual identities to behaving in terms of their shared social identity and its accompanying norms and values. It is also implied that, having no formal mean of communication, crowd members infer the stereotypical norms that define their group identity from the behaviors of those perceived as typical crowd member.

A direct consequence of the social identity model is that crowd behavior can be predicted by understanding social identity, and hence, we stress on crowd profiling and preparation.

The elaborated social identity model (ESIM) incorporates all the elements of the social identity model but focuses on the interaction between in-groups and out-groups and the formation of a collective identity and the resultant changes. It is believed that the way in which a group identifies themselves determines their intentions and actions. Therefore, it follows that a change in the social position during a crowd event should lead to a change in the social identity, ultimately determining the actions endorsed by a crowd.

More specifically, the ESIM believes that two features of group interaction are necessary for a behavioral change, and most likely conflict, to occur during crowd action:

- An asymmetry between the way in which the in-group (the crowd) perceive their social position and the way in which the out-group (the organization controlling the crowd) perceive the in-group's social position. For example: if the crowd views themselves as pacific protesters trying to deliver a message, while the police view them as troublesome, there is a discrepancy in the perception of the collective identity, thus increasing the likelihood of a conflict.
- An initial asymmetry of power relations between the in-group and the out-group. For example: if the out-group (e.g., the police) has the power to act against what they perceive to be illegitimate behavior of the in-group (the crowd), this will lead the police to not only view the crowd as troublesome, but also treat the crowd as such.

According to the ESIM, if the above two conditions occur during a crowd event, then the two likely consequences are as follows:

- The perception of the out-group may become a self-fulfilling prophecy. For example: if police perceive all crowd members as dangerous and act accordingly against them, the crowd is likely to unite against the hostile treatment and recognize themselves as the legitimate opposition to the police.
- Social relationships within the crowd will also be transformed. Under the circumstances of the crowd, barriers between different groups within the crowd (most notably the peaceful majority and the troublesome minority) will be overpowered by the unitary action of the crowd against the police, for example, resulting in a new more inclusive categorization where a larger number of individuals become troublesome.

A direct implication of the ESIM is that the crowd control style and force should be always adjusted to the type of crowd to avoid imbalances in perception among crowd members. This suggests that organizers (or the police) must try to facilitate and actively communicate with the crowd and differentiate between people behaving legitimately and illegitimately.

The "self-policing" approach originated from the above considerations. In this approach, the crowd itself marginalizes inappropriate behaviors, thus maintaining and reinforcing a non-violent social identity. This can only emerge if the crowd interprets organizers' (or police) actions as legitimate, i.e., facilitating rather than controlling.

Place Scripts

This relatively recent theory (originating in the 1990s) assumes that individuals typically follow rules to guide their behavior. Under normal circumstances, individuals' understanding and adherence to these rules enable them to function effectively. These rules, often represented as scripts, or sequences of behavioral patterns, allow individuals to automatically engage when in a particular environment or when experiencing a particular event. Scripts are also used to help individuals interpret the behavior of others, in addition to guiding their own behavior.

An important characteristic of these scripts is that once ingrained are remarkably resistant to change, even in extraordinary circumstances such as emergencies. Considerable effort must be applied in order to abandon their schemas.

Therefore, it can be deduced that in an emergency situation, it is unlikely that individuals will have a suitable schema to guide their actions. Consequently, they typically refer to their scripts for the particular environment under normal circumstances, despite the inappropriateness of these scripts. Thus, the more familiar people are with a particular setting, the more at risk they may actually be in emergencies.

2.3.2.3 Factors Potentially Influencing Individual Behaviors in Crowds

Now that the most important theories have been discussed, we may consider some aspects related to them and discuss the moderators affecting crowd behavior. In this regard, we should mention that all the theories considered so far and most of the discussion of this chapter consider crowds as a collective uniform mass moving as a single unit. Although social influence is a powerful force bonding people in a crowd, it can affect different people in different ways and some people more powerfully than others. In short, the crowd membership is typically not homogeneous; rather, crowds are composed of individual members, each of whom may differ in their susceptibility to such social influence. This susceptibility depends on a number of variables that can be used to moderate the effect of the crowd's social influence on the behavior of its individual members.

Two different kind of moderators can be distinguished: stable moderators and situational moderators. Stable moderators act on certain people that will always have a higher or lower level of susceptibility to social influence compared to others. On the other hand, the efficacy of situational moderators may depend on the context as the same person may be susceptible depending on the situational context. All the moderators in crowds who influence individual behavior are listed and discussed in Table 2.6.

In addition to the above factors, crowd managers should be particularly aware of the so-called triggers, i.e., elements that can turn a manageable, well-behaved crowd into an unruly, uncontrollable crowd. According to Berlonghi [6], these triggers include the following:

- Operational circumstances (e.g., event cancelation, train delay, or lack of parking)
- Event activities (e.g., loud noises or special effects)
- Performers' actions (e.g., violent or offensive gestures toward the crowd)
- Spectator factors (e.g., cheering or throwing objects)
- Security or organizers' factors (e.g., abuse of authority or excessive force)
- Social factors (e.g., rioting, gang activity, or racial tension)
- Weather factors (e.g., rain, heat, humidity, or lack of ventilation)
- Natural disasters (e.g., floods, earthquakes, or typhoons)
- Human-made disasters (e.g., structural failures or release of toxic chemicals).

2.3.3 Crowd Behavior in Emergencies

Although this book mainly focuses on managing crowds (under normal conditions), which translates into preparing for a crowd event or planning a pedestrian facility, it is also important to be aware of crowd behavior in emergencies. As seen above, some factors may trigger crowd reactions that are difficult to control, possibly leading to an emergency. Knowledge of the typical behaviors of people in emergencies may help in the event that things get worse due to unavoidable circumstances.

Table 2.6 Moderators in regard to the influence of crowds on individual behavior [2, 3]

	Description
Stable moderator	**Gender**
	There is robust scientific evidence that in general, men are more aggressive than women. It is a logical implication that crowds of men, or those that are male-dominated, are more likely to behave in an aggressive manner than crowds of women. Officials managing crowd events should, therefore, be aware of the greater potential for male-dominated crowds to behave in an aggressive manner and prepare accordingly.
	Personality
	Although little is known about how the personality traits of individual crowd members affect their susceptibility to crowd influence it is believed that (a) collectively, emotional stability, agreeableness, and conscientiousness are positively related to conformity and (b) collectively, extraversion, and openness are negatively related to conformity.
Situational moderator	**Identifiability**
	Several types of collective behaviors occur as a result of the anonymity that the presence of many other people confers upon the members. Antisocial behaviors are believed to occur because of the combined effect of arousal and anonymity. Thus, removing anonymity by making individual crowd members identifiable should counter antisocial behaviors. The use of closed-circuit television (CCTV) or spotlights for troublesome areas of a crowd may help identify as well as verify the identity of the crowd members, for example, those buying tickets for an event.
	Social identity
	Every person is simultaneously a member of multiple social groups with the salience of these different identities varying depending on the situation. Hence, collective crowd behavior that can be attributed to members sharing a common social identity is more likely to occur in environments that are more conductive to fostering a shared social identity among crowd members.
	Environmental familiarity
	People develop place scripts, or schemas, for venues or routes with which they are highly familiar, and once ingrained, these schemas are remarkably resistant to change even during emergencies. Therefore, people who are highly familiar with particular venues or routes are more likely to behave as individuals, rather than as a collective crowd. This implies that those people are not to be treated as a collective entity moving in mass.
	Intoxication
	Alcohol intoxication is known for leading to aggressive behavior via the powerful interaction of such intoxication with a masculine social identity. Under such a condition, defense of male honor often acts as a trigger. Further, reduced balance leads to erratic walking gait, increasing collisions with crowd members. Collisions represent a perceived invasion of personal space (and act as a trigger for increased violence). To address such dangers, drinking restrictions and the close monitoring of highly intoxicated members could help in managing crowds.

2.3.3.1 Relevant Theories and Facts

"Panic" is a concept that is typically used to describe a crowd's response to emergency situations. Old (and now widely disregarded) theories suggested that when faced with an emergency situation, social bonds between the members of a crowd dissolve, resulting in mindless, instinctive, irrational, and self-centered behaviors that rapidly spread through the crowd as a social contagion. The concept of panic is often cited to blame the crowd in the aftermath of a disaster, but scientific evidence shows that traditional panic theories are largely wrong and that the opposite is actually true. It is now known that behavior in emergencies and disasters has a predictable and relatively consistent set of characteristics. In many emergency situations, crowd behaviors remain fairly organized and structured, with members of the crowd exhibiting helping behaviors, alongside a collective concern and cooperation. If, in relatively rare occasions, panic does arise, it typically remains confined to individuals, as opposed to spreading through the crowd.

Some theories suggest that when faced with an emergency such as a threatening situation, individuals are motivated to move toward familiar places. This proximity to familiar places and people is thought to have a calming effect, reducing the fight-or-flight instinct. For instance, studies have found that family groups do not break down in emergencies but try to evacuate together and remain united as a group. It is also often found that alternative routes are typically overlooked or insufficiently used as individuals move toward familiar routes, generally the one normally used if people are familiar with the place or the one used for entering in the case of new users.

The most recent theories argue that crowd behavior is effectively modified by the presence of an emergency, but pro-social behaviors become stronger with helping, cooperation, and coordination displayed even among individuals who do not know each other. It is generally believed that the common experience of a threat or an emergency can transform a physical crowd into a psychological crowd, with a shared social identity. The salience of a shared social identity provides crowd members with the perceptions of unity and expectations of mutual support while also helping to reduce stress levels. In this regard, increased social support in emergencies is reported to be associated with reduced stress levels, increased optimism, and lowered levels of depression, and it also moderates possible post-traumatic stress disorders [2].

2.3.3.2 Key Factors of the Evacuation Process

In general, any evacuation can be seen as a process where three key factors are involved: interpretation, preparation, and action [2]. The evacuation time is, thus, the sum of the time necessary for the three operations—the time taken to recognize the danger (interpretation), the time taken to decide the most appropriate course of action (preparation), and the time taken for individuals to actually move toward the exit (action).

Interpretation

In the initial stage of the evacuation process, people attach meanings to the warnings issued. Therefore, communication and accessibility of information are vital for an efficient evacuation. Some even argue that systems of communication should be prioritized to the design of physical features (e.g., exit width).

Because of time pressure and other stresses, people process information in a different way during emergencies as compared to normal situations. Hence, warning must be given with regard to several important criteria. For warnings to be effective, they must be specific, comprehensible, timely, historically valid, come from a credible source, convey the nature and extent of the danger, enable rapid verification, and provide cues to help people prepare for action.

Preparation

Leader figures, belonging to the organizers or the crowd itself, play an important role preparing crowd members for evacuation. The (spatial) position of those leaders influences both the speed and accuracy of crowd movements. Careful consideration must be given to the number of individuals within the crowd who should be made aware of the location of emergency exits.

Action

Since emergencies are relatively rare, individuals are typically unfamiliar with the most appropriate form of action in such situations. Public disposition will let them believe that a situation is normal for as long as possible. Hence, people behave as usual for as long as possible, thereby delaying evacuation.

People usually behave according to scripts or schemas that are developed over time and that familiarize them with the environment. Since these schemas are very hard to break, it is vital that evacuees are provided with clear information and specific instructions [10]. A consequence of these "scripts" is that people typically prefer to leave same way as they came in. Following in terms of exit choice is usually proximity, meaning that a good distribution of emergency exits is needed to minimize the distance traveled by individuals. Finally, herding behavior is also relevant to choosing the exit as people tend to follow the majority.

The above considerations show again the importance of communication in evacuations. Timeliness, accuracy, clarity, and credibility of communication (in multiple forms as opposed to a single alarm) too are highly influential during action as well as during all phases of an evacuation.

2.4   Quantitative Crowd Characteristics

While it is important to understand the qualitative aspects of crowd behavior in order
to effectively manage large groups of people, the quantitative aspects are of primary
importance with regard to practical applications. In particular, when engineering
and technical solutions are involved, it is essential to define crowds in terms of
numbers, and therefore, we need to discuss what are the fundamental properties
quantitatively describing crowds. Most of the discussions in the upcoming chapters
will deal with the quantitative aspects of crowds, and therefore, it is essential to
introduce the most common measures. We should nonetheless remind readers that
even when measures based on crowd properties are available, the qualitative aspects
cannot be neglected. A suspicious and dangerous behavior observed in a group of
people represents a warning signal even if numbers are within tolerable limits. With
regard to the following discussion, it is essential to remind the readers that quantitative
crowd properties are simply an attempt to put into numbers what is seen qualitatively.
However, since numbers cannot always reveal every qualitative aspect, it is wise to
adopt a critical approach regarding the quality of quantitative indicators and their
limitations.

2.4.1   Speed, Density, and Flow

Pedestrian speed and density, together with the related flow, are among the most
important quantities of crowds. We will start first by considering speed and density
since they are among the simplest and yet important properties. A discussion of the
flow, which requires particular considerations, will be presented later.

2.4.1.1   Speed

Pedestrian speed simply indicates how fast a person is walking. In the case of crowds,
the speed is taken as the average value relative to the whole group of people. The
typical walking speed of pedestrians is known to change depending on a variety
of factors, but under unobstructed conditions, it generally lies in the range of 1.3–
1.5 m/s (some old texts use the units m/min instead of m/s, and km/h is almost never
used for pedestrians). When the free flow speed (under unobstructed conditions) of
a population comprising a sufficiently large number of people is measured, a normal
distribution is typically obtained (see Fig. 2.3), implying that few people walk very
fast and few very slow, and the walking speeds of most of the people lie in the
1.3–1.5 m/s range.

Some of the most relevant factors influencing walking speed and their effects are
listed in Table 2.7. For example, ambient temperature is known to have a negative
effect on walking speed, which means that when it gets warmer, people tend to walk

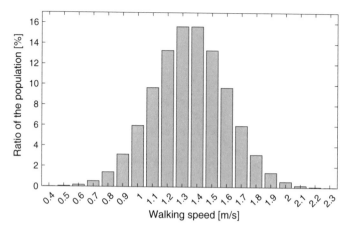

Fig. 2.3 Typical distribution of pedestrian walking speed. Most of the people usually walk at speeds of 1.3–1.5 m/s

Table 2.7 Factors influencing the walking speed of pedestrians [11–13]

Factor	Influence	Confirmed?
Age	Speed increases until about 20 years age, then decreases	Yes
Gender	Men walk faster than women	Yes
Purpose	People walking for work-related purposes walk faster than tourists	Yes
Time of the day	Changes usually observed at lunch time and in peak hours	Partially
Temperature	Faster when cold, slower when hot	Yes
Crowd density	Speed decreases with an increase in crowd density	Yes
Lifestyle	Countryside walking speed lower than that in cities	No (controversial)

slower, and on cold days, the walking speed is usually higher. Table 2.7 also provides an indicative evaluation of how certain is the relationship between a given factor and walking speed. For example, some studies showed that people in rural areas tend to walk slower compared to urban population, but there is no consensus on this particular aspect.

The influence that the steepness of the path has on walking speed needs a separate discussion. Speed clearly drops when the path gets steeper, as shown in Fig. 2.4. However, a peculiar behavior is observed for descending paths. For moderate descent rates (up to about 10%), speed increases as people need less effort to walk. However,

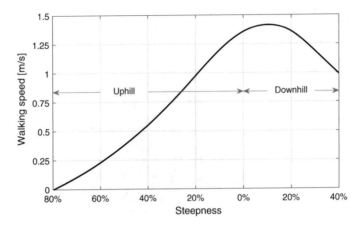

Fig. 2.4 Typical effect of path steepness on pedestrian walking speed [11]. A walking speed of 1.35 m/s is assumed here for flat surfaces (0%)

when the descent rate further increases, fear of falling becomes predominant, and people slow down to avoid accidents.

A similar behavior is observed on stairs although the slope is typically constant for most stairs with only slight variations from place to place (the angle of stairs is typically between 30° and 40°). Thus, in the case of stairs, only the ascent and descent needs to be considered (as the angle is almost constant). Walking speed is typically faster when descending, but it is interesting to observe that locations close to the wall tend to have a higher speed when descending as people get a sense of security by the presence of the handrail (they could grab it if they are about to fall down). Therefore, descending speeds in the central section of stairs tend to be comparatively small.

2.4.1.2 Density

Crowd density is simply defined as the number of people in a particular area. It is obtained by dividing the number of pedestrians by the surface area. It is typically measured in units of people per square meter and is abbreviated as person/m^2 or simply m^{-2}. In this text, we will use the m^{-2} notation (without specifying "person" every time) for simplicity.

For people who are not familiar with pedestrian traffic, the concept of crowd density might sound new, and it can be difficult to relate a particular value to a specific condition. Therefore, a few examples of densities in typical crowds observed in daily lives or during accidents may be helpful. These examples are obviously only indicative and are intended to provide an idea of the orders of magnitude observed in pedestrian crowds.

- **Less than 0.5 m^{-2} (or around 0.1 m^{-2}):** There is complete freedom of motion, and people can walk in the desired direction without having to consider other pedestrians. This condition is encountered, for example, in large uncongested public plazas or residential areas.

- **0.5–1 m^{-2}**: The freedom to determine walking speed (pace) and direction is restricted, and people need to consider others to avoid collisions. At this density, emergent behaviors such as the ones described earlier may form; for example, lanes may spontaneously form in corridors.
- **1–2 m^{-2}**: Walking at a constant speed becomes difficult, and continuous speed adjustments are required. At this density, pedestrians may partially move intermittently, but walking is still possible and there is no need to stop.
- **2–3 m^{-2}**: Continuous walking is very difficult, and progress is made by shuffling. Visual field is restricted, and judgments are only possible based on neighboring pedestrians. This condition can arise in queues or waiting areas.
- **Around 6 m^{-2}**: This is the maximum density sustainable for medium–long time. Packed trains in congested cities usually reach this value during the morning rush. Although this density represents a very unconformable level, it can be physically sustained for long periods of time. However, at this density, psychological tolerance may go beyond acceptable limits if the situation does not improve. Also, shock waves are observed in the crowd if people try to move.
- **Around 8 m^{-2}**: This is the maximum density typically reported for controlled experiments under safe conditions. Experiments under these conditions are usually performed with specially trained people (e.g., firemen or professional soldiers) under close supervision of personnel responsible for safety and only for a short time [14].
- **Over 10 m^{-2}**: At this density, causalities will occur almost certainly. This value is not uniquely defined, and sources vary regarding this physical "maximum" of crowd density. Values describing this dangerous situation are typically obtained by the analysis of video footage relative to crowd accidents (like the ones reported in the following chapter). Some authors reported densities of up to 15 m^{-2} in locations where people lost their lives [15].

Figure 2.5 also gives an idea of which condition corresponds to a particular crowd density. Further note that crowd density depends on the size of the individuals. So, in a country/region where people tend to be overweight, even low densities may already imply a congested situation. On the other hand, in countries where people tend to be smaller by constitution, a quite high density may still be considered acceptable.

A final remark regarding crowd density concerns more practical aspects related to its estimation and measurement. The images shown in Fig. 2.6 should help understand the issues that may arise in practice when crowd density needs to be estimated in large and heterogeneous areas. Since by definition, crowd density is simply people's count divided by the surface area, any surface can be used to quantify it. However, determining how large an area should be to accurately represent local density and applying this area for management purposes is not always a straightforward task [16]. As the pictures in Fig. 2.6 show, defining a density for a whole infrastructure may not be accurate. For instance, people tend to gather close to access points (entrances, exits, or gates), thus resulting in a very nonuniform density. However, when the area

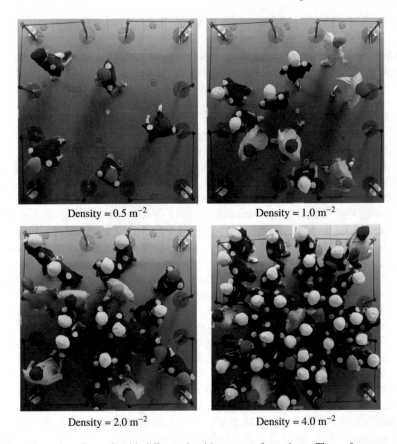

Density = 0.5 m^{-2} Density = 1.0 m^{-2}

Density = 2.0 m^{-2} Density = 4.0 m^{-2}

Fig. 2.5 Examples of crowds with different densities as seen from above. The surface area of the room used for this example was about 10 m^2 (i.e., the room had sides of roughly 3.2 m) and people wore caps of different colors; smaller colored markers were used to distinguish the shoulders

used to measure density is too small, the variations in people's count (and thus, density) could be large, and it would be difficult to monitor changes effectively.

2.4.1.3 Flow

Pedestrian flow represents the number of people transiting over a specific section in a specific time. It is typically obtained by counting the number of people passing over a particular checkpoint, which is usually a virtual line perpendicular to the motion of the crowd, and then dividing this number by the length of that line and the time taken for counting. Pedestrian flow, consequently, is expressed in units of persons per meter per second, often abbreviated as 1/(m·s) or (m·s)$^{-1}$.

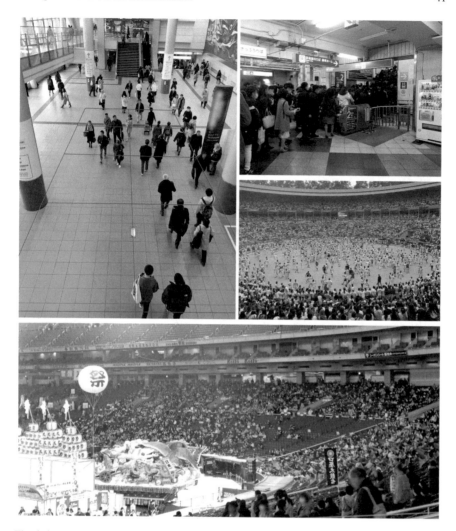

Fig. 2.6 Example of situations in which defining a correct area to count people and determine crowd density is not a trivial problem. In general, the crowd density should be representative of the situation observed and should not be too high or too low

To further clarify the concept, we can consider a real case, such as the snapshots relative to people walking in a corridor as shown in Fig. 2.7. In the 3.5 s represented in the example, 18 people transited through a 3-m section in both directions. This will consequently lead to the total flow shown below:

$$\text{Flow} = \frac{18}{3.5 \text{ s} \cdot 3 \text{ m}} = 1.71 \ (\text{m} \cdot \text{s})^{-1} \tag{2.1}$$

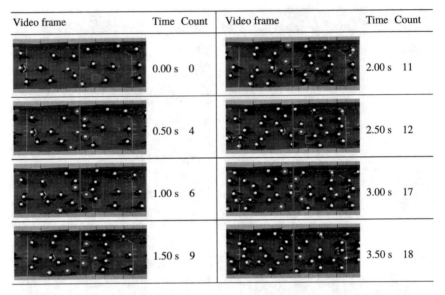

Video frame	Time	Count	Video frame	Time	Count
	0.00 s	0		2.00 s	11
	0.50 s	4		2.50 s	12
	1.00 s	6		3.00 s	17
	1.50 s	9		3.50 s	18

Fig. 2.7 Obtaining the flow of people walking in a corridor in two opposite directions. A snapshot is captured every 0.5 s, and people passing across the red line are counted between consecutive snapshots (only people who completely cross the line are counted). Red circles indicate the counted people. The corridor width is 3 m. Thus, the resulting flow is 1.71 $(m \cdot s)^{-1}$

As in the case of crowd density, for estimating pedestrian flow too, it is essential to be able select a transit line representative of people's motion and to count people transiting over a time that is neither too long nor too short. In Fig. 2.7, people density tends to get higher in the last snapshots, and hence, so a shorter time might be more appropriate to grasp observed changes in flow (this will, however, lead to larger fluctuations in estimated flow).

However, in some situations, it is not always possible to define a line where people are to be counted (e.g., the ground of the arena shown in Fig. 2.6). In such cases, the fundamental equation linking flow with density and speed may be used:

Flow = Density × Speed

This fundamental equation can be used also to estimate density or speed when flow is known. For example, we can estimate that crowd density in the frames shown Fig. 2.7 is about 1.2 m^{-2} (knowing the people count and corridor's surface area), and this allow us to compute the velocity by dividing the flow by density:

$$\text{Speed} = \frac{\text{Flow}}{\text{Density}} = \frac{1.71 \, (m \cdot s)^{-1}}{1.2 \, m^{-2}} = 1.43 \text{ m/s} \tag{2.2}$$

Pedestrian flow is an important property for designing pedestrian facilities, and it is used in architectural and building norms. The (maximum) flow considered in designing a pedestrian facility is also defined as "capacity." When a building is designed at capacity, it means that every part of it should have a flow never exceeding capacity, and this principle should guarantee safe motion and eventually safe evacuation. The capacity may vary depending on the purpose of the facility and local regulations, but generally a capacity between 1.0 and 1.5 $(m \cdot s)^{-1}$ is employed in most standards.

Capacity plays an important role because it can determine the number of exits and the width of corridors in facilities, and choosing the appropriate value is of upmost importance. When capacity is set high, construction costs can be reduced, but comfort and more importantly safety may be at risk. Also, setting a high capacity may hinder future expansions as there is little room for modification. In general, it is always better to fix the capacity as low as possible to ensure that comfort and safety are ensured and that future modifications are easier to implement.

2.4.2 Fundamental Diagram of Pedestrian Traffic: Theory and Limitations

We have now discussed important pedestrian quantities such as speed, density, and flow and the concept of capacity. However, to complete the discussion on quantitative crowd properties, it is necessary to discuss how these quantities are related with each other and also how is the capacity determined.

In addition to the previously presented equation (the "fundamental equation"), pedestrian speed, density, and flow are linked by the so-called fundamental diagram, which is a mathematical and physical concept often employed in transportation. The fundamental diagram has two variations: the speed–density fundamental diagram and the flow–density fundamental diagram.

As the name suggests, the speed–density fundamental diagram shows the relationship between walking speed and crowd density. The speed–density fundamental diagram is simply obtained by measuring how the speed of people changes when the crowd gets denser. Although this is a simple concept to understand, obtaining universal and reliable figures of speed for various densities is not always straightforward. For example, Fig. 2.8 (left) shows measurements obtained by different researchers over the years and in different places.

As seen in Fig. 2.8 (left), for a similar density, the values obtained for speed are different, partially reflecting the factors that can affect walking speed [23]. However, even if the differences among datasets are somehow large, a general behavior is observed: when crowd gets denser, the walking speed decreases. This characteristic behavior is usually referred to as the speed–density fundamental diagram of pedestrian traffic and is schematically given in the right panel of Fig. 2.8. Using this diagram, the crowd speed can be estimated when its density is known. Of course, the value obtained for a given density will not be absolute, as differences are possible because of several factors. However, the calculated crowd speed can help estimating how slower/faster a crowd will be when the density increases/decreases.

Although the speed–density fundamental diagram is useful when crowd properties are to be estimated, it does not allow defining a limit or a capacity to be used in design. In fact, when the crowd becomes denser, the speed continuously decreases, and the density limit that ensures smooth motion of pedestrians is not clear. The maximum density observed when speed becomes zero (also called "jam density") is only a physical limit of the crowd, meaning that crowds denser than $10\,\mathrm{m}^{-2}$ cannot exist as there is no place to pack people. However, this is a very dangerous condition, and as we discussed earlier, people are likely to die under these densities. As a consequence, limits for acceptable density are to be set at a much lower value.

Using the simple equation explained above (again, the so-called fundamental equation), the speed–density fundamental diagram can be converted into a flow–density fundamental diagram, yielding the curve shown in Fig. 2.9 (left panel).

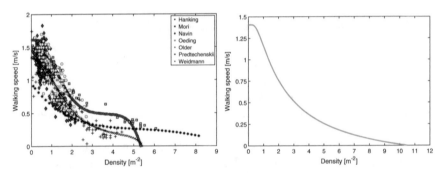

Fig. 2.8 Left: measurement of crowd speed depending on its density according to several researchers [11, 17–22]. Right: a typical representation of the speed–density fundamental diagram for pedestrian flow; walking speed quickly decreases as the crowd density increases

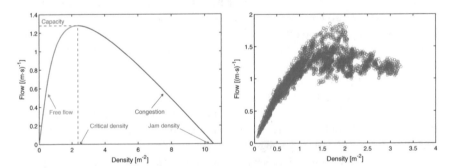

Fig. 2.9 Left: typical shape of the flow–density fundamental diagram. The most important terms related to it are also shown in the figure [24]. Right: flow and density values measured for people walking in a corridor (similar to Fig. 2.7) [25, 26]. The "typical" shape of the fundamental diagram is seen, but variations are large. Source: the right figure was generated by the authors using open data from the Pedestrian Dynamics Data Archive (Forschungszentrum Jülich)

The flow–density fundamental diagram Fig. 2.9 (left panel) has an interesting and important property: the flow increases at low densities, but a quick deterioration occurs when the density exceeds a certain limit, which is typically defined as the "critical density." The maximum flow observed at the critical density is the previously discussed capacity.

For densities below the critical value, "free flow" is typically observed. Under the free flow condition, people can move without slowing down. When density approaches the critical limit, people may have to pay attention to others to avoid collisions, but do not need to stop or slow down. As the flow–density fundamental diagram shows, a rapid change in flow occurs when the density is close to the critical value. Hence, although maintaining the flow below the capacity is mandatory, it is preferable to maintain a safety margin since changes close to the critical density tend to be abrupt and rapid crowd control is required.

This representation of the fundamental diagram also explains why most of the regulations employ a capacity value between 1.0 and 1.5 $(m \cdot s)^{-1}$ (and why a capacity lower than the theoretical limit set by the fundamental diagram is generally better).

When density exceeds the critical value, congestion occurs, and people have to slow down or stop because they cannot walk at their desired pace. It is important to observe that congestion is a deteriorating process. When some people have to slow down, others behind them too will have to slow down and eventually stop to avoid collisions. This will increase the density as the accumulating people will further decrease the overall walking speed. Therefore, if people keep coming at a constant rate, density will steadily increase, leading to a dangerous situation. Hence, for safety purposes, crowd management should ensure that the critical density and capacity are never exceeded. Temporary overshoots are possible (as explained in Chap. 7), but such overshoots should be considered as an exceptional situation that will only occur because of unpredictable circumstances.

Finally, it is important to remember that as in the case of the speed–density fundamental diagram, the flow–density version too is subject to several factors, and the line shown in Fig. 2.9 (left panel) is obtained only in theoretical representations. When measurements are performed in the real world (by obtaining flow and density for people walking in a particular place), the typical profile is still obtained, but defining critical density and capacity is more difficult. This is also a good reason for always using conservative values in design: variations relative to human factors always need to be taken into account.

Further, note that the fundamental diagram and the way in which it has been defined in this text generally holds true for those cases in which it is possible to measure the flow in a clear manner. For example (comparing also the graphs in Fig. 2.10), in the case of corridors, it is easy to draw a virtual line to count the passing pedestrians [27]. But when people move fairly randomly in multiple directions (take for example the central hall of a large train station), flow measurement becomes difficult, and the features of the fundamental diagram are partially lost [28, 29]. These considerations do not have any impact on the importance of the fundamental diagram in understanding people movements and defining a division between free flow (not congested) and congestion. It is simply necessary to remember that as applications move further away from the original theory, some of the theoretical considerations could lose their validity. Using conservative values for capacity and safety standards ensures that evaluation errors do not affect pedestrian safety.

2.4.3 Level of Service (LOS)

The so-called level of service (LOS) is related to pedestrian density and flow and originates from the nature of the fundamental diagram. The LOS is an important method to classify quantitative aspects of crowds. The LOS (for crowds) was introduced by Fruin in 1971 [30] and is still in use in several institutions to judge the quality of pedestrian spaces and design them. Although the method was originally applied for vehicular traffic and only targeted a limited number of facilities (highways or local roads), it is now widely used in traffic management, and it is now also used to grade structures such as crosswalks, roundabouts, and pedestrian spaces (this last based on the proposal by Fruin).

The fundamental idea of the LOS is that the quality and comfort of pedestrian spaces can be categorized based on density and flow. For each facility, Fruin determined the comfort perceived by pedestrian users using density and flow and assigned alphabets to ranges, with A being the best standard and F being the worst. Table 2.8 presents an example for the LOS of walkways and stairways taken from Fruin's original work. A schematic illustration for some of the LOS is also provided in Fig. 2.11.

For example, the LOS of a walkway with a density $0.5\,m^{-2}$ will be classified as C. All categories of the LOS are well below the critical density considered earlier when discussing the fundamental diagram. This is because high densities are never considered when designing facilities accommodating pedestrians on a daily basis. In fact, the turning point of congestion will be classified roughly as F, which is above acceptable standards of design.

Although the methodology used in the LOS is the same for a large number of facilities, the values assigned to each level are obviously different. This is clearly seen in Table 2.8 when comparing the values for walkways and stairways. Since the way in which people move on stairways is different from that on flat walkways, different combinations of density and flows are used.

Here, it is important to note that the values used in the table for LOS have undergone a number of revisions (and alternative methods have been proposed [31]) and that they are corrected yearly (the reference is normally the "Highway Capacity Manual" [32]). Hence, LOS published in old editions may not be completely equivalent to that in the newest releases, but changes are usually minimal.

The LOS is an important concept employed in pedestrian traffic, and it also plays an important role in dealing with pedestrian spaces. Since traffic engineers are prone to present their studies using the concept of LOS, it is important to be familiar with the concept and to understand that while it is shown in a rather qualitative way (a

Table 2.8 Level of service (LOS) for flat walkways and stairways according to Fruin [30]

	Type	Density [m^{-2}]	Flow [(m·s)$^{-1}$]	Description and example
A	*Stairways*	<0.31	<0.38	• Virtually unrestricted walking speed • Minimum maneuvering needed to pass other pedestrians • Unrestricted crossing and reverse movements
	Walkways	<0.54	<0.27	Example: A wide plaza on a quiet day, a train station main hall during the early morning, or a residential area.
B	*Stairways*	0.31–0.43	0.38–0.55	• Normal walking speeds, restricted only occasionally • Occasional interference in passing other pedestrians • Occasional interference in crossing and reverse movements
	Walkways	0.54–0.72	0.27–0.38	Example: A transportation facility at off-peak time with few trains/planes arriving, or a business area on weekends/public holidays.
C	*Stairways*	0.43–0.72	0.55–0.82	• Partially restricted walking speeds • Restricted passing movements, but possible with maneuvers • Restricted crossing and reverse movements • Reasonably smooth flow of pedestrians
	Walkways	0.72–1.08	0.38–0.55	Example: A transportation terminal under normal conditions and with steady and constant movements of people.
D	*Stairways*	0.72–1.08	0.82–1.09	• Restricted and reduced walking speeds • Passing other pedestrians rarely possible without conflicts • Severely restricted crossing and reverse movements, conflicts unavoidable • Momentarily flow stoppages are possible intermittently
	Walkways	1.08–1.54	0.55–0.71	Example: The most crowded space of a large pedestrian infrastructure during normal operation (off-peak and no particular congestion/jamming issues).
E	*Stairways*	1.08–2.15	1.09–1.37	• Restricted walking speeds, occasionally reduced to shuffling • Passing other pedestrians impossible without conflicts • Severely restricted crossing and reverse, conflicts unavoidable • Flow interruptions and stoppages becomes frequent
	Walkways	1.54–2.69	0.71–0.93	Example: Sport stadia or rail facilities where large crowds form for a short time when people leave the stadium or disembark from trains.
F	*Stairways*	>2.15	>1.37	• Walking speed reduced to shuffling • Passing, crossing, and reverse movements are impossible • Frequent and unavoidable physical contact • Sporadic flow on the verge of complete stoppage
	Walkways	>2.69	>0.93	Example: Pedestrian facility during a complete breakdown in traffic flow. This level can only occur in queues and cannot be a part of a design where people are assumed to walk.

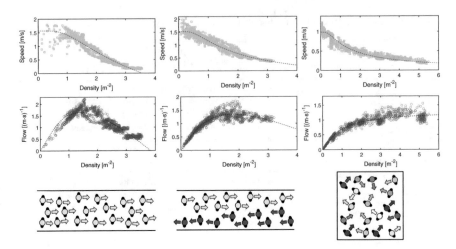

Fig. 2.10 Fundamental diagram obtained by analyzing different types of pedestrian facilities. Left: a corridor where people walk in the same direction [25, 26]; center: a corridor with people waking in opposite directions [25, 26]; and right: people walking randomly in a delimited area [27]. As seen, the shape of the fundamental diagram changes when the motion of the crowd becomes more complex. Source: some graphs in the figure were generated by the authors using open data from the Pedestrian Dynamics Data Archive (Forschungszentrum Jülich). Diagrams reprinted under Creative Commons CC BY license from [29]

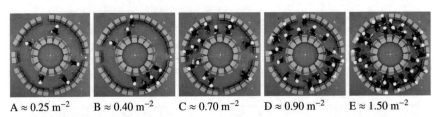

$A \approx 0.25 \text{ m}^{-2}$ $B \approx 0.40 \text{ m}^{-2}$ $C \approx 0.70 \text{ m}^{-2}$ $D \approx 0.90 \text{ m}^{-2}$ $E \approx 1.50 \text{ m}^{-2}$

Fig. 2.11 Schematic representation of density and its equivalent level of service (LOS) from A to E for an infinite walkway (a loop walkway). Total surface of the walkway considered here is about 20 m^2. Courtesy of Akihiro Fujita

letter from A to F), there are quantitative criteria and specific theories determining its application.

References

1. Canetti, E.: Crowds and Power. Macmillan (1962)
2. Challenger, R., Clegg, C.W., Robinson, M.A., Leigh, M.: Understanding Crowd Behaviours: Supporting Evidence. UK Cabinet Office, pp. 1–308 (2009)
3. Challenger, R., Clegg, C.W., Robinson, M.A., Leigh, M.: Understanding Crowd Behaviours: Guidance and Lessons Identified. UK Cabinet Office, pp. 1–134 (2009)

4. Zeitz, K.M., Tan, H.M., Grief, M., Couns, P., Zeitz, C.J.: Crowd behavior at mass gatherings: a literature review. Prehospital Disaster Med. **24**(1), 32–38 (2009). https://doi.org/10.1017/S1049023X00006518

5. Momboisse, R.M.: Riots, Revolts, and Insurrections. Thomas Publisher, Charles C (1967)

6. Berlonghi, A.E.: Understanding and planning for different spectator crowds. Safety Sci. **18**(4), 239–247 (1995). https://doi.org/10.1016/0925-7535(94)00033-Y

7. Gorrini, A.: Empirical Studies and Computational Results of a Proxemic—Based Model of Pedestrian Crowd Dynamics. Ph.D. thesis, University of Milano-Bicocca (2014)

8. Helbing, D., Buzna, L., Johansson, A., Werner, T.: Self-organized pedestrian crowd dynamics: experiments, simulations, and design solutions. Transp. Sci. **39**(1), 1–24 (2005). https://doi.org/10.1287/trsc.1040.0108

9. Moussaïd, M., Perozo, N., Garnier, S., Helbing, D., Theraulaz, G.: The walking behaviour of pedestrian social groups and its impact on crowd dynamics. PloS one **5**(4), e10047 (2010). https://doi.org/10.1371/journal.pone.0010047

10. Proulx, G.: How to initiate evacuation movement in public buildings. Facilities (1999). https://doi.org/10.1108/02632779910278764

11. Weidmann, U.: Transporttechnik der fußgänger: transporttechnische eigenschaften des fußgängerverkehrs, literaturauswertung. IVT Schriftenreihe **90** (1993). (in German)

12. Finnis, K.K., Walton, D.: Field observations to determine the influence of population size, location and individual factors on pedestrian walking speeds. Ergonomics **51**(6), 827–842 (2008). https://doi.org/10.1080/00140130701812147

13. Poapst, R.: Characterizing Pedestrian Traffic by Hour-of-Day Periodicities in Commercial Zones. Ph.D. thesis, University of Manitoba (2015)

14. Feliciani, C., Zuriguel, I., Garcimartín, A., Maza, D., Nishinari, K.: Systematic experimental investigation of the obstacle effect during non-competitive and extremely competitive evacuations. Sci. Rep. **10**(1), 1–20 (2020). https://doi.org/10.1038/s41598-020-72733-w

15. Murosaki, Y.: Crowd avalanche at the Akashi fireworks show. Accident Prevention Newsl. (Yobō Jihō) **208**, 8–13 (2002). (in Japanese)

16. Duives, D.C., Daamen, W., Hoogendoorn, S.P.: Quantification of the level of crowdedness for pedestrian movements. Physica A: Statistical Mech. Appl. **427**, 162–180 (2015). https://doi.org/10.1016/j.physa.2014.11.054

17. Hankin, B., Wright, R.A.: Passenger flow in subways. J. Oper. Res. Soc. **9**(2), 81–88 (1958). https://doi.org/10.1057/jors.1958.9

18. Oeding, D.: Verkehrsbelastung und dimensionierung von gehwegen und anderen anlagen des fussgengerkehrs. Dipl.-Ing., Strassenbau und Strassenverkehrstechnik, Technische Hochschule Braunschweig Institut fur Stadtbauwesen (1963). (in German)

19. Older, S.: Movement of pedestrians on footways in shopping streets. Traffic Eng. Control **10**(4) (1968)

20. Navin, F.P., Wheeler, R.J.: Pedestrian flow characteristics. Traffic Eng. Inst. Traffic Engr. **39** (1969)

21. Predtechenskii, V.M., Milinskiĭ, Ivanovich, A.: Planning for Foot Traffic Flow in Buildings. US Department of Commerce and the National Bureau of Standards (1978)

22. Mōri, M., Tsukaguchi, H.: A new method for evaluation of level of service in pedestrian facilities. Transp. Res. Part A: General **21**(3), 223–234 (1987). https://doi.org/10.1016/0191-2607(87)90016-1

23. Ishaque, M.M., Noland, R.B.: Behavioural issues in pedestrian speed choice and street crossing behaviour: a review. Transp. Rev. **28**(1), 61–85 (2008). https://doi.org/10.1080/01441640701365239

24. Daamen, W.: Modelling Passenger Flows in Public Transport Facilities. Delft University Press (2004)

25. Zhang, J., Klingsch, W., Schadschneider, A., Seyfried, A.: Ordering in bidirectional pedestrian flows and its influence on the fundamental diagram. J. Statistical Mech.: Theor. Exp. **2012**(02), P02002 (2012). https://doi.org/10.1088/1742-5468/2012/02/P02002

26. Zhang, J.: Pedestrian Fundamental Diagrams: Comparative Analysis of Experiments in Different Geometries, vol. 14. Forschungszentrum Jülich (2012)
27. Feliciani, C., Nishinari, K.: Measurement of congestion and intrinsic risk in pedestrian crowds. Transp. Res. Part C: Emerging Technol. **91**, 124–155 (2018). https://doi.org/10.1016/j.trc.2018.03.027
28. Zhang, J., Klingsch, W., Schadschneider, A., Seyfried, A.: Transitions in pedestrian fundamental diagrams of straight corridors and t-junctions. J. Statistical Mech.: Theor. Exp. **2011**(06), P06004 (2011). https://doi.org/10.1088/1742-5468/2011/06/P06004
29. Feliciani, C., Nishinari, K.: Investigation of pedestrian evacuation scenarios through congestion level and crowd danger. Collective Dyn. **5**, 150–157 (2020). https://doi.org/10.17815/CD.2020.45
30. Fruin, J.J.: Pedestrian Planning and Design. Tech. rep, Metropolitan Association of Urban Designers and Environmental Planners (1971)
31. Talavera-Garcia, R., Soria-Lara, J.A.: Q-plos, developing an alternative walking index. A method based on urban design quality. Cities **45**, 7–17 (2015). https://doi.org/10.1016/j.cities.2015.03.003
32. Transportation Research Board: Highway Capacity Manual 6th Edition: A Guide for Multimodal Mobility Analysis. Transportation Research Board (2016)

Chapter 3
Analysis of Past Crowd Accidents

Abstract Analyzing under what circumstances crowd accidents are likely to occur and how they can be avoided is important to ensure safety. The information provided in this chapter can help to prepare for the imminent risks of crowd accidents. These risks can be determined by comparing given circumstances to those that caused crowd accidents driven by external (environmental) and internal (crowd intrinsic) factors. We analyzed over 100 crowd accidents and classified spatial structures and crowd flows associated with the accidents. Moreover, we evaluated how and why crowd density increases to be able to manage it for crowd accident prevention. We introduced crowd domino and crowd avalanche by classifying crowd accidents based on their physical characteristics. Both of them are triggered by the fall of someone in the crowd, although they demonstrate different transmission mechanisms. In addition, statistical analysis of the crowd accidents that occurred over the last 120 years was performed to clarify the likelihood of their occurrence and help design appropriate planning and control crowd density to prevent them in the future. A brief description of crowd mood and the presence of competition were also discussed since they can contribute to worsening the preliminary conditions. In regard to crowd management, communication between stakeholders is particularly important as a lack of coordination among them has been a common aggravating factor in the past.

3.1 Introduction

There is a saying that goes "Hope for the best; plan for the worst." When management designs an event with this idea in mind and a crowd accident occurs, it is likely because of deficient assumptions about the worst-case scenario and optimism that leads to this deficiency. In other words, careful planning rather than misleading optimism can minimize the risk of accidents.

In the 1980s, there was no effective crowd management measure; thus, hundreds of people had unfortunately lost their lives in crowd accidents. These tragedies have led to the formulation of recurrence prevention measures (e.g., Green Guide, which sets regulations in stadium design and management [1]). Over the last 30 years, no fatalities related to crowd accidents have occurred at football games in the UK owing

© The Author(s), under exclusive license to Springer Nature Switzerland AG 2021   51
C. Feliciani et al., *Introduction to Crowd Management*,
https://doi.org/10.1007/978-3-030-90012-0_3

to the introduction of strict regulations and reconsidering the design of stadiums. The history of crowd accidents shows that learning from them can help establish efficient practices in crowd management.

Here, we analyze the major crowd accidents that occurred in past centuries to determine how they were induced and provide a fundamental understanding of the issues that require attention to prevent crowd accidents. In this chapter, we are not going to analyze each of them individually, but we limit our investigation to analyzing the documentation obtained and showing the differences among accident contexts and types. Details of each accident analyzed in this review are provided in the Appendix of this book in the form of a table.

In addition, we explain the motion and the conditions of the crowd and the environment under which each accident occurred. Discussing the definitive causes of each accident and criminal and civil responsibilities is beyond the scope of this book. Nonetheless, newspaper articles and official reports provide undeniable sources to be informed about the details of crowd accidents. Additionally, official reports, pictures, and/or videos can offer specific information about the location, time, type of crowd motion observed, and in some cases, factors leading to a potentially dangerous high crowd density. Spatial and environmental circumstances and crowd motion have been analyzed as they commonly induce crowd accidents and are of utmost importance for designing facilities, guidance, flow lines, and security measures to achieve crowd safety.

This chapter offers a macroscopic perspective while concerning the causes of each accident since the consequential conditions led by external and internal factors can be considered as a result of failure in planning or on-site management.

3.2 Objectives of This Chapter

This chapter is intended to familiarize readers with the mechanisms and the circumstances leading to crowd accidents to prevent their occurrence. Readers are expected to understand how external (environmental) and internal (crowd intrinsic) factors contribute to critically increasing the crowd density to a dangerous level. Although accidents sometimes occur under a combination of many simultaneous events, the planning of the facility, event, and flow lines ultimately determine the occurrence of a disaster. Notably, coordination among the stakeholders plays a critical role in tackling a risky situation.

3.3 Crowd Incident Mechanisms

Mechanisms that lead to crowd accidents have remained controversial, as briefly stated above, and various investigations performed to establish liability in trials fell short of clarifying the causalities. In addition, a number of terms often associated with crowd accidents are widely used by various media without a common definition. Such situations are making it difficult to understand the mechanism leading to fatalities when accidents occur.

"Stampede" is often used in media reports and also commonly used in scientific literature, although its usage is often misleading and sometimes takes meanings not implicit in its original definition. According to some dictionaries (e.g., Oxford, Cambridge, Collins, Merriam Webster), "stampede" is defined as a sudden collective move that is usually intended to describe animal behavior and partially implies fear or panic. However, in media reports, it is often associated with fatalities and used regardless of whether panic existed or not (in the previous chapter, we mentioned that this is relatively rare in crowds). Because of its controversial nature and often improper use, in this book, we refrained from using "stampede."

Similarly, we avoided using "trampling" or "crushing," which are also very often employed in media reports and scientific publications. Trampling (by definition walking or stepping heavily on something or someone) and crushing (pressing something very hard so that it is broken) are the reasons for the outbreak of casualties in crowd accidents. Most of the casualties occurred because some people have forcibly fallen inside the crowd and were trampled by many others. However, in this book, we focused on what happens just before the accident rather than postmortem examination. Since trampling and crushing are often employed as general terms to indicate crowd accidents without unification, we tried not to use these terms as much as possible. Regardless, we employed dictionary definitions if unavoidable. In addition, several definitions have been used to describe different types of crowd accidents, such as "collective crowd collapse" or "crowd turbulence", which is included in this book.

In this book, we will align to the analysis performed by the official investigation committee on the Akashi Pedestrian Bridge Accident [2] (the details of which are provided in the Appendix and later in this chapter), which occurred in 2001 in Japan. This incident and the following investigation triggered the police to make crowd handling regulations in the following years. Most of the casualties have died of suffocation by thoracic compression caused as a result of being trampled over by a crowd or trapped underneath a pile of fallen people. The investigation committee introduced crowd domino and crowd avalanche as the ultimate causes of fatalities in crowd accidents during the process of their investigation trying to clarify the mechanism of how this mortal condition had formed.

3.3.1 Crowd Domino

Crowd domino, as the name suggests, is similar to a row of dominos toppling over. It is triggered by someone at the back of the crowd falling by some reason and knocking over those in front, and the effect of the fall cascades through each successive person (Fig. 3.1). This effect can occur even at relatively low crowd densities of 3–5 m^{-2} and causes people to fall over from the rear of the crowd toward the front in a linear manner. It can also occur when the pressure from the rear of a crowd is comparatively small, such as when people are queuing [3]. The cause of the first fall in the chain is not only by the physical force of the crowd pressure behind them but can be a variety of events, including tripping after stumbling or sudden illness. For example, if we look at a queue of people going down a flight of stairs, one person may lose their footing and fall forward, which causes the person below them to fall into the person in front of them, causing a series of people to fall onto each other in sequence. As this type of incident can be caused by an individual fall, it is difficult to avoid it through crowd management, but proactive use of handrails on stairs and dividing stairs' flight into shorter flights interspersed with planar sections can help to mitigate potential risks of crowd accidents. Furthermore, it is also fundamentally important to avoid queue formation in stairways.

3.3.2 Crowd Avalanche

In contrast to crowd domino, crowd avalanche (schematically illustrated in Fig. 3.2) occurs when many people are pressed together in a high-density crowd. Many historical crowd incidents are considerably classified in this category. It is therefore important to ensure that crowd densities do not become too high, and activities to achieve this purpose can be said to form the core of crowd management.

The physical contact between people forms a network of forces that interact with each other when they are closely packed together in a crowd. This means that the pressure force travels through the crowd. While in this situation, a large crowd pressure is generated when an entire crowd moves in a certain direction because everyone tends to move and may push others in the same direction. This generates an unstoppable pressure for people at the front of the crowd, causing them to try to escape to areas of lower crowd density to avoid suffocation. This forms an even higher crowd density, while simultaneously making the whole mechanical network extremely unstable. In turn, this causes a phenomenon called crowd turbulence due to its resemblance with the motion of fluid in unstable conditions. In this state, the contact between people forces them to move in various directions without their intention. In this type of ultrahigh-density crowd, an "arching state" occurs, and

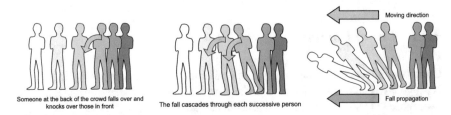

Someone at the back of the crowd falls over and knocks over those in front   The fall cascades through each successive person   Moving direction   Fall propagation

Fig. 3.1 Crowd domino mechanism: The illustration goes from left to right in order of time

several bodies may float off their feet. This is when a person surrounded by a large group of people is involuntarily held up by strong contact with the bodies around them, and their feet are lifted off the floor. When this occurs to a large number of people, empty spots are created in various places, and the mechanical equilibrium within the crowd becomes unstable. Additionally, the people who are floating may be suddenly carried in different directions against their own volition, and this is the precursor state for a crowd avalanche. When they can no longer be supported by their surroundings and fall to the floor, the crowd surrounding them is no longer under a pressure balance from all directions and thus collapses due to the missing support. Due to its resemblance to snow avalanches, this type of fall is referred to as a crowd avalanche. In terms of crowd density, this effect occurs in situations with more than $10\,\mathrm{m}^{-2}$, and the falls are characterized by falling from the surrounding crowd into the newly formed void. This phenomenon also occurs as a result of the instantaneous change in mechanical balance when an architectural structure suddenly collapses under the pressure of an ultrahigh-density crowd.

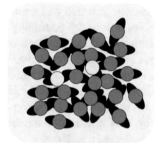

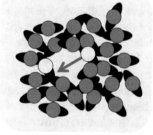

① Under extremely high density, people experiences strong contact with the bodies. Then, the "arching state" outbreaks where some people are involuntarily held up and their feet are lifted off the floor.

② As people are moved by collective crowd forces, empty spots may randomly form in a given location.

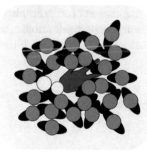

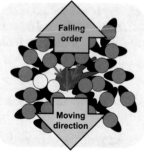

③ People close to empty spots will rapidly lose balance and fall in the open space.

④ People around will in turn lose balance and successively fall over into the person already on the ground, creating a sort of avalanche.

Fig. 3.2 Crowd avalanche mechanism: Events 1–4 describe the chain of events in the same order

Past crowd incidents that have been described in various sources as having been caused by different mechanisms may have actually been, upon closer inspection of the circumstances surrounding the incident, caused by a crowd avalanche. For example, the accident that occurred at Yahiko Shrine (Japan) in 1956 where 124 people lost their lives (details will follow later) or the one that occurred in 1954 when a large crowd attempted to visit the Imperial Palace in Tokyo (Japan), which resulted in 16 fatalities, were both ultimately caused by crowd avalanches. Another example of a crowd avalanche that was caused by the sudden collapse of a structure is the disaster which occurred at the Burden Park stadium in the UK in 1946. A more recent example occurred during the 2010 Love Parade in Germany, for which an extensive documentation and several videos are available [4]. If a crowd avalanche occurs in a high-density crowd, the collapse forms a void by changing the mechanical balance, and this instability propagates in various directions. This can lead to further crowd incidents or secondary disasters in other locations. Furthermore, crowds cannot predict accidents and may not be aware of what is happening at the time of accidents, leading them to speculate about the situation. As a result, confusion and inaccurate information can spread through the crowd, where visibility is extremely limited, causing further concern and anxiety. These environmental and emotional factors can significantly change people's behavior, leading to the possibility of a chain of incidents. During the Akashi Pedestrian Bridge Accident, a second crowd avalanche occurred several meters away from the first incident in the opposite direction to the movement of the crowd. Furthermore, many people at a considerable distance from the site of the original incident were injured. Also, at a 2005 incident at the Mandhardevi Temple in India, a confused crowd trying to flee the scene of an initial incident caused an electrical short circuit nearby, causing a fire and subsequent explosion that led to further confusion and severely increased casualties.

It is not just crowd avalanche that must be addressed for crowd management but also anxiety, discomfort, and danger that may not lead to a major incident. It is beneficial to analyze and learn from both past failures and successes in crowd management. However, very few materials are available for cases that does not end in criminal proceedings, and scientific analyses of the subject have remained underdeveloped, which means that there is a need for further research on this topic.

3.4 Classification and Analysis of Crowd Incidents

3.4.1 Causality of Crowd Incidents

Now, let us take a broader perspective and consider the circumstances and factors that create the conditions for crowd accidents. This analysis is based on a review of the major crowd incidents that occurred since the start of the twentieth century and are listed in the Appendix of this book. Interested readers may take a closer look for details.

We should note again that the occurrence of crowd incidents is highly correlated to crowd density. In fact, it is reported that "in terms of crowd density, $2\,m^{-2}$ is usually considered to be a critical crowd density for ensuring safety. If the density of a crowd reaches $3\,m^{-2}$, immediate countermeasures are required; thus, it is preferable to intervene at lower densities so that this value is never reached" [2]. These numerical conditions have been established by the Supreme Court of Japan as the judicial precedents of the criminal trial of the Akashi Pedestrian Bridge Accident (crowd densities above $2.69\,m^{-2}$ exceeded acceptable standards in the LOS presented in the previous chapter). Thus, factors that increase the crowd density are critical as they facilitate the occurrence of crowd accidents.

Even so, crowd incidents often occur as a result of complex chains of actions and events, and it can be difficult to use the limited information available to trace all of the causal relationships back to their original cause. It is not possible to establish a chronological series of events until after an incident occurs, and in very few instances, camera images were able to provide a proper record of events. Therefore, we often estimate what happened by investigating the scene of the incident and listening to the testimony of those involved (although visibility is difficult in a packed crowd, and testimonies concern only a local vision of the accident, thus requiring to interview many). Eventually, the relationship between three factors must be established to understand the causes of an accident: the "external" environment of the site of the incident, the "internal" state of the crowd, and the crowd management system. The management system is the most difficult factor to analyze as this is where human culpability for the incident lies.

Accordingly, in this chapter, we examined environments and crowds as they can be objectively analyzed to some extent. We interpret an incident as a phenomenon that occurs due to the interaction between the environment and the crowd and examine the direct contributory factors that lead to higher crowd densities. Of course, if there are deficiencies in the management systems put in place by stakeholders that contributed to the incident, we also consider them as appropriate.

The above factors are summarized in Fig. 3.3, which shows that the environment intrinsic "external" factor and the crowd intrinsic "internal" factor contribute to high crowd densities and shows the influence of the human factor of management on both of these elements. Then, we will look in particular detail at the factors caused specifically by the environment and the crowd so that we can attempt to construct a management system that can eliminate these issues.

Firstly, in terms of the environment, physical structures, and the conditions under which they operate are important, and many crowd incidents occur in dead ends, stairways, enclosed spaces or doorways, and constricted segments. As for the factors that are linked to the crowd itself, flow patterns, the purpose of gathering, and other causes can all be intricately linked to the occurrence of many incidents.

Although, in general, it is usually possible to distinguish between external and internal factors, they sometimes partially influence each other. For example, a corridor will restrict crowd motion to one or two directions but whether people will ultimately move in one or two directions depends on their interactions, showing that flow patterns are mostly related to crowd internal factors but can be forcibly influenced by the environment. Further, people waiting in a queue could restrict the motion of the rest of the crowd, thus creating an artificial boundary. In that sense, the crowd itself contributes to changing the environment. For these reasons, the relationship between internal and external factors is given using a dotted line in Fig. 3.3. In most cases, both external and internal factors can be taken independently, although their interactions sometimes exist.

In addition, we should also be aware of factors that cannot be easily linked to the environment or the crowd, such as sudden changes in the weather or the outbreak of violence. For example, if there is a sudden downpour, the crowd may simultaneously run in search of shelter. Furthermore, earthquakes, fires, and loud noises are difficult to control, which pose a serious threat to crowd safety. In some cases, people trying to escape from acts of terrorism have become caught in a crowd avalanche with fatal consequences. It is necessary to be prepared for the worst including this kind of unexpected uncertainty rather than hope for the best, e.g., by securing evacuation routes and planning evacuation guidance. We will discuss this topic in greater detail as part of the planning processes covered in Chap. 8. This chapter, however, deals with crowd incidents that could be controlled.

Finally, crowd incidents are considered to have an ultimate single direct cause out of all the possible factors that could contribute to their occurrence: the ultrahigh-density crowd. However, to prevent the reoccurrence of similar incidents, it is necessary to trace the causal relationship that exists between all of these factors, which, in turn, poses the problem of how they can all be effectively managed at once. This is also a difficult question to answer. The following aims to provide a detailed explanation of the issues, citing various actual contributory factors and giving examples from historical incidents.

3.4.2   External Factors (Environmental)

In this section, the locations of crowd incidents listed in the Appendix are analyzed with respect to the spatial structures and their environment. (Note that only the

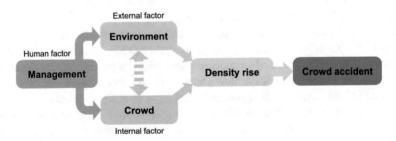

Fig. 3.3 Framework for factor analysis of crowd incidents

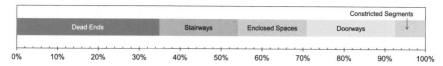

Fig. 3.4 Spatial structures in which incidents are likely to occur. Note that only accidents in which the spatial structure was clear have been considered to create this graph

cases in which this information has been clearly reported are adopted unless stated otherwise).

People choose and utilize various spaces based on the functionality to help them achieve their respective goals. These include, for example, staircases to enable them to get to the ground, bridges that allow them to cross rivers, and emergency exits that they can use to quickly evacuate buildings. The crowd condition for any given space is determined by its utility and functionality. For example, bridges tend to have moving crowds, while crowds must stop in front of fences. Accordingly, when a large number of people occupy the same space, they tend to have a sense of the use value of that space, which greatly affects the flow and density of the crowd. Therefore, when analyzing the causes of a crowd incident, it is important to identify the space in which the incident occurred, as its spatial structure can offer clues that help to analyze the situation at the time of the incident.

A particularly important spatial structure is the "bottleneck," stipulated here to indicate spaces in which the flow rate is reduced due to external factors. These are commonly seen in almost every infrastructure accommodating pedestrians, where paths are narrowed due to obstacles or movement is restricted by tunnels, bridges, staircases, steep slopes, entrances and exits, ticket gates, and so on. When a crowd passes through this type of area, its density increases, and subsequently, its average walking speed decreases, reducing its flow rate, which correlates with a higher risk of accidents. Although they are not strictly spatial structures, areas in darkness, and slippery paths can be considered bottlenecks in the broad sense of the word as they impose their own restrictions on the flow of people. In an accident, which occurred in 1999 in Austria during a sport event, when spectators left the arena, many people fell on the dark and slippery slope outside, resulting in six people getting killed and another 38 being injured [5].

If we look at an overview of the cases considered in this book, we can see that the majority of the incidents occurred in dead ends, stairways, enclosed spaces, doorways, and constricted segments, in the order of frequency, as shown in Fig. 3.4. Additionally, some environmental circumstances can obstruct their footage or cognition, such as slippery or ragged floors, bumps on the floor, darkness, backlighting, smoke, unpleasant noise or smell, meteorological temperature or humidity, rain, strong sunshine, etc., leading them to the pre-incident state.

3.4.2.1 Dead Ends

Spatial structures that prevent a crowd from moving forward are referred to as dead ends, which include artificial structures and obstacles, as well as natural features of the environment such as rivers and cliffs. In our daily life, a corridor with a locked door, an elevator, and a toilet, which have only one doorway, are considered in this category. Furthermore, a pedestrian crossing or railroad crossing can form a temporary dead end during a red light. Additionally, the crowd itself functions as a hindrance to movement when considered from the perspective of those who are inside it.

When people know the place they are heading to is a dead end, they would not go forward unless they have a specific purpose. However, incidents have occurred in which crowds have moved into dead ends despite being aware of the lack of exits ahead. At a rock concert in 1991 in the USA and the Roskilde Festival held in Denmark in 2000, excited crowds went forward into dead ends (there is only a stage in front and hindrance on the left and right side of the crowd), killing three and nine people, respectively. In 2004, a crowd flooded a concession stand for souvenirs in India, resulting in an incident.

On the other hand, emergency evacuations are typical examples of when crowds unknowingly move into dead ends. Incidents occurred when emergency exits at the end of passageways were locked or closed, or the exit door was inward opening when crowds attempted to flee from fire or violence, escape from security forces or were driven to move due to misinformation. Among these incidents, we may include the one occurring at the Italian Hall (USA) in 1913, the disaster at the Glen Cinema (UK) in 1929, the accident at the Estadio National (Peru) in 1964, the tragedy at Gate 12 of the Monumental Stadium (Argentina) in 1968, the one at a stadium in Kathmandu (Nepal) in 1988, the accident at the Accra Sports Stadium (Ghana) in 2001, the incident at the E2 nightclub (USA) in 2003 or the accident at the Al-Aimmah Bridge (Iraq) in 2005, and so on. Surprisingly, these incidents have occurred repeatedly for over a century. Additionally, although it was not an emergency evacuation, an incident occurred when a crowd flow equivalent to an evacuation rushed into a dead end in 1989 at the Hillsborough Stadium in the UK, leading to 96 deaths and 766 serious injuries.

3.4.2.2 Doorways

Doorways (entrances and exits) are narrow sections that connect two spaces to prohibit access to unallowed visitors. On this scope, doors and other obstacles are usually installed at their location. Doorways tend to be significantly smaller than the rest of the available space. From the perspective of crowd flows, entrances and exits are typical bottlenecks, but they differ slightly in that their intended function is to completely block the flow of people.

Generally, for most mass facilities (e.g., stadiums, arenas, or religious buildings), the perceived value of the interior space is higher than that of the exterior space. When seen from the perspective of people outside coming in, the doorway is referred to as entrances, and they are exits when seen from the opposite perspective. For fans of a particular artist or football team, for example, the inside of a venue holds an extremely high value, while the concert or the match is being held and that value cannot be obtained at any other time. Because of this, the gathered crowd seeking this value with having potential fear of the possibility of losing it tends to be selfish, have a strong shared identity, and think in terms of maximizing this value rather than losing it. This is thought to be the behavioral principle that is responsible for crowds rushing to entrances. This is not just limited to the moment that doors are opened. Even during quiet intervals, if the crowd suddenly perceives that they will lose something of great value, they will rush in simultaneously.

At a rock concert held in the USA in 1979, an incident was caused by the crowd rushing into the entrance before the opening of the venue as they believed the concert had started earlier than planned. In 1991 in Mexico, a large number of pilgrims rushed into the entrance of a church to receive blessings from God, causing a crowd incident. Similar incidents also occurred in Saudi Arabia in 2004, twice in India in 2005 (food relief was being provided to families in need after a natural disaster), in the Philippines in 2006, and in China in 2007, among others.

3.4.2.3 Stairways

Stairways interconnect different floors along the vertical distance; thus, they often tend to be narrower than other areas of pedestrian passageways. In addition, they also tend to reduce the walking speed of people transiting through them to about half of what would be possible in the same space on flat land [6]. This means that both crowd density and crowd pressure acting from behind tend to be high. In the predominant form of accident that occurs in stairways, one person falls, and this causes a successive fall in the front. Simultaneously, the crowd at the back of the initial fall would also successively fall into the created gap when many people move in the same direction.

Although it could not be determined whether the accident was caused by crowd domino or avalanche, the tragedy that occurred in 1943 at the Bethnal Green Tube Station (UK) appears to have been a case of crowd avalanche, as reports noted that "a woman holding a child fell and the backward crowd collapsed" (another accident also occurred in Italy in 1942 under similar circumstances). Additionally, in the accident that occurred at Yahiko Shrine (Japan) in 1956, the collapse happened on the stairs to the shrine's gate, but records noted that "those who fell at the top were prone and had their feet pointing toward the gate and their heads pointing to the bottom of the stairs. Many people at the bottom ended up lying on their backs, with their feet pointing toward the gate." This situation was likely caused by a combination of crowd domino and avalanche happening at the same time. Furthermore, the conditions that lead to this type of incident not only occur in emergency situations in which a crisis is unfolding (where people are prone to rush) but also happen in situations where there are regular time constraints, including when exiting religious and sporting venues.

3.4.2.4   Enclosed Spaces

These are spaces in which part of the crowd becomes temporarily segregated from the rest and the number of people who can enter or exit is significantly smaller than the total number of people. Usually, only part of a larger crowd can enjoy something they value in these spaces, while other people stay outside the limited area. Classical examples for enclosed spaces include stadiums in which spectators watch sport games or concert halls filled with fans. However, station platforms are also classified as enclosed spaces due to their structural characteristics.

In general, crowds are contained in enclosed spaces, and significant density changes cannot occur. However, there is still a risk of crowd turbulence caused by local high-density states swelling through the crowd or by the crowd simultaneously taking unexpected action. At a rock concert in the UK in 1988, a "swell" occurred in the crowd, which was probably caused by crowd turbulence, leading to an incident. Additionally, a crowd avalanche can occur when the boundary of the enclosed space is a fence or a similar structure that can easily fall over and collapse under crowd pressure. Examples of this occurred during a football game in the UK in 1946 and religious events held in India in 1954 and 2008. Although the chain of events is different, a similar accident occurred in South Africa in 1991 as "peaceful" spectators tried to flee violence during a football match but were pushed against the fence, which, in contrast to the 1946 accident in the UK, did not collapse.

In certain cases, enclosed spaces may be created by the crowd itself without external structures being involved. This can occur when the outer part of a crowd rushes from multiple directions to a single point, thus restricting those in the center from leaving and creating a spatial structure with the properties of an enclosed space. During the tragedy that occurred in the Lan Kwai Fong area of Hong Kong in 1993, more than 15,000 drunk people gathered at the intersection of four entertainment districts to watch the countdown on New Year's Eve. The converging flow of people overcrowded the center of the intersection, leading to the death of 21 people. As was the case here, crowds themselves can act as moving walls that inhibit the movement of other sections of the crowd.

3.4.2.5   Constricted Segments

In terms of crowd flow lines, constricted areas are parts where the width of the area is narrower than those of other places. Constricted segments are similar to doorways in that they connect spaces, but they do not have the intended function of completely blocking the flow of people.

In urban infrastructure, tunnels, bridges, and pedestrian overpasses are considered in this category. When seen from a micro perspective, vending machines, kiosks, and pillars placed on pavements, and carry bags as moving obstacles may limit the space of a path, creating constricted segments.

From a crowd flow perspective, the open part at the front of the constricted area is the inlet, and the other side is the outlet. As the crowd enters from the inlet, its density increases, and its moving speed decreases, starting to satisfy the conditions of crowd accidents. Furthermore, the crowd behind that has yet to reach the constricted area continues to move forward without decreasing its speed. This can cause a further increase in density in the segment as well as the probability of crowd accident. Besides, crowds may jam at the entrance to the constricted segment, which carries its own risk of accidents.

If the outlet of one constricted segment connects to the inlet for another, this leads to even higher crowd densities and further risks. The footbridge of the Akashi Pedestrian Bridge Accident mentioned at the beginning of this chapter had a structure that tapered from the station forecourt to the bridge and then narrowed again from the entrance of the bridge to the exit stairs (details are discussed later and schematically represented in Fig. 3.8). This means that people on their way to the firework display were unable to cross the bridge even after the display had ended. The crowd avalanche was caused when another opposite-directed crowd moved toward the station trying to access the stairs to the bridge, causing a counterflow. Other accidents that occurred in constricted bridge areas, such as the one occurring in Taiyuan (China) during a light show in 1991 and the incident that occurred in 2004 during a lantern festival in Miyun (China) were caused by counterflow on the bridges themselves.

3.4.3 Internal Factors (Crowd Intrinsic)

Internal factors are crowd intrinsic factors, which appear as a result of collective interactions within the crowd. They are influenced by physical, psychological, and physiological factors, while external factors are fundamentally limited by geometrical constraints related to the structure. When many people with the same purpose simultaneously move or act, they form a crowd and make some specific type of flows. In this section, the flow patterns that appear to be responsible for increasing the crowd density to a potentially dangerous level are classified, followed by a discussion on factors driving the crowd to collective motion.

3.4.3.1 Flow Pattern

The flow pattern of a crowd is deeply connected to the nature of the incidents when they occur. In this section, we will provide a detailed discussion while also including examples for each type of flow pattern as we go through.

As an example, a stationary crowd is the one that is orderly queuing in a line or watching a match while sitting or standing still. When people are seated, the maximum crowd density is determined by the seating arrangement, but there can be a danger of higher densities when a crowd is discourteously queuing or standing. When there is overcrowding in the latter situations, people in the crowd try to move slightly in search of space. This can result in crowd turbulence where the distribution of local density changes windingly, as described earlier. Additionally, crowd turbulence can occur even in a stationary crowd when members of a crowd come into contact with each other in an excited state, as is common at rock concerts. The previously discussed incident that occurred during a rock concert in the UK in 1988 was the result of this type of turbulence.

However, these cases are rare, and most historical crowd incidents occurred in crowds that are moving rather than stationary. Therefore, it is necessary to pay attention to the flow pattern of the crowd as it moves. The study of the past crowd incidents has led to a conclusion that crowd flow patterns at the time of incidents fall into one of the following classes: one-way flow, counterflow, confluence, intersection, entanglement, rushing-in, scattering, aggregation, and packing. The types of flow are listed as follows:

- **One-way Flow (Unidirectional Flow)**: This is a type of flow in which everyone in the crowd moves in the same direction toward the same destination. The higher the density of the crowd is, the more likely it becomes for dangerous situations to occur due to stagnation. A crowd swarming toward the stage during a rock concert is also included in this category in a broad sense.

- **Counterflow (Bidirectional Flow)**: Two crowds move in one-way flow toward each other from opposite directions. Because strong interactions occur between people from both directions, when lanes cannot be formed, the risk of deadlock is high, potentially leading to very dangerous situations.

- **Confluence**: This pattern occurs when two crowds in one-way flow move from different points to the same destination and meet at a certain point along the way. The point of confluence and the area in front of it are inherently dangerous for both flows that are joining together.

- **Intersection**: In this form, two crowds in one-way flow that are traveling from different points to different destinations meet at a given point. The point of confluence is inherently dangerous for both flows involved.

- **Entanglement**: This flow pattern involves two or more one-way flows of crowd coming from different points in different directions but with individuals choosing their own destinations in the intersecting space. The point of entanglement is inherently dangerous for everyone involved.

- **Rushing-in**: Multiple crowds come from different directions at once, and all come together at a single point to form a new one-way flow. The crowds before they come together differ from those in confluence in that they are not clearly defined one-way flows before they meet. This pattern causes density to rise sharply at a single point. The danger is inherent at the affluence point and in the crowd flow in front of it. There have been incidences where the opening of gates at the beginning of an event has led to accidents caused by this flow.

- **Scattering:** This pattern involves multiple crowds scattering from a central point simultaneously. The density in the center drops sharply. The behavior in this pattern starts at the central point, but the reaction is delayed for those further away from the middle. This means that "crowd walls" are formed at points away from the epi-center, causing areas of high-density and high-pressure that are moving outward, which carries a danger of causing accidents. This pattern has caused incidents when a crowd has tried to escape from violence or the threat of terrorism.

- **Aggregation**: In this pattern, crowds come from all directions to concentrate in a single spot. This is similar to rushing-in, but the newly formed crowd does not form a new one-way flow. Those who have achieved their goals at the center of the crowd try to return to the perimeter, which causes local collisions between the center and the rest of the crowd. The high-density at the center is compounded by the complicated nature of the resultant flow, causing a high risk of accidents.

- **Packing (Stationary standing)**: Stationary standing crowds should also be regarded as a form of crowd flow. In this pattern, there is a high density of people standing in an enclosed space. Turbulent crowd flow in which the local distribution of density changes within the crowd causes a risk of accidents. Other crowd flows (such as counterflow and entanglement) can locally form this pattern, which can also lead to accidents.

Figure 3.5 illustrates the statistics of past incidents based on crowd flow type. We can see that some patterns are more likely to cause accidents than others. The figure shows that one-way flow has been present in most incidents, followed by counterflow, scattering, rushing-in and aggregation, and packing.

We can now consider the crowd flow patterns in relation to the external factors, which have been discussed earlier. As can be seen from Fig. 3.6, one-way flow patterns tend to cause issues in dead ends and stairways, counterflow tends to cause problems in constricted segments and stairways, scattering and packing cause incidents in enclosed spaces, and all flow patterns except packing cause problems in doorways.

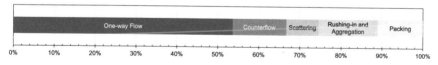

Fig. 3.5 Rates of occurrence for various flow patterns in incidents. Note that only accidents for which the flow pattern was clear have been considered to create this graph

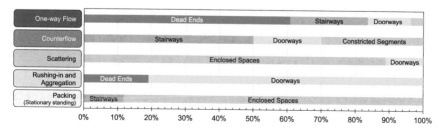

Fig. 3.6 Spatial structures in which incidents occurred, by crowd flow pattern

The identification of how these crowd flow patterns are formed at the moment of the incident is complicated because crowd management, environmental factors, and preceding flow patterns are mutually related. We will discuss the problems on the management side in detail later, but to show concrete examples in relation to the topics discussed here, we will look at the following cases in which ultrahigh crowd densities leading to the incidents was caused by the interactions of several flow patterns.

- **Lan Kwai Fong Accident (Hong Kong, 1993)**
  During this accident, that occurred in an area of Hong Kong famous for its nightlife entertainment, a large number of drunk people gathered organically to enjoy the New Year countdown at an intersection around the center of the district. A continuous flow of people came to gather at the crossroads in the run-up to the countdown. At this time, each road had a one-way flow that merged at the intersection. This meant that it was extremely difficult to escape from the rising density at the intersection itself as the crowds of people coming in from all sides acted as walls. In other words, the four crowd walls created by people coming from the four respective roads virtually formed an enclosed space, which caused the center of the crowd to become static and overcrowded. Once the countdown had ended, the crowd in the middle of the intersection began to move, causing crowd turbulence, and eventually, a crowd avalanche occurred shortly after the New Year started. In addition, the site of the incident was on a slope that had become slippery with liquids such as alcohol, and there were several sections with stairways nearby. The flow pattern formed in this case was complex rather than a linear series of one-way flow, confluence, and aggregation. In addition, the spatial structure and the environmental factors played a complex role in the incident. It is also likely that the flows of four respective roads were one-way flow, and that their destinations were overcrowded, making movement effectively impossible; thus, partly a dead end existed, which are circumstances of a large number of incidents. As a consequence of the accident, crowd control measures have been put in place in that area in the following years, allowing only one-way access with a no-turning rule.

In contrast to this, both the 1956 incident at Yahiko Shrine (Japan) and the previously discussed Akashi Pedestrian Bridge Accident are examples of incidents that resulted from a single type of crowd flow pattern. In both cases, counterflow was responsible for the blockage on the stairs to the shrine and the pedestrian bridge, respectively. The crowd in both incidents pushed into the available space from front and back with no leeway for movement to left or right, causing the extremely high crowd density that led to the incidents. An overview of both incidents is given below.

- **Yahiko Shrine Accident (Japan, 1956)**
  During the New Year's festivities held at Yahiko Shrine over the end of the year and the start of the new one, about 2,000 rice cakes were thrown from the roofs of the gate into the worship hall, following the firework of New Year's beacons. After this event, the crowds flowed out from the worship hall through the gate forwarding to a train station, simultaneously with an opposite-directed crowd trying to get

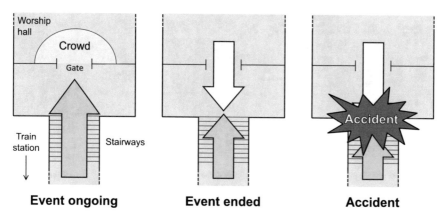

Fig. 3.7 Dynamics of the crowd accident at Yahiko Shrine

into the venue for regular New Year celebrations. Two crowds collided, forming a counterflow; then, the incident occurred on the stairway (as illustrated in Fig. 3.7). Many of the people who fell at the top of the stairway were prone and had their feet pointing toward the gate, and many people at the bottom ended up lying on their backs, with their feet pointing toward the gate. There were attendees from both crowds among the 124 people killed. Another 91 were injured in the accident.

- **Akashi Pedestrian Bridge Accident (Japan, 2001)**
  The accident occurred on a pedestrian bridge that connected the railway station with the fireworks venue. Pedestrians continued to arrive at the station throughout the display and attempted to cross the pedestrian bridge. The outflow from the bridge was extremely small in comparison to the inflow because the staircase on the venue side halved the available space and the entanglement of the flowlines at the bottom of the staircase narrowed the outflow. In addition, the firework display could be seen from the bridge, which meant the crowd stopped each time the fireworks were set off, leading to high-density stagnation for the duration of the event. As the display came to an end, spectators began to return to the railway station and the concession stand area adjacent to it, causing a counterflow in the staircase as they began to climb (see Fig. 3.8 for an illustrative representation). Once the firework display was over, the stagnation on the bridge increased even further, causing the incident. A total of 11 people were killed, and 247 people were seriously injured. Importantly, the point of the accident was not at the point where the two crowd flows collided but at its vicinity.

These two incidents that occurred in Japan share many similarities. Firstly, they were both caused by a collision between two crowds that were moving in opposite directions. People pushed into the collision area from both directions, leading to a high-density, high-pressure crowd. The second similarity is in the spatial structures involved. The incidents occurred on stone steps and a pedestrian bridge, respectively, but both structures shared the same feature that there was no way for the crowd to

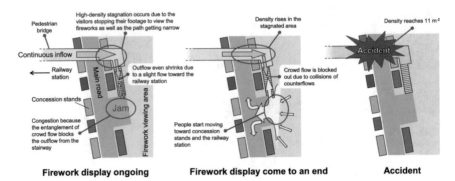

Fig. 3.8 Relevant moments for the accident during the 2001 Akashi Firework Display

escape left or right, further increasing the crowd density along the crowd flow lines. The third similarity is the characteristics of the events themselves: even after the main events (rice cake distribution or fireworks) had finished, other sub-events (shrine visits and concession stands) continued. When this type of event structure occurs, the crowds coming out from the main event and the crowd entering sub-events can have the macroscopically opposite direction flow. The final similarity is in the timing of the incidents, which both occurred immediately after the main event had ended.

From the examples considered above, it can be intuitively understood how dangerous counterflow can be, but we should nonetheless remind that most incidents occur in one-way flow and/or in spatial structures such as dead ends, as shown in Figs. 3.4, 3.5, and 3.6. For accident risk analysis, we need to consider not only crowd flow patterns but also crowd emotional status, spatial structures, and event design. Some of these aspects will be discussed in the remainder of this chapter.

3.4.3.2 Purpose of Assembly

The characteristics and state of crowds can differ greatly, depending on the characteristics of the event, and the type of incident can also change in relation to this. In particular, the attributes of gathered crowds depend greatly on their purpose of assembly, and it is necessary to take into account factors, such as age, gender, cultural background, psychological state (or mood), and the existence of a shared identity when managing a crowd. In order to understand the states and characteristics of an incident, it is necessary to understand the characteristics of the event and why the crowd gathers. Therefore, the states and characteristics of crowd dynamics at the time of the incident are analyzed using general knowledge and prior experience.

For example, events such as bargain sales for the promotion of supermarkets or the distribution of limited numbers of goods have quantitative limits on their value, which means that crowds are likely to rush and flood because of competition and act aggressively. Therefore, incidents are most likely to occur at the entrance to the event, just after opening. In addition, when people perceive an opportunity value to an event but cannot enter at the originally scheduled start time (such as a concert or a football game), they are more likely to flood as they seek to get access to locations or places that have particular importance for them. At events such as fireworks festivals and New Year events, crowds perceive value in being at the right place at the right time since they know that what they come to see is only available at a specific moment and is better seen from a specific place. This is likely to lead them to take even more aggressive actions to pursue their goals.

On the other hand, at a concert, the nature of the crowd differs depending on the artist performing, the type of music being played, and the number of people who can be accommodated. Crowds who are attending classical concerts with dress codes are often sedate, while crowds attending rock concerts are often excited. Excited crowds tend to act simultaneously at slight provocations. Audiences at classical concerts tend to sit quietly, while the opposite is true for people watching a rock concert. If we look at accidents that occurred during concerts in the list provided in the Appendix, they are all rock concerts at venues with standing arenas. Crowds at the back of rock concerts tend to move forward toward the stage as they get excited by the music, causing an increase in crowd density that can lead to accidents. Furthermore, an excited crowd moves in unison to the music, creating turbulence, and this could be particularly dangerous if it occurs in areas with high crowd densities near the stage. There are several cases of crowd incidents at concerts since the late 1980s, most of which occurred at the front of the standing area.

Some spectators at sporting matches, especially football games, can become mobs and act violently when they are unsatisfied with unfavorable decisions against the team they are supporting. These types of fans that are referred to as hooligans require special attention, and strict measures are taken to control them at football games, especially in European countries. In particular, effective physical boundaries are set between fans cheering for rival teams so that they do not interact and cause conflict. Accordingly, there have been several historical crowd incidents that occurred because spectators were reportedly trying to escape from a mob of hooligans, such as Heysel Stadium (Belgium) in 1985 or a similar one that occurred in India in 1980 (which is also referred to as the "Football Lovers' Day").

Finally, we should mention that there has also been a large number of crowd incidents at religious events. Crowds that come together in a gathering having a sacred value often act in a state of excitement because a given place or time has particular importance in the frame of the religious tradition. These crowds are sometimes in a sort of trance state and may even require psychological preparation to withstand unfavorable conditions [7]. Thus, they are sometimes unable to realize the tangible danger of the incident.

3.4.3.3 Time Constraints and Competition

As we have seen so far, most crowd incidents involve crowds acting simultaneously as a result of some form of time or quantitative constraint. For example, when there are a limited number of items being distributed over a given period of time, or temporal factors at play such as the start time of a match or the departure time of a train, this can become a factor that drives people's collective actions. This driving force can be thought of as a judgment of value such that whether an opportunity, experience, profit, or right is lost or not. The simultaneous actions that crowds take can include both cases where the action is performed ahead of a predetermined time, and when the predetermined time arrives.

For instance, in a 2004 accident in Saudi Arabia, around 8,000 people gathered at a major furniture store for limited distribution of gift certificates and, as the store opened, the crowd rushed in killing three people. This was because the crowd was aware that the number of vouchers that were available for distribution was fixed and flooded because of competition. A similar incident occurred when a supermarket in China held a 20% off sale on cooking oil in 2007 (cooking oil prices had been soaring in that period). Further, when there is an emergency evacuation from a fire, an outbreak of violence, or a natural phenomenon, crowds simultaneously perform the same action as quickly as possible under extremely tight time constraints to not lose their lives or become injured, the conditions of which are similar to those of a nonemergency-driven competition.

In addition, it is worth pointing out that even if an event that requires emergency evacuation does not occur, an individual's casual utterance can become a rumor and spread rapidly, becoming misinformation that leads the crowd to act, ultimately leading to an accident. As an example, when the Brooklyn Bridge (New York, USA) opened in 1883, a person in the crowd shouting that the bridge would collapse caused a panic that led to a crowd incident that killed 12 people. Another example is the disaster that occurred at the Shiloh Baptist Church (USA) in 1902, where the mishearing of the word "fight" as "fire" caused a mass evacuation of the crowd, killing 115 people. More recently, at a religious event held in Iraq in 2005, panic spread when one person in the crowd shouted that another person had explosives, and people fought each other to escape, killing nearly 1,000 people. The combination of competition and misinformation can lead to dramatic cases. In 2005 in India, when food relief supplies were given to people after a natural disaster, 4,500 people gathered while rumors spread that supplies were limited to 1,000 families. As the facility opened, people rushed in, eventually killing 42 despite the fact there were enough supplies for 45,000 families. There are many other cases in which floods of people who did not want to miss an opportunity have caused accidents at times such as New Year's countdowns, the end of firework displays, or just before the departure times of buses and trains. In 1934, an accident occurred at the Kyoto Railway Station (Japan) and was caused by a crowd of families rushing the platform who wanted to see military recruits at their departure. Even at religious events, if a particular act will need to be performed at a particular time and place, there is a high possibility of the occurrence of accidents. There have been incidents at the stoning of the devil, part of the Hajj pilgrimage, in Mecca (Saudi Arabia) in 1994, 1998, 2001, 2003, 2004, and 2006, killing over 1,000 people.

3.5 Role of Crowd Management

Here, we shall consider the role played by crowd management itself. Firstly, we should consider why crowds have taken potentially hazardous actions. It can be argued that the flow patterns that formed at the time of these incidents are often the result of inappropriate crowd management systems. This can be either because the management side actively did something, or because they failed to do something else. Such action and inaction are of the same level of responsibility in crowd management, and particularly the duty of care is owed by all individuals involved, regardless of the degree of involvement.

Some of the incidents we have looked at could have been avoided if some of these factors were present. However, generally speaking, many factors are necessary for the operation of events, and excessive measures against risks may negate events at all. Table 3.1 summarizes acts that are directly related to past incidents. It should be noted that the possibility of creating a potentially dangerous high-density crowd is immanent in these acts. Thus, particular care is needed when these operations are planned or acted. It is often the case that many of these factors are correlated with each other; therefore, potential risks appear either vaguely or cannot be recognized at the moment when the preceding acts are carried out. This occurs because the correlation with succeeding acts is not existing yet. The knowledge from this chapter comes into play at this time, to help one to recognize the risk within these preceding acts, and to foresee the potential consequence created by the correlation of preceding acts with the planned succeeding acts.

Arguably, if crowd management stakeholders create a potentially dangerous high-density crowd through action or inaction, although it is foreseeable, by not taking appropriate measures, any resultant incident is human-related. This is the fundamental principle behind negligence liability. Therefore, management should act upon various environmental and crowd factors, as shown in Fig. 3.3. For example, if a crowd of people who are packed into a dead end cannot escape because a facility manager has locked (or forgot to unlock) an emergency exit, the facility manager's action (inaction) is a human factor on the management side. If the emergency exit had not been locked, the crowd could have escaped to the outside, and the incident could have been avoided. Moreover, in a case where a counterflow causes an incident

Table 3.1 Managerial reasons leading to specific flow patterns

Action-related	Inaction-related
Sudden relaxation of access controls, opening of shops, starting or ending a show, religious ceremonies, provision of poor guidance and/or wrong/misleading information, operation of free buses, simultaneous arrival of trains, forced exclusion by security forces, police enforcement, air raids, etc.	Leaving excited crowds without guidance, unsupervised density increase, do nothing to stop the spread of misinformation, etc.

because the on-site event supervision did not properly regulate or guide the flow of people, this is also a human factor as the counterflow could have been prevented with appropriate management. The important point to highlight here is that there must be proper cooperation between management stakeholders. At the trial that followed the Akashi Pedestrian Bridge Accident [2], it was found that the organizer, security guards, and police had continued to work on the crowd security plan until the day of the event. However, effective measures to prevent congestion had not been taken, and no specific answers were given in regard to aspects such as the type of control methods to deploy in the event of congestion, the type of situation that would trigger requests to the police for assistance, and the form of cooperation that should take place between the organizer and the local police. It can be said that lack of communication and cooperation among the organizer, security guards, and the police was a management failure.

Similarly, a lack of coordination among stakeholders seemingly played a role in the Love Parade Accident [4]. It is alleged that a combination of multiple factors ultimately caused the accident, but many details have remained unclear. Although the criminal trial has been discontinued due to the statute of limitations, the prosecutor admitted that the combination of the minor negligence of the stakeholders was responsible for the accident, where the level of negligence of each is minor guilt not exceeding the level of conviction. Seven out of ten defendants have accepted the prosecutor's claim and paid fines.

Furthermore, what we can perceive from these cases is that when a number of different organizers and event management are present, problems can easily occur at the intersection of their management areas if mutual and meaningful communication is missing. Stakeholders must, therefore, share information and discuss potential issues in advance to form a consensus and clarify the boundaries of responsibilities

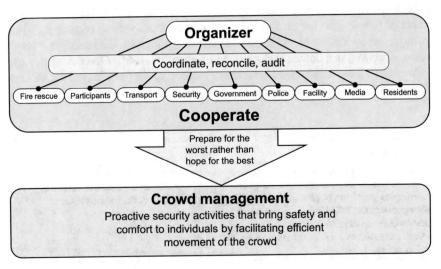

Fig. 3.9 Importance of stakeholders' cooperation to prevent accidents

in order to reduce the likelihood of accidents and to design an event at which visitors can feel safe and comfortable. The Japanese and German cases are in some sense at the opposite ends of the spectrum in terms of centralizing (decentralizing) responsibilities, although three entities were convicted in the former case. In dealing with crowds, a decentralized management structure that shares or imposes responsibilities is not preferable.

As highlighted in Fig. 3.9, the favorable relationship of the stakeholders in the frame of crowd management is that the event organizer stays at the top of the relationship hierarchy rather than a parallelly structured relationship and has the duty to coordinate, reconcile, and audit subsequent stakeholders to make sure all parts involved in management fully understand the scope of their individual responsibilities. Subsequent stakeholders are expected to cooperate with these processes at the same time. This does not necessarily contradict profit-making in the sense that the entity that directly receives part of the profit from the event must share the appropriate level of the responsibility. Prior to all of these, as a major premise, all stakeholders have to prepare for the worst scenario rather than hope for the best. Although this management structure may be controversial, it would be possible to deploy an external and confirmed organization for professional auditing on the crowd safety issue.

References

1. Great Britain: Department for Culture and Media and Sport: Guide to Safety at Sports Grounds. The Stationery Office (2008)
2. Osaka High Court of Japan, April 6, 2007: Saikō Saibansho keiji hanreishū (2010). Available at LEX/DB 25463707
3. Helbing, D., Buzna, L., Johansson, A., Werner, T.: Self-organized pedestrian crowd dynamics: Experiments, simulations, and design solutions. Transp. Sci. 39(1), 1–24 (2005). https://doi.org/10.1287/trsc.1040.0108
4. Helbing, D., Mukerji, P.: Crowd disasters as systemic failures: analysis of the love parade disaster. EPJ Data Sci. 1(1), 7 (2012). https://doi.org/10.1140/epjds7
5. Wagner, U., Fälker, A., Wenzel, V.: Fatal incidents by crowd crush during mass events.(un) preventable phenomenon? Der Anaesthesist 62(1), 39–46 (2013). https://doi.org/10.1007/s00101-012-2124-z (in German)
6. Weidmann, U.: Transporttechnik der fußgänger: transporttechnische eigenschaften des fußgängerverkehrs, literaturauswertung. IVT Schriftenreihe 90 (1993) (in German)
7. Lohner, R., Muhamad, B., Dambalmath, P., Haug, E.: Fundamental diagrams for specific very high density crowds. Collective Dyn. 2, 1–15 (2018). https://doi.org/10.17815/CD.2017.13

Chapter 4
Pedestrian and Crowd Sensing Principles and Technologies

Abstract Although it is possible to define crowd's properties in a quantitative way, measuring these quantities ultimately relies on sensors. Nowadays, there are multiple ways to collect quantitative data from crowds of people. Images from cameras can be analyzed to extract people's position or related information and additional technologies such as distance sensors allow to obtain similar quantities in an alternative way. The widespread use of smartphones and electronic devices also allows to get information such as people's position or the density in a given area without the need to install dedicated sensors. By exploiting wireless communication functionality of electronic devices, it is also possible to understand what are the most typical routes of people ranging from small structures such as museums or shopping malls up to large areas covering entire cities or regions. While the possibilities given by modern technologies seem unlimited, each sensing method comes with potentials and limitations. Understanding how each technology works and what are its advantages and disadvantages is important for successfully grasp crowd properties in relation to everyone's need and constraints. This chapter will review sensing technology from a practical perspective, which also accounts for privacy issues, while also propose a methodology to select the solution best fitting one's conditions.

4.1 Introduction

Over the last decades, there has been a steady increase in technologies that can be used to detect, count, track, and monitor pedestrian and crowd activity in public spaces and it is now even technically possible to identify individuals. It is, therefore, important to know the most relevant technologies and understand the differences between them in order to choose the type of sensor that is most suited to the environment where its use is envisaged.

However, before going into the details of sensing technologies for crowd management, it is important to add a few remarks on the general purpose of sensing and its meaning, in particular, in view of the recent improvements in information technology (IT). In the context of this chapter, sensing is simply an alternative expression for the concept of measurement. In other words, by measuring a property of some object/person, it is possible to translate that property into numbers and track changes and/or compare it with other similar objects. Typically, a direct measurement is not possible, and indirect methods are used to quantify physical properties.

Hotness/coldness is a typical example that can be used to clarify the above discussion. This property is commonly measured in terms of temperature, which cannot be measured/sensed directly. In fact, the old thermometers used mercury or similar materials and translated changes in their density into a change in the height of the column inside the bulb, which was then read as temperature using the scale provided over the glass. Although this is a simple and practical approach, this old method of measuring temperature has the disadvantage of being difficult to digitalize and difficult to read and record temperature automatically for remote locations. Digital access to measurements is important as it enables establishing automatic warning systems and implementing single measurements into a wider system.

Hence, modern sensors measure temperature by sensing changes in the electrical properties of materials that can be readily fed into a computer and converted into digital numbers, which are easy to process and store. However, this approach has some limitations when temperature needs to be measured over a large range. For instance, thermocameras use the infrared wavelength to measure the surface temperature of objects from a long distance and over a large area.

In brief, as we have seen, in the case of temperature, although it is a physical property, its direct measurement is not possible, and there are different methods to quantify it and make it available in numbers.

In the case of pedestrians and crowd, similar remarks are necessary, as the presence of one person cannot be measured directly. Instead, we need to get rid of indirect approaches to quantify relevant properties for pedestrian crowds. In particular, most of the current sensing technologies employed in pedestrian monitoring (and the ones discussed in this chapter) are related to one or several of the characteristics of human beings:

- People have a very particular shape, making them a unique object different from animals and the surrounding background. In particular, the round head, the two eyes and ears with the nose in the middle, and the body silhouette are a quite useful set of properties to detect humans, and in some cases, also guess more subtle information such as age or gender (going as far as identifying one person). However, depending on the conditions, it may be impossible to see the eyes or distinguish the clear silhouette of one person, and thus, detecting humans from their shape alone could have some limitations (as we will see later by discussing technologies related to computer vision).
- People have a quite unique size. Generally, the height is around 160–170 cm, their depth (in the bust direction) is around 30 cm, and their width (along the shoulders) is around 50 cm [1]. Regardless of the details (such as the characteristics discussed above), this particular size may be useful to detect the presence of humans when it is not possible to use standard cameras showing in colors and details the physical aspects of people. This property (together with some shape-related properties) are used by three-dimensional (3D) distance sensors.

- People have a typical weight of about 55–65 kg (worldwide average is around 60 kg). Although there are clear differences between individuals (and more generally among gender and countries), the more the number of people sampled, the more it is likely that the average will be close to the overall population average. For instance, the weight of one person may be useful for systems where a weight sensor is already employed, for example in elevators or train carriages. In addition, the way in which that specific weight is applied on the ground may also help in estimating foot location, ultimately allowing human detection and count.
- People have a typical body temperature, usually around 36–37°C. This makes them different from the surrounding objects, which are usually colder (this is especially true for indoor spaces where the ambient temperature is usually kept at 20–25°C). Considering both the surface of the human body and its temperature, it is possible to count humans or at least detect their presence (if a place is completely empty or not) also without light. In addition, people breathe; which translates in the absorption of oxygen and the release of carbon dioxide (CO_2) into the air, thus making places filled with people resulting in a higher concentration of CO_2.
- Finally, there is one property that is more loosely related to human nature, but it is becoming more and more useful for detecting human activity: the use of smartphones and electronic devices (smartwatches, wireless headphones, etc.). In particular, the use of smartphones has rapidly spread throughout the globe, and most individuals own a mobile device to make phone calls and access the internet. In other words, detecting the presence of such a device can be regarded as detecting the presence of one person and counting the number of devices in a particular place can help estimating the number of people being there. Also, as we will see later on, modern smartphones contain a number of sensors that may help estimating the specific activity one person is involved in. In addition, as most devices contains a GPS module, their position is directly available worldwide.

By exploiting the human properties listed above, it is possible to detect the presence of humans and go as far as determining one's identity. In general, in the frame of pedestrian sensing, there are five spatiotemporal properties that can be detected and, depending on the sensor used, one or more may be obtained [2].

- **Presence**: *Is someone present?* Knowing whether one or more people are present in a given space is important during rescue operations or for surveillance. This is generally the most fundamental information on crowds and can be represented in a purely binary manner: someone is there or nobody is there. For this reason, it is also the easier to get from sensors, since almost all the properties listed above could be used on this purpose.
- **Count**: *How many people are present?* While presence is important, usually, knowing the number of people is also necessary, especially in the frame of crowd control. Although generally easy to obtain, to count people, the human presence has to be numerically quantified, thus requiring more detailed information from sensors.
- **Location**: *Where are those people?* The number of people is important, but since crowds are usually heterogeneously distributed in space, knowing individuals'

position is preferred. When position is concerned, the complexity of the task further increases. Sensors able to cover a wide surface with a sufficient detail are needed, but the reward of this difficult task are density maps, which represent an important information for crowd management.

- **Track**: *How did those people move?* To better grasp crowd properties, the ability to extract people's trajectories is also relevant. This is obtained by "following" people and connecting their successive locations over time. In this way, it is therefore possible to obtain velocity and understand how people move inside a structure. However, this brings further difficulties, since it may not always easy to follow individuals, especially if crowds are packed.
- **Identity**: *Who are those people? Is Anne there?* The most advanced sensing techniques can also extract individuals' identities, allowing to track individuals over non-interconnected spaces or non-subsequent time periods and determine whether a specific person is within the crowd. Identity does not necessarily relate with private information, and very often a generic ID is assigned to a person to allow following her/his movements through different areas or over long time periods. However, while identity detection allows to further refine tracking and may be needed in specific applications, privacy could become an issue, and it is important to check with regulations and laws to avoid violations.

In this chapter, we discuss how human properties can be exploited to obtain the above-listed features and ultimately measure crowd properties. It is nonetheless necessary to remind readers that human sensing is a huge research area developing at a very fast pace. For example, in medical sciences, gait analysis is used for patients' rehabilitation, and markers are often placed on the body to monitor movements with a high level of accuracy. Also, it is possible to detect presence of humans by sensing seismic vibration of the ground [3].

Covering all kind of human sensing methods is beyond the scope of this book, and we will limit ourselves to those methods that are relevant for crowd management. In other words, we focus this chapter on the methods allowing to estimate the most important crowd properties (i.e., speed, density, and flow) without the need to install special sensors/trackers on people and/or owing to a minimal involvement of monitored individuals. More concretely, we will focus on methods to estimate count, location, and track people, since presence is usually not sufficient to manage crowds and identity is often not strictly needed and may also lead to the violation of people's privacy.

4.2 Objectives of This Chapter

At the end of this chapter, readers should be able to understand the basic working principle of the different sensors involved in detecting pedestrians and the properties that they use for this purpose. Readers should be able to understand the differences between each sensor and grasp their potentials and limitations. In particular, people involved in the task of crowd management should be able to choose the sensor that better suits their environment. Sensors that work well indoors may not work outdoors, and brightness/lighting conditions may be an issue depending on the technology used.

With this said, we want to emphasize that presenting the details of each sensing technique and providing a list of the different products goes beyond the scope of this book and would also be difficult considering that many solutions are customized to fulfill client's needs and are not available to the general public.

However, a background knowledge allowing one to distinguish between different products based on their working principle is important as it allows one to understand if the given product is suitable for the envisaged application.

In this chapter, we tabulate a summary to facilitate the task of choosing the right sensor/solution, though this is only indicative as modern and complex crowd sensing solutions usually employ a combination of different technologies (termed as "sensor fusion" and discussed at the end of this chapter). We will also briefly discuss the technologies that are currently under development (or limited in use), but may become relevant in the near future.

4.3 Computer Vision

One of the most commonly employed solutions to count, track, and analyze pedestrian activity in public spaces is the use of images from (surveillance) cameras. This type of application is defined within the wider field of "computer vision," which aims at recognizing elements inside an image and getting detailed information using computerized algorithms [4–6].

For the sake of completeness, we wish to start with few remarks on how videos are made and explain some technical details of digital video recording. What is important to know is that videos are made up of images (called frames) taken at a fixed interval (see Fig. 4.1 for an example). Typical cameras used for surveillance takes 10–60 frames per second, which means people's movements are smoothly recorded even when people walk very quickly. Also important is the number of pixels (points) that an image is composed of. The more the number of pixels, the more "fluid" is the image, and details are easier to recognize. Most modern cameras used for surveillance

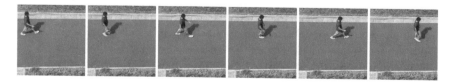

Fig. 4.1 Different frames showing a person walking from left to right. Six frames per second are shown in this example (the full sequence lasted 1 s), with the person walking at normal speed

in public spaces work in the HD range (1920 × 1080 pixels), although old models may have lower resolutions (but typically above the 640 × 480 standard).

For pedestrian dynamics, the type of algorithms employed within computer vision can be roughly divided into three main categories: detection/tracking, optical flow, and density estimation. These solutions employ images from cameras as the input to analyze pedestrian activity, but the type of information obtained by the subsequent analysis is different. The various approaches will be described in detail in the following sections.

4.3.1 Detection and Tracking

As the name of the section suggests, the detection and tracking algorithm has two main activities that (typically) are performed independently: people detection and continuous tracking.

First, in each frame, people are detected inside the image. Several techniques are available to detect presence and position of people within a given image. Without going into details, it should be mentioned that there are fundamentally two approaches that are often employed on this scope: "traditional" computer vision and deep learning algorithms [7]. Although the final outcome is the same (i.e., detect people in the image), it may be necessary to add a few words on the differences between both approaches.

Traditional computer vision methods first extract summarized information from an image, a step called "feature extraction," and later use these information to determine whether there is a human in there and where is she/he located. Typically, the presence of a contour representing a human silhouette is used on this purpose although other body parts may be used. This kind of approach is generally computationally faster and easier to employ, but the growing computational power is shifting the attention toward a more recent approach where the feature extraction step is no more required.

Deep learning (a special class of machine learning, sometimes also described as an AI method) allows to simply recognize people in images by training a computer with the use of several thousands (or millions) of pictures showing single individuals. In this approach, it is not possible (or very difficult) to know why a person is recognized as such. People are simply recognized because the computer has been trained using images of human subjects. The same approach could be used for example to recognize specific animals, cars, or other vehicles. Despite being computationally more demanding and requiring to perform the training operation (although already trained datasets are available), this approach has the advantage to allow more specific recognitions, considering for example gender, but going as far as the identity of a person.

Regardless on the approach used, typically either a box representing the individual (the so-called "bounding box") or a point referring to a particular part of the body is obtained after human detection (both are also possible). Figure 4.2 presents the two different representations for the frames given in Fig. 4.1. Both methods effectively

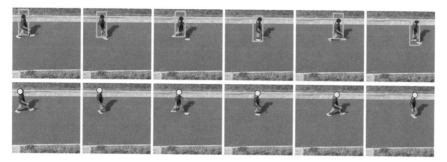

Fig. 4.2 Pedestrian detection using different representations. The algorithm given above searches for the full person silhouette, while the example provided below recognize patterns having a particular color and shape corresponding to people's head. Both examples are relative to the frames presented in Fig. 4.1

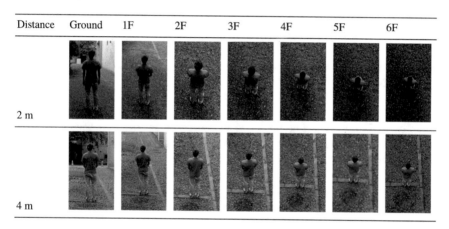

Distance	Ground	1F	2F	3F	4F	5F	6F
2 m							
4 m							

Fig. 4.3 Images of a standing person taken from different horizontal distances and heights. The body silhouette changes greatly when distance and angle is increased. Also, the lighting conditions and contrast have a big impact on pedestrian recognition (which is particularly clear for pictures taken from 5F and 6F)

allow to distinguish the person from the background and define his position. Obviously, each representation has its own limitations, but capabilities depend largely on the product, and the selection of computer vision solutions should be based on the evaluation of individual products.

However, there are some common aspects that need to be carefully considered when evaluating the performance of computer vision sensing technologies. As presented in Fig. 4.3, the shape and size of the human body change depending on the distance from the camera, both vertically and horizontally.

Images taken from great heights (such as the 6th floor of a building) only show a round head and an elliptic shape for the shoulders, while images taken from the same floor as the standing person also show feet, legs, and arms. Hence, algorithms that work well for azimuthal position may not work well at a low-angle perspective.

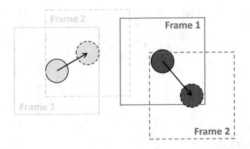

Fig. 4.4 Principles of pedestrian tracking. Typically, a search area is defined to connect pedestrian positions between two subsequent frames. Yellow and red dots represent different people

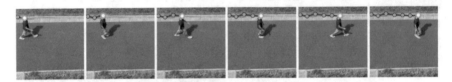

Fig. 4.5 Example of tracking pedestrian position over time. The frames correspond to Figs. 4.1 and 4.2, and the pedestrian's head is used to track the position

Therefore, while testing a computer vision solution, several scenarios need to be considered also taking into account future deployment conditions. Also, algorithms that are developed to target a particular size may not be able to detect close and/or far people for images taken at low angles where people may have different sizes within the image (see also Figs. 4.12 and 4.13).

While pedestrian detection may be sufficient to get a count of the people staying in a given place, usually it is useful to track the positions of people to understand what are the most commonly used paths or how people navigate inside a given space. As briefly stated earlier, pedestrian tracking is the task of connecting each pedestrian in each frame with the same person in the next frame. Figure 4.4 schematically presents this process.

Usually, a search area where a pedestrian is expected to move between two frames is defined. The search area for the yellow pedestrian of Fig. 4.4 is given along with her/his position. Knowing her/his position in frame 1, the same pedestrian is searched inside the area during the next frame, and both positions are linked. An example of pedestrian tracking is shown in Fig. 4.5 for the frames used earlier as an example. In this case, the head is used as a marker, and a red line is shown connecting the different detection points. We should also remark that tracking is only needed when people are detected as boxes or points without properties. If, for instance, identity or characteristics for each individual are known, tracking becomes much simpler as there is no need to search in the surrounding areas.

The tracking task seems straightforward when Fig. 4.5 is considered since only one person is present, and occlusion never occurs. Figure 4.6 presents a more realistic image of the conditions occurring when real crowds are to be tracked in a public

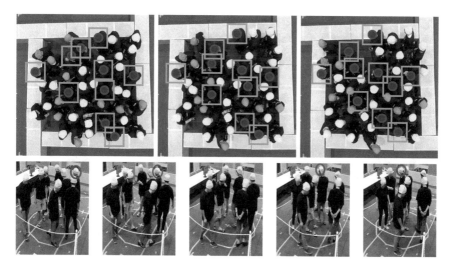

Fig. 4.6 Principles of and difficulties in pedestrian tracking. In the above series of pictures, the number of people is high, making it difficult to connect positions of people between the different frames (1 frame per second is taken here to emphasize the problem). The search area for blue caps is provided as an example. In the series of picture in the lower panels, occlusion occurs (people are covered by others), making it difficult to continuously track their positions. Frames are shown at a 0.5 s interval in the lower series of images. In both series of images, colored caps were used as markers allowing to easily detect and track people, although obviously, this is possible only in supervised experiments

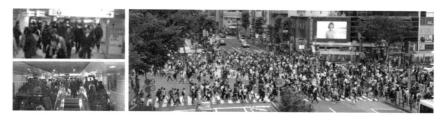

Fig. 4.7 Examples of situations where detection and tracking could be challenging or not possible at all. Top-left: low resolution (120 × 52 pixels), bottom-left: high occlusion and unfavorable light exposure, right: excessive number of people, insufficient resolution, and high occlusion

space. The high number of people and occlusion makes it difficult to relate positions of people between successive frames [7, 8]. Increasing the number of frames per second could help make tracking easier, but occlusion can only be solved by finding a good camera positions (and sometimes there are no ways to avoid it at all).

However, even the most efficient and performant detection and tracking algorithms may fail under extreme conditions.

Figure 4.7 presents some conditions where detecting and tracking people is very difficult if not impossible. In general, the number of people (or their size inside the image), the resolution of the video, and the conditions where the videos are taken determine the success or failure of detection-based computer visions algorithms.

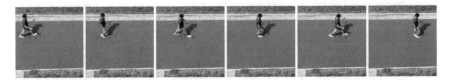

Fig. 4.8 Optical flow applied on the frames shown in Fig. 4.1. Direction of motion is clearly recognizable

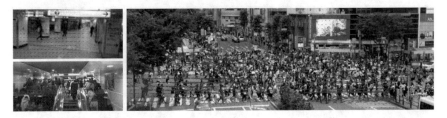

Fig. 4.9 Long-time application of the optical flow on the scenarios presented in Fig. 4.7. In all the cases, the general dynamics of the crowd is clearly recognizable

4.3.2   Optical Flow

When detection is not possible on the individual level, an alternative approach that allows getting a limited but still useful amount of information from crowd videos can be adopted: the so-called optical flow [9, 10]. The optical flow is a method that can be employed to any sort of videos but is particularly suitable for those with moving objects, such as pedestrians or vehicles. Here, we should mention a first practical difference from the approach described above: while pedestrian detection is possible also for single static images, optical flow only works with videos (or sequences of images) since moving objects are the target. While nowadays videos are almost entirely used in computer vision, this difference should be kept in mind if optical flow is considered as a potential solution.

The optical flow allows us to determine the direction and speed of objects moving within the video. Explaining details of this technique is beyond the scope of this text, and interested readers may find some references at the end of this chapter [9, 10], but the frames of Fig. 4.8 should help understand the outcomes obtained. The series of images is the same as that was used in Figs. 4.1, 4.2, and 4.5. The arrows indicate the direction of motion of the person shown in the images. As can be seen, there is more than one arrow per person, but it is generally sufficient to understand that something (a person in this case) is moving in that specific region in that particular direction. However, depending on the algorithm and parameters used, the number of arrows may be reduced as needed to get a better representation.

The optical flow is particularly useful and suited for situations where sudden changes are not seen and people move along typical routes for a (relatively) long time. Figure 4.9 presents the long-time results for the optical flow applied to the

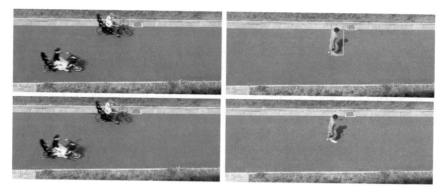

Fig. 4.10 Optical flow (applied on the lower images) does not have a detection process (performed on the images at the top), and therefore, bicycles are not distinguished from people

scenarios given in Fig. 4.7. The direction of motion is averaged over time intervals of 10–20 s. In all the cases, it is possible to grasp some information on the direction of movement and the areas that are occupied by moving people. Although actually counting the number of people and getting their trajectories is not possible, in some cases, estimating the speed and direction of people can be sufficient to judge crowd conditions and analyze pedestrian navigation within public spaces.

One of the biggest limitations of the optical flow approach is the impossibility to distinguish objects, as shown in Fig. 4.10. When a pattern detection approach is used, people are correctly recognized while bicycles are not (or both may be distinctively recognized using machine learning), but when the optical flow approach is used, all moving objects are seen in the same way, regardless of whether they are walking pedestrians or moving bicycles.

Also, we should remind that optical flow only measure speed and direction of moving objects, so if a crowd is static little can be known about its conditions, except the fact that motion is not observed.

4.3.3 Density Estimation

Finally, there is an additional approach that is worth mentioning in the frame of computer vision applied on crowd management: density estimation. In some cases, there is no need to extract trajectories or detailed information about pedestrians, but only their total number is needed or crowded areas need to be identified. On this purpose, there are special algorithms that allow to count the number of people or obtain the surface occupied by people, thus providing a rough estimate on crowd density [11–13].

Again, also for density estimation, each algorithm relies on quite different principles (some are quite simple approaches based on the so-called "background sub-

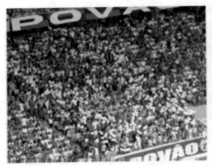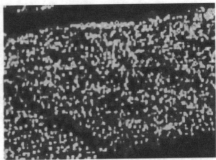

Fig. 4.11 Example for an algorithm estimating crowd density. Unoccupied or hidden areas are shown in blue (such as the access stairs or supporters' flags) and the portion occupied by pedestrians is given in lighter colors (from green to red). Courtesy of Future Standard Co., Ltd.

traction," others rely on more complex machine learning methods with an example provided in Fig. 4.11), and it is beyond the scope of this chapter to provide details. However, it is nonetheless useful to know about the existence of this alternative class of algorithms, as density is often one of the most important crowd properties and while trajectories are more appropriate to determine collective behavior, safety is more typically related to density (as already discussed through this book).

4.3.4   Advantages/Disadvantages

Computer vision has the clear advantage of being a very versatile technology employing quite inexpensive hardware (in regard to image acquisition). Also, numerous cameras can be used for this purpose, and so it is possible to control the costs of a sensing system based on computer vision and easily scale the requirements based on the surface one is planning to manage/control. In addition, since these approaches are based on computer software, it is also possible to employ computer vision by using cameras already in place. One would need to buy a sufficient amount of computing power to deal with the images generated from a camera without having to install any new sensor. In addition, it is also possible that cloud solutions will appear in the future, thus drastically reducing the initial investment.

However, as computer vision directly works on people's images, there are concerns about privacy, and even if institutions can guarantee privacy (by keeping images in their internal storage only for a short time or refraining from storage at all), and there is a legal framework allowing to work on pedestrian information, people may be discouraged from going to places where a large number of surveillance cameras are employed (although cameras could also help making people feel safe in some contexts and can remove the "cloak of anonymity" as discussed in Chap. 2).

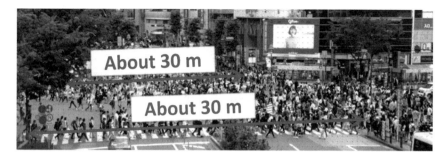

Fig. 4.12 Although the real world has a three-dimensional nature, it is represented as bidimensional in figures. Hence, computer vision approaches need careful calibration depending on the scenario where they are used

In addition, detection/tracking approaches require considerable computing power (thus partially increasing overall hardware cost due to the need of expensive computers), but more efficient algorithms and more powerful machines are reducing the costs for such applications. The optical flow approach is less computationally expensive, but as we have seen, it provides limited information. On the other hand, in the case of the optical flow, computing power is not related to the number of people in the scene. In contrast, as already seen from the examples of Figs. 4.5 and 4.6, tracking is more difficult when the number of people increases, and it requires larger computing power, translating into higher costs. Density estimation lies somewhat in the middle, requiring less computational power than detection/tracking, but it is not as efficient as the optical flow (although, again, differences among single products may be large).

Another important point to be considered when dealing with computer vision is perspective. Although this cannot be considered a disadvantage as it is relatively easy to get rid of it, it is important to not overlook this aspect when evaluating a computer vision solution. In fact, although the real world has a three-dimensional nature, images only contain bidimensional information. In other words, positions of people in images are given by their horizontal and vertical positions, but in the real world, a third position, depth, is present. As Fig. 4.12 shows, both arrows are relative to the same size (the crosswalk width) in the real world, but the distance (in pixel) inside the image is different (the distance you can measure on the book).

Figure 4.13 also shows a similar problem related to perspective (and partially lighting and contrast). The person in the image has the same height in all the frames, but he clearly gets bigger as he approaches the camera. To correct the perspective and get correct positions for pedestrians in images, a calibration process is necessary (and calibration has to be performed for every camera individually). Although this is not a difficult task and most of the computer vision solutions have calibration tools, it is an aspect that is worth keeping in mind. This may not be a problem for infrastructures where very few changes are done after the sensing system is installed, but may become

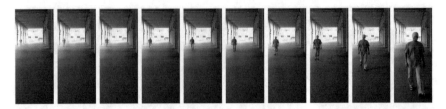

Fig. 4.13 Comparison of people size in different frames taken at constant intervals. Because of the perspective, silhouette size changes, thus necessitating a three-dimensional calibration to correctly work with computer vision algorithms (changes are clearly larger as the person gets closer to the camera). Lighting and contrast could be also an issue here

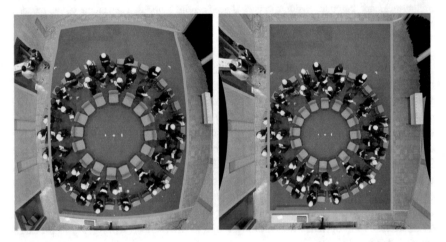

Fig. 4.14 Image distortion before and after correction. Cameras using wide angle lens require particular attention as the distortion may be particularly strong, causing problems during conversion from digital to physical units

problematic for buildings with continuous layout changes (exhibitions halls, concert halls, etc.)

As a result of a successful calibration, computer vision algorithms can translate pedestrians' positions given in pixels within digital images to real-world positions, providing the location of that person in the monitored environment.

Finally, with regard to perspective, some cameras may have a very strong deflection because of the lens used. In this case, a further "calibration" step is required to adjust lens curvature and get accurate positions of pedestrians, like the case shown in Fig. 4.14.

As shown in Fig. 4.15, lens deflection can have an important influence on people detection and tracking. This was already clearly seen for the examples provided in Fig. 4.3, although in Fig. 4.15 the changes are very large within the same image: while only the head and shoulders are seen around the center of the image, the feet and legs are visible in areas far from the center. Hence, if the location of the head is

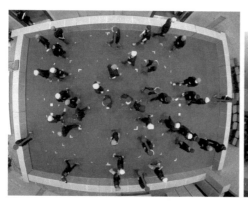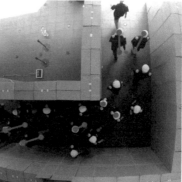

Fig. 4.15 Effect of image distortion of body height and positions of the head and feet

used as the pedestrian position, detection is accurate around the center but inaccurate (without proper calibration) near corners.

To conclude, although computer vision is making rapid progresses and automatic calibration features may appear in the future, the bidimensional nature of the input limits the amount of information gained. For instance, it is difficult to determine the height of people, and although it is already possible to get personal information by reading people's faces, privacy concerns limit the application of surveillance cameras for pedestrian and crowd sensing. Nonetheless, price and versatility definitely play in favor of computer vision. In addition, recent solutions can overcome privacy concerns by processing images within the camera and transmitting externally only non-privacy sensitive data.

Finally, it should be mentioned that perspective issues related to the use of images could be overcome by employing stereo cameras, in which a three-dimensional representation of the world is provided. This allows getting rid some of the problems related with computer vision, but algorithms get more complex and privacy remains as a potential obstacle. In regard to the use of 3D information, more details will be provided in the next section while presenting distance sensors.

4.4 Distance Sensors

Privacy issues related to the use of computer vision solutions are partially solved by employing so-called distance sensors that work with anonymous information and are much easier to calibrate and prepare for a new environment.

Distance sensors are electronic devices that can measure the distance between the sensor and objects located in their sensing range. Working principles vary with the manufacturer and product, though most of them use invisible light (mostly infrared light or lasers) to measure distance from objects. Explaining the working principles

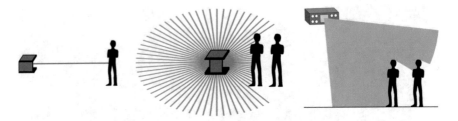

Fig. 4.16 Differences between 1D, 2D, and 3D distance sensors (from left to right)

of such sensors is beyond the scope of this book, but readers should understand the difference between different sensors and the kind of information such sensors use to detect people and eventually track their position.

In general, it is possible to distinguish distance sensors in three categories: one-dimensional (1D), two-dimensional (2D), and 3D sensors. Sensors employing a laser ray and operating on two or three dimensions are often referred as LiDAR or LADAR, although both definitions are generally vague.

The 1D sensors measure the linear distance between the sensor and the closest object (see Fig. 4.16). These sensors usually employ an (invisible) laser light, and only a single number is provided as the distance. These kinds of sensors do not allow recognizing people, but can be used to count people passing through a door or a corridor. When nobody is present, the distance between the sensor and the closest object is either constant or "infinite" (above the sensing range). When a person passes through the laser ray, the distance decreases to later increase again, and a count is triggered. Obviously, when the crowd is dense and people keep transiting, counting each individual is difficult, but setting the laser at a proper height or using an array of lasers could help making these problems smaller.

To overcome the limitations of single ray distance sensors, 2D scanners are often used. In 2D applications, the laser is rotated or moved within a given angle (typically at high speed) to get a distance map of nearby objects over a surface (a schematic example of such an application is given in Fig. 4.16) [14]. The scanning direction and scanning method can be changed depending on the context to get the most information from the situation, but it is generally difficult to locate people with this method, although it becomes easier counting transit events. Pedestrian sensors used in low-risk environments (e.g., in self-driving vehicles moving at low speed in warehouses or in robotic vacuum cleaner) typically employ a 2D sensor to detect the presence of obstacles (such as people passing by) and stop the vehicle. In this context, using a 2D distance sensor is sufficient since it is not necessary to count people or get their accurate position, but the main and only goal is to provide a warning message indicating an obstacle.

Distance sensors employed for pedestrian detection are usually 3D sensors, which allow us to obtain a 3D map of the surrounding area [15]. Figure 4.17 shows the basic output of 3D distance sensors: an image in which each point represents the distance between the sensor and the object is provided, and it is later used to detect and track

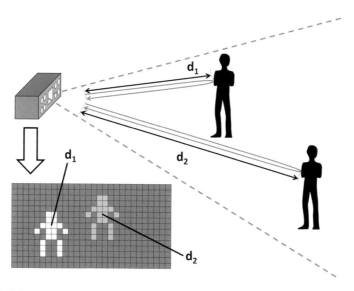

Fig. 4.17 Schematic example of people detected using a 3D distance sensor

people. 2D sensors in which the laser is rotated on multiple axes or multiple lasers are used at the same time also allow obtaining a 3D representation of the space, although depending on the degree of freedom on each axis and the number of lasers used, a fully 3D representation may not be possible.

In contrast to computer vision algorithms, distance sensors allow us to measure the physical distance between the sensor and the objects. In this regard, distances d_1 and d_2 in Fig. 4.17 will be provided in meters or centimeters without having to calibrate the sensor (or only the orientation angle, which is easy to obtain, will have to be given during the calculation).

Although the 3D distance map provided by these kinds of sensors already allows us to recognize people and track their positions (see also Fig. 4.18), tracking and detection algorithms for distance sensors usually convert the distance map into an azimuthal view, which allows us to recognize people using the distance from the floor and their shapes.

As Fig. 4.18 shows, once an azimuthal distance map is obtained, it is easier to recognize people as they are closer to the sensor compared to the floor and have a typical shape made up by their head and shoulders. In this regard, distance sensors can also be used to obtain the height of people, thus allowing us to distinguish adults and children more systematically.

Figure 4.19 shows an application of a 3D distance sensor in a real scenario. The image in the left panel represents the image obtained with a normal camera; the image in the middle panel is the distance map obtained using the sensor, which is later translated into the azimuthal representation that is finally used to detect and track people. The height of each person is also shown. Algorithms employed to

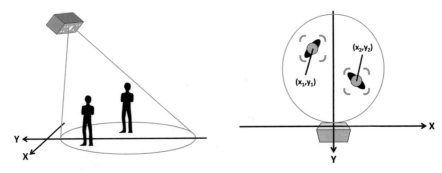

Fig. 4.18 Schematic illustration of how detection and tracking of pedestrians with 3D distance sensors works

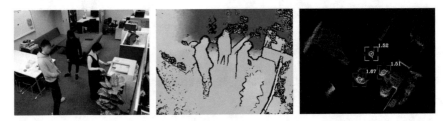

Fig. 4.19 Example of a real application of 3D distance sensors to detect and track people in public spaces. Left: image obtained using a conventional camera, center: distance map gained from the sensor, and right: the representation used to track pedestrian positions (height is given next to each person). In the central image, the color scale represents distance from the sensor, while in the image on the right, it represents height from floor

detect people using 3D distance sensors are similar to those used in computer vision: some looks for specific features of human body, others rely on training computers using 3D representations of thousands of individuals.

Further, 3D distance sensors provide additional information that cannot be obtained or are difficult to obtain using computer vision, for example, body orientation and arm-pointing direction. Once people are detected, tracking algorithms similar to the ones employed in computer vision are used to continuously track people (by "connecting" the dots).

4.4.1 Advantages/Disadvantages

One of the biggest advantages of distance sensors is that they directly measure distance and typically do that in a three-dimensional manner, thus simplifying the calibration process required for computer vision. In addition, more detailed information such as body orientation and arm-pointing direction is made available. In addition, only anonymous data are used (see Fig. 4.19), thus reducing the privacy issues related to the use of images in computer vision. In addition, the amount of data processed by distance sensors is much smaller than that used for computer vision, thus reducing both computational time and computational requirements. Finally, since distance sensors work using light emitted by the sensor itself (laser in most of the cases), they can work in darkness and are only slightly influenced by variable lighting conditions (although strong solar irradiation could be an issue, thus limiting outdoor use in some cases).

Among the disadvantages of distance sensors is their relatively high cost, especially for 3D sensors. Also, the installation costs can be high, as the technology is relatively new and only partially standardized. In addition, the sensing distance typically ranges around 10 m [16] (although this is rapidly increasing, and sensors reaching 50 m or more are being developed), and hence, a large number of sensors are required to monitor relatively small areas [17]. Finally, by missing visual clues, distance sensors do not allow obtaining human characteristics such as gender or age and their use to gain customer profile or detecting recurring customers is limited.

4.5 Localization Technologies (GPS, Indoor Positioning, Etc.)

Sensors presented so far have to be installed at facilities and operate by capturing the presence of pedestrians based on their physical properties. However, as already stated at the beginning of this chapter, there is also the possibility of directly detecting the presence of pedestrians by using the devices they carry.

In particular, Global Positioning System (GPS) sensors are found in a very large variety of electronic products: smartphones, smartwatches, and also some laptops. In addition, GPS bracelets are commercially available and some countries (e.g., Saudi Arabia) are considering (and partially already testing) asking people participating in particularly dense mass events to carry one of those devices to store relevant information and track the positions and density of people [18].

In this section, we will consider all technologies related to device localization. GPS is the most common one of such technologies, but over the years, several systems have been introduced to allow localizing devices even in indoor places using the strength of wireless antennas [19]. Providing a list of the different technologies used for both outdoor and indoor localization will be of little use, since most smartphones and electronic devices already have them integrated to obtain the precise location as output in a large number of places (especially in airports, train station or exposition halls).

In this regard, since localization devices directly provide the position of one person, there is no need to explain the technical background of this technology, but it is sufficient to mention a few aspects related to it. First, one should remember that if pedestrians are using localization systems, it does not necessarily mean that it is possible to get their position. In order to track people and obtain their position, a communication infrastructure is necessary, with mobile devices sending the pedestrian position to a remote location where data are analyzed (this is particularly true for GPS, which uses a communication protocol different from mobile networks). This means that in case of network problems, people could still get their position (although may not be able to load maps or related content), but those positions cannot be collected or their collection could be difficult.

In addition, and this affirmation holds true for all methods that aim at detecting mobile electronic devices, it is always difficult to guess how big is the proportion of the crowd that is using them. High-tech oriented business neighborhoods may have a high percentage of users of electronic devices (and maybe people there carry multiple devices), while kindergarten may have a lower percentage, thus mistakenly leading to a lower/higher estimation. In general, it is also difficult to say how large is this percentage as it may depends on time of the day and day of the week.

Finally, the use of mobile devices owned by pedestrians makes them a part of the solution as well as a part of the problem. Detection is in fact dependent on the battery level of their devices. Should the battery level decrease (e.g., during nightlong concerts), many users will turn the GPS or other functions off, thus limiting the possibility of tracking them.

4.5.1 Direct and Indirect User Involvement

After having discussed mainly technical and practical aspects related to localization services, a few words are necessary on user involvement. Although for field studies or in particular events, it would be possible to ask participants to carry a localization device or install an application to track their movements (direct involvement), location information are also automatically transmitted when people use navigation tools or access to certain applications requiring the localization feature (indirect involvement). When users are directly involved, it is usually possible to get better and more complete information as position is continuously streamed. In case of indirect involvement, information may be only shared with third parties when a specific app is used or a "locate me" button is pushed. However, more people are likely to use a navigation tool or check-in through an application in a busy city center compared to rural areas, thus providing a very clear image on the macroscopic pedestrian density over moderate periods of time.

Companies collecting this sort of data through indirect user involvement are therefore able to provide information in regard to crowd motion (see Fig. 4.20 for an example). In addition, although collected data are anonymous, age group, and gender are often shared along with the position (users are often asked to provide them when registering to a service, and it is confirmed whether they agree to the terms and conditions), thus allowing geographical and temporal profiling of the crowd. Usually, this sort of data are available with a consistent delay (hours, but more commonly days), thus making their use on the scope of crowd control difficult, but they could become useful when planning events and the disruption to the local community need to be assessed.

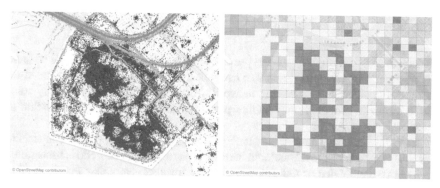

Fig. 4.20 Visualization of location data obtained through the use of smartphone applications, labeled here as "indirect user involvement". The map on the left shows details of users' activity, while the one on the right summarizes those results in the form of a density heatmap. Source: courtesy of Agoop Corp. with contributions from OpenStreetMap

4.5.2 Advantages/Disadvantages

A clear advantage of the use of localization technologies is the low infrastructure costs for facility operators. The amount of data to be processed is limited, and assuming pedestrian will use their own smartphones, there is virtually no cost for sensors. Also, there are no limitations on the area that can be sensed, and pedestrians can be tracked everywhere that communication facility is provided. Finally, device localization works under any condition, light or darkness, and can be also normally used during natural disasters, thus allowing one to obtain the positions of people to be evacuated or to detect areas where people are still trapped.

On the other hand, a big limitation related to most of these technologies (in particular, for GPS) is that they typically only work outdoors. As already mentioned, recent improvements have now made it possible to locate devices indoors using the signal strength of antennas, but this type of service is not always guaranteed. Also, the position accuracy is typically in the range of 10 m (1 m in the best case), thus making it difficult to obtain the precise position of pedestrians in public spaces (normally, it is also difficult to detect the side of the street on which someone is walking). Finally, a partial disadvantage is the need for the cooperation and permission of people in obtaining their positions, but this typically holds true only if direct involvement is sought. While this limitation could be overcome by acquiring dataset prepared by firm specialized in location data collection (through indirect involvement), costs tend to be high and generally data are not provided on real-time.

4.6   Instrumented Detection

Although localization systems can provide simple and useful information to facility operators, they require devices to transmit user position, implying the need for both user consent and a working network. Instrumented detection partially solve those problems, although they cannot provide as equally accurate information as localization services.

Each time a smartphone or any antenna-equipped electronic device connects to a wireless network or to a Bluetooth hardware, an alphanumeric code is transmitted to identify that device or the user using it. For instance, an alphanumeric number (either the MAC address or the so-called UUID) is transmitted every time someone connect to a WiFi network or when pairing/transmission is performed with a Bluetooth device. This code is not related to personal information, and it is simply a "machine number" used to distinguish each device uniquely. On the other hand, the phone number is usually employed to identify users connected to a specific antenna. Although scale and approach is typically different (details will be discussed later), these "identification codes" allows tracking the route traveled by people by tracking their devices.

Figure 4.21 shows how device detection is typically used and the information that can be obtained from this approach. Assuming one device (thus, one person) is detected at point A at 12:00, and later, the same device (thus, the same person) is detected at point B at 12:05, it is possible to guess that it took 5 min to go from A to B. Although the travel time may represent a simple information, it can help estimating the congestion along a specific route. However, to obtain accurate travel time estimations in complex urban environments, a large number of detection point may be required. As the example of Fig. 4.21 shows, when only two locations are used, it is not possible to know whether the long or the short route was taken by the given person. Hence, device detection is usually employed along major arterial roads such as bridges or tunnels that people have to pass.

Having explained the general principles, to go further into details, we now need to distinguish between tracking performed through information shared with mobile phone carriers and device tracking based on short-range electromagnetic signals (WiFi, Bluetooth or RFID). In regard to that, Table 4.1 may be useful to understand those differences further explained in the forthcoming discussion.

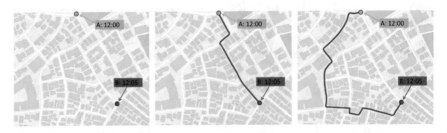

Fig. 4.21 Example of the typical use of instrumented detection for crowd monitoring. Image generated from the authors based on a map with contributions from OpenStreetMap

Table 4.1 Comparison between different methods used for instrumented crowd detection

	Mobile phone	WiFi	Bluetooth	RFID
Typical outdoor range	Several km	100 m	30 m	1 m
Typical indoor range	N/A	50 m	15 m	1 m
Individual tracking	Possible	User intervention needed		
Anonymous detection	Possible	Possible	Possible	Possible

Values given have to be considered as an order of magnitude and may largely change due to the environment (e.g., urban/rural area or wall thickness)

4.6.1 Mobile Network Antennas

Nowadays antennas used for mobile communication cover the almost entirety of land surface, with only remote areas being unserved. In the USA alone, about 400,000 cell sites are installed with roughly 300 millions of smartphones being in active use [20] (thus 90% of the population). Also, the more densely populated is an area, the higher the number of antennas needed.

Considering that each phone has a unique number, it is therefore possible to monitor how people move within a city or a country by tracking the antennas used by the person as she/he moves from place to place. Although, this technique is very often used to estimate travel behaviors [21, 22], it is also routinely employed to monitor changes in population (density) observed for example in business or leisure districts or to much larger scales [23].

In addition, since age and gender of users is provided at the time of service subscription, it is usually also possible to profile a population in a given area and time. Although resolution for mobile data may be course (especially in rural areas), the large number of users allow a rather precise profiling, which can be useful to identify efficient ways to guide/inform/control crowds based on the characteristics of the local population.

4.6.2 Bluetooth, WiFi, and RFID Tags

Antennas used for mobile communication are useful to monitor crowds on a large scale, but if details on a lower scale are needed, short-range communication protocols can be used. In particular, WiFi, Bluetooth, or RFID may be used on this purpose. However, when these technologies are used, active involvement of users is needed. In fact, although a cell phone will automatically connect to the closest antenna without the need of action from its owner, connection to WiFi or Bluetooth devices has to be initiated by the user.

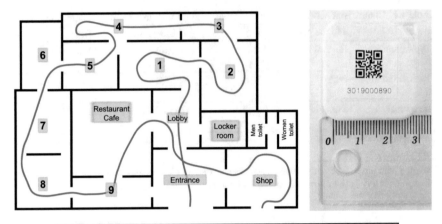

Order	Location	Dwell time	Order	Location	Dwell time
1	Entrance	3 min	8	Exhibit 6	Not detected
2	Lobby	1 min	9	Exhibit 7	8 min
3	Exhibit 1	12 min	10	Exhibit 8	5 min
4	Exhibit 2	7 min	11	Exhibit 9	4 min
5	Exhibit 3	4 min	12	Cafe	1 min
6	Exhibit 4	9 min	13	Lobby	Not detected
7	Exhibit 5	5 min	14	Entrance	1 min

Fig. 4.22 Example of the typical use of Bluetooth devices for crowd monitoring. The picture at the top shows a common BLE beacon employed in crowd sensing and the table below the result representing the behavior obtained for an individual. If transition from one place to another happens too fast, detection may not be possible

In fact, due to privacy concerns and specifically to avoid people being tracked without their consent, ID associated to WiFi or Bluetooth devices are either hidden or changed frequently, and users cooperation is required get them tracked. Therefore, if WiFi or Bluetooth is chosen, individuals to be tracked typically need to install a specific application or carry a device that sets a unique and static ID making their tracking possible. Considering the transmission range of WiFi and Bluetooth, both are suited to track the way in which people move indoor, especially in buildings with clear divisions between single areas, such as museums, shopping malls, or offices [24–29].

Figure 4.22 shows an example for a typical indoor use of Bluetooth devices to monitor visitor activity. Selected visitors (or all of them if possible) will need to carry a device that is used to record the order in which exhibits are visited and the time spent on each area. Collected data remains anonymous as long as visitors are not asked to provide some information about them or the beacon used is associated, for example, to their tickets (which may have data in regard to gender or age, especially if bought online).

In addition than providing traveled route and time, similarly to what presented for mobile phones, it is also possible to get an estimate for density and congestion by counting the number of devices transmitting though WiFi or Bluetooth in the vicinity [30, 31]. When only the count is concerned, it is possible to perform it without user intervention. In fact, although the ID associated to each device may change over time, thus preventing them from being tracked without their consent, the presence of devices nearby is detectable. While it is not possible to get the exact number of people (as some may not use electronic devices or may have WiFi and Bluetooth turned off), it is possible to get reliable estimates of changes over time. For example, if the number of devices at a given time is twice that at a different moment, one can assume the number of people doubled.

Radio-frequency identification (RFID) are electronic chips that can be used as digital tags to identify objects. When objects tagged with a RFID pass in the proximity of a scanner, their ID number can be read and the object recognized. RFIDs are used as digital keys to open lockers or for vehicle toll collection in traffic management. Their use is also possible for pedestrian recognition and detection, resulting in applications very similar to the scenarios presented above for WiFi or Bluetooth. The main differences to the latter cases is that RFID must be necessarily given to the tracked individuals and detection distance is typically small, often requiring people to take the tag close to the scanner. For this reason, RFID use is typically restricted to specific studies or in the case of access control requiring high security.

4.6.3 Advantages/Disadvantages

To discuss advantages and disadvantages of instrumented detection, some distinction is required on the technology involved.

If mobile phone network is employed, a clear advantage lies in the fact that active involvement of users is not necessary. Position is automatically provided to the mobile phone carriers as people move and different antennas are used to connect to the network. So, as long as a phone is turned on, its position can be easily estimated within a few kilometers (often even less). Also, the availability of aggregated information on phone ownership (gender, age, etc.) in a specific area makes this approach particularly convenient when profiling is needed. However, these sort of data are usually collected from a limited number of companies and cost tend to be high. Also, level of detail is coarse making mobile phone data only useful to study movements in cities or neighborhoods.

On the other hand, WiFi and Bluetooth can be easily employed to study dynamics inside a building, and it is possible to buy or independently develop such systems. Also, cost are generally proportional to the number of scanning units employed, thus allowing one to have a control on costs (if budget is limited only critical areas may be monitored). However, when tracking is sought, the need for user cooperation is a clear disadvantage requiring human resources to instruct visitors or targeted individuals and increasing hardware cost. While density estimation has the advantage of being possible also without active user involvement, the number of devices that are detectable with this method is typically low, making in turn accuracy also low.

Finally, it should be reminded that for both approaches, device position is not directly provided, but estimated through the antenna connected to a specific device. Hence, usually only an estimate is provided and is limited to travel time and/or relative number of people. Another disadvantage in relation to travel route estimation was discussed in the example of Fig. 4.21, a complex network requires many devices, thus increasing the hardware costs and making route estimation more difficult and therefore computationally more expensive.

4.7 Alternative Methods

In addition to the methods presented above, there are also alternative solutions that are often overseen or not considered besides being very effective for particular cases. This section will introduce some of the most common and also some emerging solutions. It is also important to consider that many modern detection solutions are a hybrid combination of different technologies (a more detailed discussion will follow), combining advantages to reduce the shortcomings of each [2].

4.7.1 Gate/Transit Counting

In many cases, detecting people's position and/or speed is not relevant, and it is enough to control people moving inside/outside the facility. For facilities such as stadiums and event venues that accommodate pedestrians on a daily basis, there are usually entrance gates that make it possible to control people moving in and out. Even when physical gates (such as revolving gates or turnstiles) are not available, there are line-counters (employing different types of technologies, such as 1D distance sensors) that allow counting the number of people passing over a line in both directions.

Gates physically counting people have a very high accuracy as people can only pass one by one. However, it is always useful to have a backup solution as counting errors accumulate if one gate is malfunctioning or if some entrances are open due to special conditions.

Seamless counting solutions are to be handled with care as the accuracy greatly changes with the product. Cheap solutions can be useful to estimate the number of customers in a shop, but may largely fail when dense crowds are to be counted or accurate figures are sought.

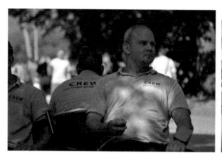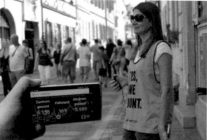

Fig. 4.23 Example of people counting passing crowds. Counting information are directly streamed through the internet to a control room where crowd is monitored. Courtesy of Stefan Leitmannslehner, Qounts Gmbh

4.7.2   Manual Counting

In some cases, no technology can guarantee sufficient accuracy, and manually counting people is the only alternative. For example, people on airplanes are still counted manually by the crew as the exact head number is sought. In this regard, a peculiarity of manual counting concerns the possibility to estimate error and/or detect issues by comparing results from different people.

In some cases, counting staff could be employed to monitor people moving in and out of festival areas. This solution, while expensive in terms of personnel costs, can be preferred to automated sensors for events lasting only one of few days, where the cost of the devices and their installation will be much higher than employing a large counting crew for just few days (see Fig. 4.23).

In addition, trained people can count with better accuracy than automated devices in different conditions, thus allowing facility operators to control the people moving in and out. In this regard, it is important to remember the importance of training, planning, and communication, since such an approach requires all the elements to be effective and successful.

4.7.3   Estimation by Total Mass

Under certain conditions, it is possible to weigh people, and therefore estimate their number. Elevators or escalators are a typical example: the torque required by the engines to move people is related to their weight and therefore their number. Trains are also an example where such an approach is possible. Carriage weight is typically available or can be made available using dedicated sensors and the difference in weight before and after a train stop allows estimating the number of people who left the platform or the train, thus giving precious information to the station's operators.

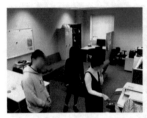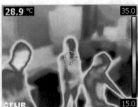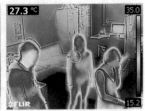

Fig. 4.24 Example for pictures of people taken using a thermocamera (left: real situation taken with a standard camera, center: temperature map, right: combination of both)

However, to ensure an adequate accuracy, the user's profile needs to be carefully studied. Average body weight varies from country to country, and facilities with a large number of travelers with luggages (train stations, airports, etc.) will have different values compared to concert venues. For instance, when people carry luggage, the weight per surface may be smaller compared to other scenarios, as the luggage weighs less than people but occupies a similar surface (especially trolleys).

4.7.4 Thermocamera

Thermocameras are special cameras that allow measuring the temperature of objects in the surroundings. Since humans have a body temperature generally higher than the environment (except very hot locations where the opposite might be true), it is possible to recognize them as regions with a particular temperature [32–34]. In particular, the head stands out being a round object close to the body temperature, while other parts of the body are colder due to clothes (see Fig. 4.24).

Although this type of technology is still partially under development (also due to the high costs of thermocameras and their low resolution), it could be a viable alternative for different reasons: privacy sensitive information is not involved in the detection process, it can work under darkness, and it can also provide some clues on the physical state of people; an application commonly seen in airports where people having fever need to be identified to prevent the spread of infectious diseases. While thermocameras alone still have limitations due to the low resolution, they are increasingly used in combination with other sensors (computer vision or distance sensors), as they provide complementary information making detection and tracking easier.

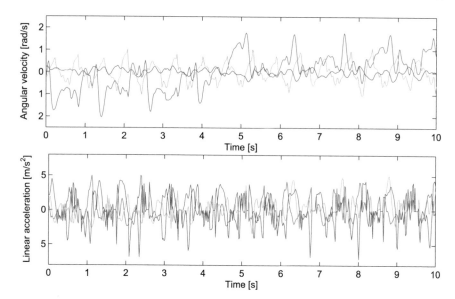

Fig. 4.25 Angular velocity and acceleration measured by an inertial sensor of a tablet when a person is walking. Each color represents one of the three different axes of the sensor [39]. Reprinted from [39], Copyright (2019), with permissions from Informa UK Limited

4.7.5   Inertial Sensors

In addition to the already presented methods performing crowd sensing by relying on the mobile devices that people are carrying, an alternative approach also deserves a short discussion: the use of inertial sensors [35–38]. Almost all electronic devices are equipped with inertial sensors, and these sensors are used for different purposes, such as to rotate the screen or to get their orientation (e.g., during video games or navigation). Inertial sensors measure the acceleration (and angular speed) of the device in a three-dimensional manner. These sensors allow, for example, counting the number of steps and estimating the distance walked (and related quantities, such as calories burned).

Figure 4.25 shows an example of the information that inertial sensors deliver. In both graphs, it is clearly visible that regular patterns are observed, with each oscillation representing a single step (this is particularly visible in the upper graph). Some of the operating systems in smartphones and smartwatches directly provide step counts by automatically analyzing sensor readings such as the one shown in Fig. 4.25. Knowing a person height, it is also possible to get a first-hand approximation of the walked distance, but this would imply a user input that may be difficult to obtain. Trajectories can be also obtained using inertial sensors (through a method known as "dead-reckoning"), but unless specialized equipment is used (such as sensors mounted on shoes), errors quickly accumulate over time, thus making inertial sensors not suitable to extract trajectories in practical applications.

Although the walked distance is a very rough estimation, the speed or pedestrian "state" is easier to estimate. Running people move their body more energetically compared to standing people, and this difference can be easily detected by inertial sensors [40]. This type of application is categorized as "human activity recognition," and an increasingly large number of algorithms are being developed for this purpose [41, 42].

For instance, using the information from inertial sensors, it is quite easy to assess if a person is standing, walking, or running. While this represents very simple information compared to that provided by other sensors, it may be enough to allow identifying congested areas (and thus, the area where many people are standing or moving very slowly).

When only speed or "state" is measured, an inertial sensor-based approach would ultimately need a localization service to obtain the position of each user and inform on crowd condition in a given area. However, quite inaccurate localization would be still acceptable under this approach: knowing that people on the fifth floor are not walking might be enough to guess that congestion is occurring there (a localization approach could not determine people's speed indoors with the same precision).

In addition, like for all localization services, user cooperation is necessary as people would need to install one application and/or agree to have their state analyzed and sent over mobile network for further processing. While the information being processed is anonymous, user cooperation cannot be taken for granted.

4.7.6 Chemosensors

Chemosensors represent a category of sensors that work by detecting specific chemicals related to human presence [43–45]. The most commonly detected chemical is carbon dioxide (CO_2), which is easy to detect and emitted by humans through their breathing process. By measuring the concentration of CO_2 in a specific place, it is possible to estimate the number of people present. Obviously, this approach is only possible in closed facilities, especially where a ventilation system is in use to move the air inside and outside the facility. Although figures provided by chemosensors are usually only an estimate, these sensors can be easily implemented in facilities having a ventilation system already in place and could therefore represent a viable solution to grasp some information on crowd size.

4.7.7 Pressure Sensors

Pressure sensors are devices that allow detecting the presence of people using special boards pressed by pedestrians while walking [46, 47]. The "trace" left by each foot is recorded allowing pressure sensors to recognize where people walked the most. Pressure sensors are simple but still provide accurate information on which area was more frequented at which time. Also, they deal with completely anonymous data and pedestrians will not notice the presence of such devices (although it is probably wise to inform them on the measuring campaign). The only drawback of pressure sensors lies in their high costs and the relatively low number of makers.

4.8 Sensing Method Selection and Comparison

In the previous sections, the working principles and main advantages and disadvantages of the different sensing solutions have been presented and discussed. In this summarizing section, we wish to provide a comparison of the different solutions and propose the criteria that may help stakeholders identify the solution that better fits their need (alternative methods will be excluded in this section as they represent minor solutions with few or no commercial products).

This section is intended to represent just the first step, in which clearly unsuitable solutions are excluded from the selection process. Once a suitable technology is chosen, each product needs to be evaluated and tested separately. It is also important to remember that quality and performances of sensors largely change with the manufacturer, and as already mentioned, hybrid solutions are being developed and becoming increasingly common. This means that, for example, a computer vision solution from a particular manufacturer may work at night because an infrared camera is combined with a normal camera. The tables provided below should help making the selection and comparison of different solution more schematic and organized, thus helping one find the best partner and getting the most from the chosen solution.

We will divide this discussion into two aspects: sensor specifications and working conditions. Sensor specifications are meant to be seen mostly as technical aspects, covering information that is provided from sensors, its nature, and the possibility to customize the system. Working conditions refer to the environment where sensors are planned to be used and the resources available. Both aspects are crucial for finding the best solution. Even the best sensors providing a large amount of accurate information cannot help in monitoring crowds under extreme conditions. In this context, a less accurate but more reliable solution may be preferred, so that at least some information can be gained even in difficult conditions.

Table 4.2 presents typical specifications for crowd sensing technologies. It is important to understand which primary information is gained from the sensor, because that information will be used to evaluate the crowd and eventually will become the input for a more complex analysis. For example, if only speed is obtained, then it is not possible to control people being in a place, but it could be still useful to grasp the level of congestion.

In relation to the information provided, also considerations in regard to privacy are important. Depending on the system employed, identity can be detected, general demographic information could be available (age, gender, etc.) or completely anonymous data are provided. Here, local laws and regulations need to be consulted. Some systems based on cameras do not allow users to see the images and only positions

Table 4.2 Important features relative to sensing systems to be considered when choosing a particular product/solution

Information provided	Position (trajectory), total count, speed, travel time, person ID …
Level of privacy	Completely anonymous … Identity detectable
Sensing accuracy	Low … High
Update frequency	Several times per second … Once per day
Processing time/Delay	Less than one second (real-time processing) … Several hours
Customization	Simple, partial, difficult, not possible

are provided as anonymous numbers. But the presence of a camera itself may be considered a breach into privacy, either due to laws, organizational rules or thorough visitors' perception. In addition, even inside the same facility, some privacy-sensitive devices (like cameras) may be allowed in some places but not in others.

Next, the accuracy and update frequency need to be considered. Some sensors may provide an information in very short intervals but with low accuracy. Others may provide data only every hour or so but with much better accuracy. Both aspects are unrelated and must be considered separately. In regard to sensing timing, one should also consider the delay between detection and data transmission. While most sensors almost instantaneously transmit detection data, some may require internal processing, and data transmitted could be relative to an observation few minutes or hours old. When only the daily customers number is required, several hours of delay are well tolerated, but for real-time processing few seconds may be already too late.

Finally, it can be useful to consider the possibility to customize a system or have a control on the kind of data transmitted. Some systems are sold as a whole (hardware and software), and customers can change settings over time. For other sensing methods, only the data can be obtained and little or no negotiation is possible to change data format or the approach taken to collect it. Also, some technologies are easier to be customized than others and may be more appropriate if there are plans to further develop sensing algorithms, either internally or through the assistance of an external partner.

Table 4.3 presents the typical working conditions that one needs to take into account to determine if a given sensor/solution is suitable for a specific environment and to monitor a particular type of crowd. Very often, the first selection criterion relates to the budget, and in this context, different costs needs to be accounted for. Further, the cost of the devices themselves should be considered. This not only includes the cost for the hardware, but also includes costs related to the software required to perform data analysis (for computer vision in particular, the cost of the software could be much higher than the one of the hardware). Installation cost also need to be considered, especially for devices that need to be fixed in large number to walls or ceilings and requires individual calibration. Depending on the sensor, network and power cables may also need to be lied down, often further increasing the costs. Finally, operating cost need to be evaluated. Particularly computationally expensive solutions may generate non-negligible electricity bills and personnel cost

Table 4.3 Points to consider in regard to available resources, working conditions, and monitored crowd involvement relative to the environment where sensors will have to be employed

Device cost	Cost of the device itself (eventually including software purchase)
Installation cost	Costs for installing the sensors and connecting them with the control room
Operating cost	Costs for operating the system (software, personnel, data transmission, etc.)
Outdoor/Indoor	Where will the sensor be used? Is it a waterproof solution required?
Lighting conditions	Will the sensor be used in dark conditions? Strong light contrast?
Fixed/Mobile	Will the sensor always be used in the same location?
	How much will background change? Will need to work on batteries?
Detection scale	How large is the area to be detected? Is a flexible approach needed?
Crowd involvement	Is user involvement possible? To which extent? Will the users cooperate?
Appearance/Noise	Is the sensor clearly visible by people? Is its presence invasive/unwanted?

for maintenance and operation need to be estimated. Depending on the product, fees may be necessary to update the software license from time to time. Also, for sensors operating in remote locations, mobile data plan subscription may be needed, which will generate monthly bills.

Next, physical working conditions are to be considered, in particular, exposure to harsh weather and environment temperature. Many electronic devices require a special protection against rain or snow, and some may need special cooling solutions to work under extreme heat conditions (or may even have to be warmed up when operating at low temperatures). Lighting is also an important aspect; not all sensors work in darkness, and artificial light may be required to create good working conditions. Also, some systems (especially distance sensors) could be sensible to strong light exposure and/or illumination contrasts.

One should also consider whether the sensor is to be used in a mobile context (e.g., during open air concerts or festivals) or will not be moved during its whole service life. If a mobile use is envisaged, then ease of calibration, power, and data network requirements are to be taken into account. In this regard, one should also consider if the sensing area changes very often, for example in exposition halls where stands could change daily, thus representing a sort of "mobile environment" where the sensor is not moved but the surrounding somehow does.

In regard to the point above, the envisaged sensing area also plays a relevant role in choosing the right solution. If sensing is performed in a small shop, several solutions are available, but when crowd within a whole city will need to be monitored only few methods allow to collect such kind of data. When sensing location change very often, one should also consider whether it is more convenient moving the sensors or opting for a large-scale solution that is available everywhere (like relying on the mobile phone network).

Another point to consider is whether it would be possible to obtain cooperation from customers/visitors. When people need to actively cooperate to get information on their number/motion, personnel is also needed to instruct them and inform them

Table 4.4 Categorization of different sensing systems depending on the information provided, the level of privacy contained in it and their accuracy

	Information provided	Level of privacy	Accuracy
Detection and tracking	Trajectory (identity)	Identity detectable	Quite high
Optical flow	Speed distribution	Depending on hardware	Medium
Distance sensors	Trajectory, height	Only height detectable	Quite high
Localization (direct)	Position (trajectory)	Anonymous	Medium
Localization (indirect)	Position (density)	Age group, gender, etc.	Low
Mobile phone antennas	Travel time (density)	Age group, gender, etc.	Low
WiFi, Bluetooth, or RFID	Travel time (density)	Anonymous	Medium

Table 4.5 Typical technical specifications in regard to information delivery speed and possibility to customize a sensing system

	Update frequency	Processing time	Customization
Detection and tracking	High	Quite fast	Simple
Optical flow	High	Fast	Partial
Distance sensors	High	Very fast	Simple
Localization (direct)	Quite high	Fast	Partial
Localization (indirect)	Low	Fast	Difficult
Mobile phone antennas	Low	Quite fast	Not possible
WiFi, Bluetooth, or RFID	Medium	Fast	Partial

on the information collected. Also, depending on the gathering purpose and the characteristics of the crowd, the willingness of the users to cooperate may largely change.

Finally, appearance and noise generated (cooling fan for computers for example) is also important, especially for sensors used in venues where esthetics and quietness are the primary aspect (consider for example museums or opera halls). In addition, while customers may have to be informed about the use of sensors in accordance to local laws, a too invasive presence of sensors may make people feel less comfortable and some may also doubt whether privacy is really guaranteed. In this regard, where possible, sensors using non-privacy sensitive data and having a weaker presence are typically preferred to sensors that require special permissions and are clearly visible by passer-by.

Tables 4.4, 4.5, 4.6, and 4.7 categorize each sensing solution based on the criteria illustrated in Tables 4.2 and 4.3. Localization systems have been divided into the approaches requiring active user involvement (carry a GPS tag or install a specific

Table 4.6 Typical costs for the sensing technology discussed in this chapter

	Cost		
	Device	Installation	Operating
Detection and tracking	Low	High	High
Optical flow	Low	Medium	Medium
Distance sensors	High	High	Medium
Localization (direct)	Low	N/A	Low
Localization (indirect)	N/A	N/A	High
Mobile phone network	N/A	N/A	High
WiFi, Bluetooth, or RFID	Low	Low	Medium

Table 4.7 Typical working conditions and related considerations for the sensing technology discussed in this chapter

	Indoor/ outdoor	Light	Fixed/ mobile	Detection scale	Crowd involvement	Appearance/ noise
Detection and tracking	Both	Needed	Fixed	Floor, building	Not required	Medium
Optical flow	Both	Needed	Fixed	Floor, building	Not required	Medium
Distance sensors	Indoor	Dark ok	Fixed	Floor, building	Not required	High
Localization (direct)	Outdoor	Dark ok	Mobile	Unlimited	Required	Small
Localization (indirect)	Outdoor	Dark ok	Mobile	Unlimited	Partial	Invisible
Mobile phone network	Both	Dark ok	Mobile	City, country	Partial	Invisible
WiFi, Bluetooth, or RFID	Indoor	Dark ok	Fixed	Building, neighbor-hood	Required	Small

application) and the ones in which position is indirectly provided by people through the use of generic applications (navigation tools etc.). Similarly, instrumented detection based on the mobile phone network was distinguished from solutions working on smaller scales (WiFi, Bluetooth or RFID).

One could start either from technical specifications or working conditions depending on the one which is more important. If working conditions are ideal and budget is not strict, then technical specifications may be more important, giving a larger selection range. Under difficult working conditions, only one solution may be feasible, and if also budget is strict, then the sensing project may have to be scaled down.

In any case, the information in Tables 4.4, 4.5, 4.6, and 4.7 should help identifying the best technology to later focus on more specific products and finally build a crowd sensing system which can satisfy the operator's needs. It is, however, fundamental to remind once again that it is very difficult to provide general indications for each sensing methods, since large differences exist between single products. For example, GPS-based system are typically employed outdoor, but can also work indoor depending on the location. Similarly, distance sensors are typically employed indoor, but some products allow an outdoor use and could be employed in a mobile context. Also, using Bluetooth or RFID on very large scale is possible, although typical applications are limited to buildings and single floors.

Finally, to conclude this section, we should also remember that it is generally desirable to employ different sensors with independent working principles when possible. This solution has several advantages: it allows cross-checking the accuracy of different solutions and detecting problems with some sensors, and it acts as a backup system for abnormal conditions (such as a phone network problem or bad lighting conditions).

4.8.1   Sensing Accuracy

Although sensing accuracy was already briefly touched in the presentation above, it deserves a more detailed discussion since it is an aspect that is often not considered with sufficient attention when selecting a particular solution. One of the problems associated with accuracy is that there is no standard to quantify it, and it would be also very difficult to define one. Commercial products are often advertized as having an accuracy of 90% or more, but they are typically tested in controlled conditions and with low crowd densities.

However, although the highest possible accuracy is generally sought, it is also necessary to remind that it may not be always required. For example, when data relative to visitor experience are needed, individual inaccuracies in determining the route chosen or the time spent at different shops/exhibits are not very relevant. Data can be collected for a large number of people over a long period, and the overall final image may result being accurate. Similarly, tracking individuals in crowded conditions is very difficult and trajectories may get easily "broken." But in such a situation, keeping the density under control is more important, and therefore, incapacity in tracking people plays a less important role toward the capacity to detect particularly crowded spots.

It is therefore important spending sufficient time to understand which quantity needs to be measured and what accuracy is needed. When both have been determined and a suitable solution identified, on-site testing is normally the best and only way to ensure set conditions are met. Since human sensing depends on a large variety of factors, even if a company/product has an excellent record for being able to successfully sense crowds in different locations, this should not be taken as a guarantee for success.

Finally, we would like to remind that sometimes the same information could be obtained with different approaches, both requiring a different accuracy. For example, let us assume the number of occupants in a stadium has to be computed. If this is performed by counting the people getting in and out, this has to be performed with a very high accuracy as error accumulates in this approach. In addition, a single malfunctioning gate could lead to a wrong estimation. If, however, cameras are used to estimate the number of people seated, a similar accuracy could be reached while also being robust toward a possible breaching at the gates. However, cameras may not be able to cover the whole stadium and may not work in darkness or foggy weather. This example shows how accuracy can change depending on conditions and highlights the need of diversifying sensing approaches to ensure a robust control on crowd's state.

4.9 Future and Emerging Trends in Sensing Technology

This concluding section is intended to list up some technologies that are still under development and/or in a test phase, but are expected to play an increasingly important role, therefore contributing to the improvement and diversification of pedestrian sensing.

4.9.1 Detection of Complex Patterns by Machine-Learning Algorithms

4.9.1.1 Feature/Object Detection

As we mentioned by introducing machine-learning methods when discussing computer vision, it is possible to train computers to recognize specific objects (humans in case of pedestrian detection). This means that if properly trained, a computer can also help recognizing objects or specific features in crowds. For example, the presence of people on wheelchair can be of particular importance, since they require particular attention, given their impossibility to overcome stairs or other physical obstacles. Also, detection of groups and their relationship can also help profiling the crowd with a better accuracy [48].

In addition, luggage detection is playing an increasingly important role in pedestrian traffic management. Since luggage takes a considerable volume of space, it is important that their presence is detected to efficiently estimate crowd density and predict pedestrian motion. Luggage detection is also important for security reasons, but generally, when luggage is considered a potential danger, a detailed screening is performed (e.g., in airports or at the entrance of stadiums). As a consequence, luggage detection for crowd control is typically intended to provide an input information to be used by crowd managers and simulation systems to evaluate potential conflicts between pedestrian and adapt figures for maximum capacity or flow. For example, if a given area is intended to accommodate 1,000 people without luggage, the figure will have to be adapted if most of the people carry one luggage, and it is therefore important that sensors are able to detect not only people, but also their luggage.

4.9.1.2 Behavioral Detection

The recent improvements of machine learning and computer vision are also making it possible to detect specific behaviors within the crowds by analyzing normal videos [49]. As for other machine learning approaches, the method is always the same, i.e. a computer is trained using videos showing a specific characteristic of the crowd (e.g., violence, panic, or enjoyment), allowing the same machine to recognize similar behavior in different videos (including real-time footage) [50–52]. Most of the research has focused on the detection of violence and low-infringement actions (pickpocketing, sexual harassment, etc.), but the same approach could be used to detect for example the degree of familiarity within the crowd (e.g., how many people are familiar with the place).

Accuracy is generally still an issue, since automatic systems sometimes recognize as critical situations ones that are not, and instead ignore actual cases that should be detected. However, the ability to detect critical situations in an automated way can help reducing the workload of crowd managers having to check several cameras.

Even without detecting accidents or dangerous situations, the same algorithms can help selecting the cameras displayed in control rooms. Since the number of cameras connected to crowd/traffic control rooms is typically much higher than the ones that can be displayed in the main screen (and also the maximum number a person can check simultaneously), there is a need to select the most relevant ones. Having an automated system performing this task can help crowd managers focusing on the most important situations and monitor the evolution of the situation from the very beginning when the risk is still low.

4.9.2 Sensor Fusion

A general trend in the context of crowd sensing regards the fusion of different sensors within a single device, combining different source of information to generate more accurate results [53–56]. The combination of a camera with a distance sensor is already a widespread solution in the industry, and several commercial products are available. There are good reasons to believe the more and more sensors will be combined in the future, for example by adding a thermocamera to the latter combination. However, we should remark that physically combining several sensors in a single device is technically feasible and relatively easy, but research is still needed on how to merge the information gained from the various sensors.

In that regard, another trend in the frame of sensor fusion concerns the creation of a sensing network, in which all the data obtained from sensors covering an area are combined to generate a detailed map of human activity [2]. Also in this context, more research is needed since it is not trivial to combine speed distribution gained from optical flow with counts from gates or large-scale travel behavior obtained from mobile phones. While this task is a difficult one, considering that a lot of sensors are already in use, exploiting this existing network can be much more rewarding than installing additional devices.

4.9.3 Emotional State and Mood Detection

The increasing use of health-related sensors is paving the path to the estimation of the inner and emotional state of people. Smartwatches are often fitted with sensors capable of reading body temperature, heart rate, and in some cases even more complex quantities such as pulse waveform, arterial blood oxygenation, galvanic skin response, and other electrical signals generated by the body (e.g., electromyography, electrocardiography, electrodermal activity, and electroencephalography). Such information can be used to understand if somebody is relaxed, excited, or under panic. This information can be useful to understand the general emotional state of the crowd and prepare targeted crowd control strategies. Emotional state can also become a warning message for a degrading situation, allowing crowd managers to prepare for potentially critical situations.

However, in addition to ethical and privacy issues, there are still technical and fundamental problems to overcome before emotional state assessment can become effective and reliable. Individual differences tend to be very large when it comes to body reaction to a similar stressor. Some people may react in a marked way when a stressful situation arises, thus indicating a potential risk for the crowd, while others may remain calm (at least when judging the biomedical signals). Initial studies showed that it is very difficult to differentiate specific areas within a crowd event in terms of the emotion felt from the crowd [57].

References

1. Yamamoto, H., Yanagisawa, D., Feliciani, C., Nishinari, K.: Body-rotation behavior of pedestrians for collision avoidance in passing and cross flow. Transp. Res. Part B: Methodological **122**, 486–510 (2019). https://doi.org/10.1016/j.trb.2019.03.008
2. Teixeira, T., Dublon, G., Savvides, A.: A survey of human-sensing: methods for detecting presence, count, location, track, and identity. ACM Comput. Surv. 5(1), 59–69 (2010)
3. Potamitis, I., Chen, H., Tremoulis, G.: Tracking of multiple moving speakers with multiple microphone arrays. IEEE Trans. Speech Audio Process. **12**(5), 520–529 (2004). https://doi.org/10.1109/TSA.2004.833004

4. Junior, J.C.S.J., Musse, S.R., Jung, C.R.: Crowd analysis using computer vision techniques. IEEE Signal Process. Mag. **27**(5), 66–77 (2010). https://doi.org/10.1109/MSP.2010.937394
5. Kok, V.J., Lim, M.K., Chan, C.S.: Crowd behavior analysis: a review where physics meets biology. Neurocomputing **177**, 342–362 (2016). https://doi.org/10.1016/j.neucom.2015.11.021
6. Hou, L., Wan, W., Hwang, J.N., Muhammad, R., Yang, M., Han, K.: Human tracking over camera networks: a review. EURASIP J. Adv. Signal Process. **2017**(1), 1–20 (2017). https://doi.org/10.1186/s13634-017-0482-z
7. Brunetti, A., Buongiorno, D., Trotta, G.F., Bevilacqua, V.: Computer vision and deep learning techniques for pedestrian detection and tracking: a survey. Neurocomputing **300**, 17–33 (2018). https://doi.org/10.1016/j.neucom.2018.01.092
8. Johansson, A., Helbing, D., Al-Abideen, H.Z., Al-Bosta, S.: From crowd dynamics to crowd safety: a video-based analysis. Adv. Complex Syst. **11**(04), 497–527 (2008). https://doi.org/10.1142/S0219525908001854
9. Zhang, X., Weng, W., Yuan, H.: Empirical study of crowd behavior during a real mass event. J. Statistical Mech.: Theor. Experiment **2012**(08), P08012 (2012). https://doi.org/10.1088/1742-5468/2012/08/P08012
10. Baqui, M., Löhner, R.: Pedpiv: pedestrian velocity extraction from particle image velocimetry. IEEE Trans. Intelligent Transp. Syst. **21**(2), 580–589 (2019). https://doi.org/10.1109/TITS.2019.2899072
11. Xiaohua, L., Lansun, S., Huanqin, L.: Estimation of crowd density based on wavelet and support vector machine. Trans. Inst. Measurement Control **28**(3), 299–308 (2006). https://doi.org/10.1191/2F0142331206tim178oa
12. Fu, M., Xu, P., Li, X., Liu, Q., Ye, M., Zhu, C.: Fast crowd density estimation with convolutional neural networks. Eng. Appl. Artif. Intelligence **43**, 81–88 (2015). https://doi.org/10.1016/j.engappai.2015.04.006
13. Saleh, S.A.M., Suandi, S.A., Ibrahim, H.: Recent survey on crowd density estimation and counting for visual surveillance. Eng. Appl. Artif. Intelligence **41**, 103–114 (2015). https://doi.org/10.1016/j.engappai.2015.01.007
14. Glas, D.F., Miyashita, T., Ishiguro, H., Hagita, N.: Laser-based tracking of human position and orientation using parametric shape modeling. Adv. Robot. **23**(4), 405–428 (2009). https://doi.org/10.1163/156855309X408754
15. Brščić, D., Kanda, T., Ikeda, T., Miyashita, T.: Person tracking in large public spaces using 3-d range sensors. IEEE Trans. Human-Mach. Syst. **43**(6), 522–534 (2013). https://doi.org/10.1109/THMS.2013.2283945
16. Seer, S., Brändle, N., Ratti, C.: Kinects and human kinetics: a new approach for studying pedestrian behavior. Transp. Res. Part C: Emerging Technol. **48**, 212–228 (2014). https://doi.org/10.1016/j.trc.2014.08.012
17. Corbetta, A., Meeusen, J., Lee, C.M., Toschi, F.: Continuous Measurements of Real-life Bidirectional Pedestrian Flows on a Wide Walkway. arXiv preprint arXiv:1607.02897 (2016)
18. Daamen, W., Yuan, Y., Duives, D., Hoogendoorn, S.: Comparing three types of real-time data collection techniques: counting cameras, wi-fi sensors and gps trackers. In: Proceedings of the Pedestrian and Evacuation Dynamics (2016)
19. Stojanović, D., Stojanović, N.: Indoor localization and tracking: methods, technologies and research challenges. Facta Universitatis Ser.: Automatic Control Robot. **13**(1), 57–72 (2014)
20. Cellular Telecommunications and Internet Association: Background on CTIA's Wireless Industry Survey (2020)
21. Rojas, M.B., IV, Sadeghvaziri, E., Jin, X.: Comprehensive review of travel behavior and mobility pattern studies that used mobile phone data. Transp. Res. Rec. **2563**(1), 71–79 (2016). https://doi.org/10.3141/2563-11
22. Sekimoto, Y., Sudo, A., Kashiyama, T., Seto, T., Hayashi, H., Asahara, A., Ishizuka, H., Nishiyama, S.: Real-time people movement estimation in large disasters from several kinds of mobile phone data. In: Proceedings of the 2016 ACM International Joint Conference on Pervasive and Ubiquitous Computing: Adjunct, pp. 1426–1434 (2016). https://doi.org/10.1145/2968219.2968421

23. Deville, P., Linard, C., Martin, S., Gilbert, M., Stevens, F.R., Gaughan, A.E., Blondel, V.D., Tatem, A.J.: Dynamic population mapping using mobile phone data. Proc. Natl. Acad. Sci. **111**(45), 15888–15893 (2014). https://doi.org/10.1073/pnas.1408439111

24. Utsch, P., Liebig, T.: Monitoring microscopic pedestrian mobility using bluetooth. In: 2012 Eighth International Conference On Intelligent Environments, pp. 173–177. IEEE (2012). https://doi.org/10.1109/IE.2012.32

25. Yoshimura, Y., Sobolevsky, S., Ratti, C., Girardin, F., Carrascal, J.P., Blat, J., Sinatra, R.: An analysis of visitors' behavior in the louvre museum: a study using bluetooth data. Environ. Plann. B: Plann. Des. **41**(6), 1113–1131 (2014). https://doi.org/10.1068/2Fb130047p

26. Abedi, N., Bhaskar, A., Chung, E., Miska, M.: Assessment of antenna characteristic effects on pedestrian and cyclists travel-time estimation based on bluetooth and wifi mac addresses. Transp. Res. Part C: Emerging Technol. **60**, 124–141 (2015). https://doi.org/10.1016/j.trc.2015.08.010

27. Oosterlinck, D., Benoit, D.F., Baecke, P., Van de Weghe, N.: Bluetooth tracking of humans in an indoor environment: an application to shopping mall visits. Appl. Geogr. **78**, 55–65 (2017). https://doi.org/10.1016/j.apgeog.2016.11.005

28. Tekler, Z.D., Low, R., Gunay, B., Andersen, R.K., Blessing, L.: A scalable bluetooth low energy approach to identify occupancy patterns and profiles in office spaces. Build. Environ. **171** (2020). https://doi.org/10.1016/j.buildenv.2020.106681

29. Centorrino, P., Corbetta, A., Cristiani, E., Onofri, E.: Managing crowded museums: visitors flow measurement, analysis, modeling, and optimization. J. Comput. Sci. **53**, 101357 (2021). https://doi.org/10.1016/j.jocs.2021.101357

30. Schauer, L., Werner, M., Marcus, P.: Estimating crowd densities and pedestrian flows using wi-fi and bluetooth. In: Proceedings of the 11th International Conference on Mobile and Ubiquitous Systems: Computing, Networking and Services, pp. 171–177 (2014). https://doi.org/10.4108/icst.mobiquitous.2014.257870

31. Kurkcu, A., Ozbay, K.: Estimating pedestrian densities, wait times, and flows with wi-fi and bluetooth sensors. Transp. Res. Rec. **2644**(1), 72–82 (2017). https://doi.org/10.3141/2F2644-09

32. Goubet, E., Katz, J., Porikli, F.: Pedestrian tracking using thermal infrared imaging. In: Infrared Technology and Applications XXXII, vol. 6206, p. 62062C. International Society for Optics and Photonics (2006). https://doi.org/10.1117/12.673132

33. Olmeda, D., de la Escalera, A., Armingol, J.M.: Detection and tracking of pedestrians in infrared images. In: 2009 3rd International Conference on Signals, Circuits and Systems (SCS), pp. 1–6. IEEE (2009). https://doi.org/10.1109/ICSCS.2009.5412297

34. Li, J., Gong, W.: Real time pedestrian tracking using thermal infrared imagery. JCP **5**(10), 1606–1613 (2010)

35. Feliz Alonso, R., Zalama Casanova, E., Gómez García-Bermejo, J.: Pedestrian tracking using inertial sensors. J. Phys. Agent **3**(1), 35–43 (2009). https://doi.org/10.14198/JoPha.2009.3.1.05

36. Höflinger, F., Zhang, R., Reindl, L.M.: Indoor-localization system using a micro-inertial measurement unit (imu). In: 2012 European Frequency and Time Forum, pp. 443–447. IEEE (2012). https://doi.org/10.1109/EFTF.2012.6502421

37. Lin, T., Li, L., Lachapelle, G.: Multiple sensors integration for pedestrian indoor navigation. In: 2015 International Conference on Indoor Positioning and Indoor Navigation (IPIN), pp. 1–9. IEEE (2015). https://doi.org/10.1109/IPIN.2015.7346785

38. Boltes, M., Schumann, J., Salden, D.: Gathering of data under laboratory conditions for the deep analysis of pedestrian dynamics in crowds. In: 2017 14th IEEE International Conference on Advanced Video and Signal Based Surveillance (AVSS), pp. 1–6. IEEE (2017). https://doi.org/10.1109/AVSS.2017.8078471

39. Feliciani, C., Nishinari, K.: Estimation of pedestrian crowds' properties using commercial tablets and smartphones. Transportmetrica B: Transp. Dyn. **7**(1), 865–896 (2019). https://doi.org/10.1080/21680566.2018.1517061

40. Mori, K., Yamane, A., Hayakawa, Y., Wada, T., Ohtsuki, K., Okada, H.: Development of emergency rescue evacuation support system (eress) in panic-type disasters: disaster recognition algorithm by support vector machine. IEICE Trans. Fundamentals Electronics Commun. Comput. Sci. **96**(2), 649–657 (2013). https://doi.org/10.1587/transfun.E96.A.649
41. Su, X., Tong, H., Ji, P.: Activity recognition with smartphone sensors. Tsinghua Sci. Technol. **19**(3), 235–249 (2014). https://doi.org/10.1109/TST.2014.6838194
42. Concone, F., Gaglio, S., Re, G.L., Morana, M.: Smartphone data analysis for human activity recognition. In: Conference of the Italian Association for Artificial Intelligence, pp. 58–71. Springer (2017). https://doi.org/10.1007/978-3-319-70169-1_5
43. Dong, B., Andrews, B., Lam, K.P., Höynck, M., Zhang, R., Chiou, Y.S., Benitez, D.: An information technology enabled sustainability test-bed (itest) for occupancy detection through an environmental sensing network. Energy Build. **42**(7), 1038–1046 (2010). https://doi.org/10.1016/j.enbuild.2010.01.016
44. Jiang, C., Masood, M.K., Soh, Y.C., Li, H.: Indoor occupancy estimation from carbon dioxide concentration. Energy Build. **131**, 132–141 (2016). https://doi.org/10.1016/j.enbuild.2016.09.002
45. Lei, W., Rong, C., Tai, C., Li, A.: Study on the relationship between the co2 concentration and pedestrian flow in a building evacuation passageway. In: Indoor and Built Environment p. 1420326X20940368 (2020). https://doi.org/10.1177/1420326X20940368
46. Murakita, T., Ikeda, T., Ishiguro, H.: Human tracking using floor sensors based on the markov chain monte carlo method. In: Proceedings of the 17th International Conference on Pattern Recognition, 2004. ICPR 2004., vol. 4, pp. 917–920. IEEE (2004). https://doi.org/10.1109/ICPR.2004.1333922
47. Lombardi, M., Vezzani, R., Cucchiara, R.: Detection of human movements with pressure floor sensors. In: International Conference on Image Analysis and Processing, pp. 620–630. Springer (2015). https://doi.org/10.1007/978-3-319-23234-8_57
48. Yucel, Z., Zanlungo, F., Feliciani, C., Gregorj, A., Kanda, T.: Identification of social relation within pedestrian dyads. PloS one **14**(10), e0223656 (2019). https://doi.org/10.1371/journal.pone.0223656
49. Lamba, S., Nain, N.: Crowd monitoring and classification: a survey. In: Advances in Computer and Computational Sciences, pp. 21–31. Springer (2017). https://doi.org/10.1007/978-981-10-3770-2_3
50. Hassner, T., Itcher, Y., Kliper-Gross, O.: Violent flows: real-time detection of violent crowd behavior. In: 2012 IEEE Computer Society Conference on Computer Vision and Pattern Recognition Workshops, pp. 1–6. IEEE (2012). https://doi.org/10.1109/CVPRW.2012.6239348
51. Mohammadi, S., Kiani, H., Perina, A., Murino, V.: Violence detection in crowded scenes using substantial derivative. In: 2015 12th IEEE International Conference on Advanced Video and Signal Based Surveillance (AVSS), pp. 1–6. IEEE (2015). https://doi.org/10.1109/AVSS.2015.7301787
52. Mohammadi, S., Galoogahi, H.K., Perina, A., Murino, V.: Physics-inspired models for detecting abnormal behaviors in crowded scenes. In: Group and Crowd Behavior for Computer Vision, pp. 253–272. Elsevier (2017). https://doi.org/10.1016/B978-0-12-809276-7.00013-8
53. Leykin, A., Hammoud, R.: Pedestrian tracking by fusion of thermal-visible surveillance videos. Mach. Vision Appl. **21**(4), 587–595 (2010). https://doi.org/10.1007/s00138-008-0176-5
54. Wu, J., Feng, Y., Sun, P.: Sensor fusion for recognition of activities of daily living. Sensors **18**(11) (2018). https://doi.org/10.3390/s18114029
55. Li, D., Lu, Y., Xu, J., Ma, Q., Liu, Z.: ipac: Integrate pedestrian dead reckoning and computer vision for indoor localization and tracking. IEEE Access **7**, 183514–183523 (2019). https://doi.org/10.1109/ACCESS.2019.2960287
56. Boltes, M., Adrian, J., Raytarowski, A.K.: A hybrid tracking system of full-body motion inside crowds. Sensors **21**(6), 2108 (2021). https://doi.org/10.3390/s21062108

57. Bergner, B.S.: The measurement of stress at open-air events: Monitoring emotion and motion utilizing wearable sensor technology. In: Traffic and Granular Flow 2019, pp. 11–19. Springer (2020). https://doi.org/10.1007/978-3-030-55973-1_2

Chapter 5
Crowd Simulators: Computational Methods, Product Selection, and Visualization

Abstract Crowd simulation is becoming the dominant way to design infrastructures where large numbers of people transit or move and to plan mass events. Simulation software range from commercial products provided with extensive documentation to open-source codes available for research and development. The commercialization of crowd simulators has allowed to produce user-friendly software requiring little expertise to be used and generating visually realistic results. However, to correctly set up a simulation scenario involving crowd, it is important to have a basic understanding on how these simulators work and what are their limitations. In addition, the large variety of models and products available to simulate crowds could become a challenge when a selection is required. In this chapter, we explain working principles of crowd simulators while also proposing a methodology to select the best product/solution fitting one's requirements. Also, we discuss the important topic of validation, proposing methods to judge on the accuracy of a particular simulation. Finally, methods to visualize the results will be discussed and compared to allow users picking up the right method depending on the simulated scenario.

5.1 Introduction

Simulation software is being increasingly used for planning and designing of pedestrian environments. A large number of commercial software packages are now available, and researchers [1, 2] and companies [3] are continuously developing new products and update existing ones every year. Differences between products can be large, and people without experience in crowd simulation may find it difficult to understand why such differences exist and what are the potentials/limitations of each product.

It is therefore important to understand the different simulation models used for pedestrian and crowd management to grasp the conditions under which a particular simulator may work well and its limitations. Commercial software programs generally have simple and practical user interfaces that allow one to quickly setup scenarios, making the differences between several products partially invisible and/or related to the ease-of-use. However, the algorithms used to model pedestrian motion

© The Author(s), under exclusive license to Springer Nature Switzerland AG 2021
C. Feliciani et al., *Introduction to Crowd Management*,
https://doi.org/10.1007/978-3-030-90012-0_5

and dynamics are typically limited to a few approaches, and understanding the working of those algorithms is important to evaluate and chose different products.

The practical aspects of the ease-of-use of user interface, availability of sufficient documentation, costs, and computational time clearly need to be considered before choosing a particular crowd simulator, but those considerations should come after acceptable candidates have been selected based on the capabilities and accuracy of the simulation results.

To close this short introduction, it is also important to remind readers that all-around almighty crowd simulators do not exist yet and will probably not appear in the near future as a unique product. At the moment, mostly aspects typical of "physical crowds" are implemented in simulators, and it will take a lot of time until the same will be able to reproduce characteristics of "psychological crowds" (the dual nature of crowds was presented in Chap. 2). As such, crowd simulators are useful in many situations, but it would be wrong to think that subtle aspects like the collective identity accounted for in crowd theories are implemented in the calculation algorithms.

Even when the above general remarks are considered, it should be reminded that each specific crowd simulator is typically based on a particular mathematical model for crowd motion and has its own strengths and limitations. It is therefore important to clearly understand the situation one needs to study to select the simulator that best matches the given condition. For example, simulators that work well under high crowd densities (like for evacuations) may not work with the same accuracy under low density conditions (e.g., in shopping malls). Similarly, simulators suited for highly competitive evacuations may not reproduce the behavior of families in shopping malls.

5.2 Objectives of This Chapter

At the end of this chapter, readers should be able to understand how a crowd simulation software works and the criteria that are necessary to evaluate its performances and suitability for a given scenario/application. It is not in the scope of this chapter to provide details on each computational algorithm, and a large number of references are provided at the end of the chapter for readers interested in details.

People dealing with the planning of pedestrian infrastructures or organization of mass events should understand the kind of results that can be obtained from crowd simulators and the kind of results that go beyond the capabilities of pedestrian models. Although any sort of scenario can be computed and results will be generated to help in the design and planning phase, it is important to not over-estimate the capabilities of crowd simulators and limit the simulated scenarios to simple but relevant situations. After reading this chapter, readers should be able to understand how to reduce the complexity of the studied scenarios without over-simplifying and still be able to perform the type of evaluations needed.

Finally, readers should become familiar with the different possibilities offered during result analysis and visualization. Each situation needs to be analyzed using a different quantity, and there is no universal and standard method to read the results of crowd simulations. Density may be appropriate for evacuations or extreme conditions, but waiting (standing) time or equivalent quantities are more suitable to assess the efficacy of advertisement or shop locations. For every-day use, the LOS is also commonly employed. Crowd simulation users should therefore understand the most appropriate methods to evaluate results and eventually consider a combination of several quantities to best study their scenario.

5.3 Types of Crowd Simulators and Space Representation

In general, simulation models used for pedestrian dynamics can be divided into three categories based on how space is defined and computed. These three types of simulators are macroscopic, network (sometimes referred as mesoscopic), and microscopic models.

5.3.1 Macroscopic Models

Although macroscopic models are less frequently used for commercial applications, it is important to know about their existence, since the study on pedestrian dynamics started with these models, and they can still be useful when investigating simple scenarios that may require a detailed investigation. Macroscopic models assume crowds of people are like a sort of fluid and compute their distribution in terms of density, pressure, or evacuation time.

We will not go into the details of macroscopic models, but rather explain their properties using the example given in Fig. 5.1, where the typical results obtained using a macroscopic model are presented. The scenario studied in Fig. 5.1 represents a crowd of people walking (from left to right) on a railway platform with a large round obstacle in the middle ("exit" on the right side is slightly smaller than the "entrance" on the left side as seen from the arrow or vector representation). In Fig. 5.1, pedestrian density (on the left) is given at different times, and their speed and direction are illustrated using arrows (on the right).

In macroscopic models, people are not represented one by one, but they are computed as a "fluid" (or continuum) having particular properties. For instance, it is not possible to know the positions of people in front of the obstacle after 120 s, but only how high is the pedestrian density over the platform in different locations (although total number could be actually computed by multiply density and surface).

Given their characteristics, macroscopic models are particularly suited for very dense crowds when people indeed move like a fluid and individual differences are minimal. Under these conditions, their properties can be described in terms of density

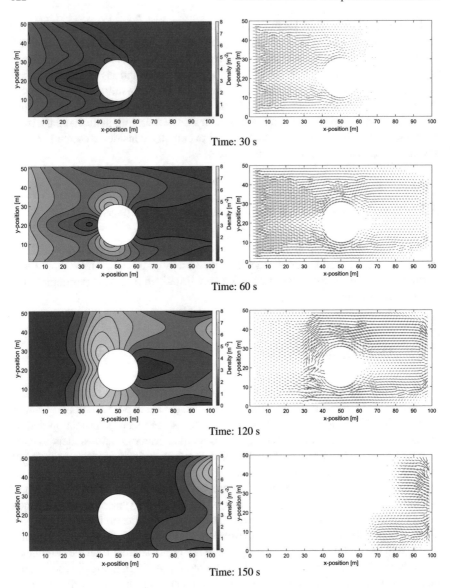

Fig. 5.1 Macroscopic simulation of a crowd of people passing thorough a railway platform with a large round obstacle. Size of the platform is 50 m × 100 m, and surface of the obstacle is 400 m². Reprinted figure with permission from [4]. Copyright (2009) by the American Physical Society

and similar distributions. However, at low densities or when the emergence of a collective behavior become evident to some extent (e.g., if there are families moving in a group), then the macroscopic description is not accurate.

5.3.2 Network Models

Network models are a class of models where people are modeled in a group and move in a simplified and compact way. Network models (as the name suggests) represent pedestrian motion as a connected grid where people move from one point (or node) to another using routes (or links) connecting them. If the scenario considered in Fig. 5.1 would have to be described using a network model, it would look something like the representation of Fig. 5.2.

In principle, network models allow representing any type of pedestrian space, with the case of Fig. 5.2 being only an example, but are generally employed to simulate large-scale scenarios.

Figure 5.3 provides some more typical examples of network models, ranging from a city center to the whole world where each node represents a single country. Network models are very versatile, and given the right assumptions, it is possible to model any type of pedestrian space or transportation network in quite a short time.

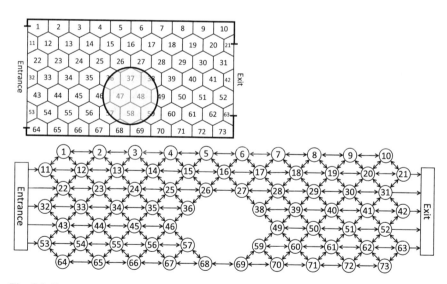

Fig. 5.2 Representation of the scenario of Fig. 5.1 using a network model (adapted from [5]). Each node represents a large section of the platform accommodating a large number of people. In this representation, each cell (or node) is 75 m² and can contain (depending on the maximum density) almost 500 people. People move from one cell (or node) to the another according to the corresponding network and precise rules governing motion

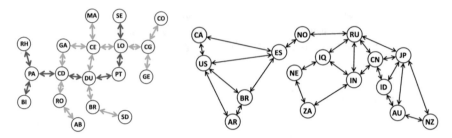

Fig. 5.3 Examples of systems represented using a network model. Left: subway network in central Tokyo (only a part of it is represented), and right: world-wide airplane network (only a very small part is given for illustrative purposes)

However, due to their simplified nature, network models give only approximative information, allowing us to understand, for example, which route is congested at what time or how the number of people change at a given station over the whole day. Network models cannot achieve the level of details given by macroscopic models and do not provide information such as people orientation or walking direction.

5.3.3   Microscopic Models

In contrast, microscopic models consider each person individually and can reproduce single pedestrian behavior similarly to reality. Figure 5.4 presents the results for a simulation performed considering the same scenario as Fig. 5.1.

As Fig. 5.4 clearly shows, a realistic picture is obtained with each person represented individually by a single point. Microscopic simulations allow setting up properties for each person individually and can therefore achieve a great level of accuracy if properly configured. However, as Fig. 5.4 shows, interpretation of the results is sometimes difficult as visual clues are the main result of this type of simulators. People density or speed will need to be computed based on individuals' positions and will sometimes require some additional steps to visualize results.

Originally, microscopic models were used only for small surfaces (such as a single room or a single floor) because a powerful computer is needed to simulate the motion of large crowds in detail. However, computational power has rapidly increased over the last decades, and it is now possible to compute the motion of millions of people individually within a reasonable time [6–9]. Therefore, nowadays microscopic models are the most used models in commercial applications and will be the ones discussed the most in this chapter.

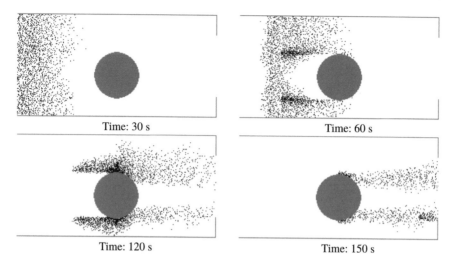

| Time: 30 s | Time: 60 s |
| Time: 120 s | Time: 150 s |

Fig. 5.4 Microscopic simulation of a group of people walking in a subway station with a circular obstacle. People walk from left to right with each point standing for one person. Geometry is exactly the same as the scenario of Fig. 5.1, but simulation conditions are slightly different (2,000 people are considered here)

5.4   State-of-the-Art Modeling Approaches

5.4.1   The Behavioral Levels and Multiscale Simulation

In the previous section, different methods were discussed in regard to space representation. Although usually a single approach is selected depending on the scale of the scenario to be simulated and the result needed, it is also possible to combine several models to consider multiple degrees of detail at the same time. But to be able to combine different models and scales, it is first necessary to understand the behavioral mechanisms that influence people motion and their need/desire to actually move.

In general, people motion can be understood through a theoretical framework made up by the so-called behavioral levels. Regardless on the scale considered, individuals will determine whether there is a need to move and how to reach their destination based on three behavioral levels defined in hierarchical order (from higher to lower) as strategical, tactical, and operational level [10–12]. Depending on the scenario considered and/or the scale of the simulation, different models may be used at each level and interactions at each level can be mutual, with outcomes at a lower level often influencing decisions at a higher level. To allow an easier understanding of the behavioral levels and grasp the interaction mechanisms, we may consider a concrete example, in which multiple scales and models will interact at the three levels. This example is schematically illustrated in Fig. 5.5.

First comes the strategic level. This is the most abstract level and determines the details of the lower levels. The strategic level defines the main goals and actions

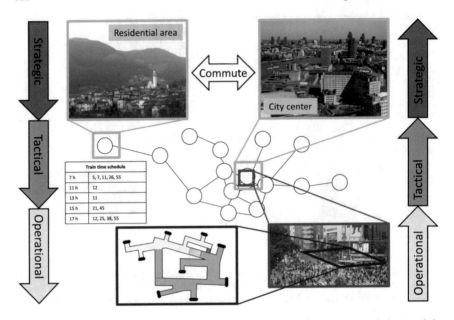

Fig. 5.5 The three levels of behavior to be considered in complex crowd simulations and the required methodological approaches

determining the need of motion. For instance, taking the example of Fig. 5.5, people living in the residential neighborhoods will need to commute toward the city center to work. In this regard, the need of each individual determines the set of actions starting in the strategic level. A more specific and everyday-life example is having to be at work by 9 a.m. for a group meeting with the colleagues. More specifically, when setting up a simulation, it is important to consider with attention who need to go where at which time of the day. This type of information is usually not computed nor modeled, but has to be given to the simulators, since computers cannot know the whereabouts of the people being simulated. However, although the strategic level is the higher level and the most abstract, it is important to consider the relation with the lower tactical level (described in detail later) where route-choice is carried out. If, for example, an accident along the commuting route will result in important delays or a complete service interruption that person may not be able to join the meeting, possibly resulting in its cancellation and leading to changes in the schedule of all people involved (with some people consequently working from home or having to take a day off). This shows how conditions can change people needs, thus requiring the creation of several what-if scenarios for simulations. In this sense, although whereabouts of people cannot be known a priori, there are statistical models [13–15] (e.g., discrete choice models [16]) that allow to estimate how travel demand will react if conditions (in particular price) are changed.

Next, the tactical level adds more details to the activity considered in the strategic level. Having defined one's need to move, in the following, route choice and time schedule are determined in detail. Using again the example of Fig. 5.5, the commute from home to work is considered taking into account the train/road network and the time schedules involved in the different sections. Coming back to the example of Fig. 5.5, commuting mode (car or train for example), departure time, station or highway entrance/exit, train line/highway, and route chosen are determined to go from home to work where the meeting will be held. If the train schedule changes or some road maintenance work is done on the way to work, considerations on the tactical level changes, although, unless large disruption occur, the strategic level remains unchanged: be at work by 9 a.m. If a whole city has to be simulated, network models are probably a valid choice since individual characteristics are less relevant in such a large scale. Also, route choice is a complex topic, and a model specifically designed to focus on this aspect may be preferred at this level. On this scope, information such as geographic maps, transportation networks, or timetables become relevant to allow a realistic simulation.

Finally, the operational level contains the details of the motion at the microscopic scale and is used to compute each single step on the way from departure to destination. For crowd simulation, in the operational level, every traveled meter is considered while determining the presence of other people and avoiding collisions with them. When crossing the street, each step and each turn is considered here, thus requiring fine details of the surrounding environment. For this reason, operational level can be only considered for facilities or neighborhoods, for which details are known and it is possible to identify user characteristics more precisely. However, to ensure that conditions set at the operational level are accurate, a sufficient understanding of what occurs on the strategic/tactical level is needed. Travelers' point of entry and exit within a facility may not largely change if total number of users does not increase excessively, but to estimate how this number will change in case of train network disruption, an accurate simulation on the tactical level is needed, which in turns requires a good statistical model to assess how decisions are affected at the strategic level. Typically, microscopic models are used on the operational level, although, depending on the need, also alternative models may be employed.

5.4.2 Procedural Steps in Setting up a Simulation Scenario

As discussed above, decisions of individuals and their relative behaviors are made via a multilevel approach with each level considered in a different way and requiring a different type of calculation. To allow a conceptual understanding of the behavioral levels and understand how changes on various scales can affect people behavior in different ways, the case of a full city was considered.

Being able to model different scales (including very large ones) is important and simulations performed in the frame of crowd management can indeed range from a single room to a whole city, but, most generally, they are performed for buildings, either for a single floor or, more often, considering several floors and their connections. More specifically, among the most commonly simulated scenarios, we may include train/metro stations, shopping malls, arenas/stadia, high rise buildings, etc. [3]. It should be also mentioned that simulations are often performed for static conditions (i.e., the flow of people moving in/out of the facility is constant). Concerning simulated scenarios, emergency evacuations are the most common, although we will not cover them here as we would like to focus on crowd management in normal conditions and also because evacuations are relatively easy to simulate: everyone will try to move to the (closest) exit. Therefore, keeping in mind what discussed above, we would like to move now into more practical aspects and consider how a simulation model is set up for a typical scenario considered in crowd management.

On this scope, we will present here the example of a subway/train station and present how the same behavioral levels can be applied on a much lower scale. This should help understanding even further the concept behind the behavioral levels and grasp the flexibility behind the concept, which allows to apply the same reasoning for a whole city but also for a single floor.

Let us consider the station schematically presented in Fig. 5.6. For simplicity, we assume that each access point can be only used as entrance or exit. Such a configuration is not common (usually gates can be used in both directions), but we can assume that an event is held on a particular day for which a large crowd is expected. Thus, the managing company want to impose some restrictions to keep the crowd under control. A simulation could help finding out if the proposed strategy is safe and/or improvements are needed.

Although, if the geometrical layout is concerned, a scenario like the one of Fig. 5.6 could be relatively easy to simulate, it is important to know the amount of people who will be moving from a specific entry into a specific exit. This modeling step

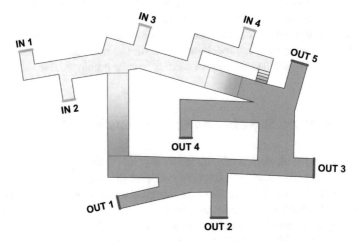

Fig. 5.6 Schematic example for a subway station to be modeled using a crowd simulator. For simplicity, we may assume access points can be used only in one direction (either entrance or exit). Floor elevation is represented using a gray scale, with darker areas being higher

represents the strategical level, which helps identifying what drives people to move in a specific direction by quantifying their need for motion.

In practice, the strategic level often consists in setting up the so-called origin–destination (OD) matrix. In other words, the user needs to instruct the software on the number of people entering from a given entrance and leaving from a given exit. For new constructions, this information need to be estimated using online surveys, mobile location data or based on what observed in similar facilities. If renovations are performed or internal layout is changed, it is usually possible to gain such information from field observations and measurements (although layout change may also influence people's habits, thus partially making current and future behavior different). In this example, we assume, as stated earlier, that changes to access point configuration are being planned in light of the upcoming event and expected motion can be estimated based on patterns observed in normal conditions. We further assume that the movements in terms of origin–destination are therefore obtained through on-site observations and surveys whose results are schematically shown in Fig. 5.7.

Based on the settings provided on the strategic level, each individual will need to select a specific route to move from origin to destination. As already discussed above, this calculation is performed in the tactical level where route and time scheduling are considered more in detail. Typically, the shortest route is used in the tactical level, but sometimes it is possible to set other criteria to define what should be the optimal route depending on conditions and usership. For example, people on wheelchair are not able to transit over staircases and may prefer a longer route if less steep (still, universal access should be always prioritized, although could be difficult for example in historical buildings). For this reason, specific weights are sometimes used to determine how disabled people evaluate each route with the one being short but also easy to move selected instead of the absolute shortest one, which may be less attractive to them [17–22]. Also, congestion along the route could contribute in modifying the decisions on the tactical level. If shortest time is the underlying criteria, then longer, less congested routes, may become the most attractive if congestion occurs along the shortest route [23, 24].

To From	OUT 1	OUT 2	OUT 3	OUT 4	OUT 5
IN 1	0.05 s^{-1}	0.05 s^{-1}	0.50 s^{-1}	0.10 s^{-1}	0.40 s^{-1}
IN 2	0.10 s^{-1}	0.10 s^{-1}	0.40 s^{-1}	0.20 s^{-1}	0.10 s^{-1}
IN 3	0.10 s^{-1}	0.10 s^{-1}	0.05 s^{-1}	0.20 s^{-1}	0.30 s^{-1}
IN 4	0.05 s^{-1}	0.30 s^{-1}	0.10 s^{-1}	0.10 s^{-1}	0.05 s^{-1}

Fig. 5.7 Example for an origin–destination matrix referring to the station given in Fig. 5.6. Note that in this case flow is given in s^{-1} as the number of people transiting in each access point is assessed regardless on the width, which is often the case while setting up simulations where it may be also possible to set up a distribution to describe time-dependent inflow patterns. (Specific) flow (as introduced in Chap. 2) may be obtained by dividing by the width of each entrance/exit

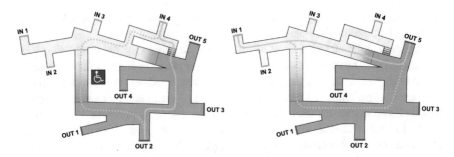

Fig. 5.8 Examples for route choice depending on pedestrian attributes and congestion. The left image shows how the shortest path could change if a person is on wheelchair or has walking impairment. The right image shows an example where a shorter route in terms of distance (solid line) could result longer in terms of time if congestion along the route occurs. Dashed route may become faster under these conditions

Figure 5.8 shows a few possible route choices for different types of pedestrians and for different conditions. Modern crowd simulators are able to perform decisions for each individual based on the simulated conditions and taking into account her/his characteristics. Ideally, tactical decisions should be updated as people move toward the various destinations, but sometimes the route is assigned at the moment of leaving the origin and each pedestrian will stay stick to the original decision.

Even when a route has been selected, there are several obstacles that pedestrians will encounter along the way, with other people being the most common ones. As already discussed, this local obstacle avoidance is computed on the operational level. Here, people interact between each other and the close environment to determine every following step. Although strategical and tactical levels employ computational methods shared with other fields (vehicular traffic in particular; consider how car navigator computes the optimal route), algorithms for the operational level are very specific for crowd motion.

An example of calculations performed on the operational level is shown in Fig. 5.9. Even if the two pedestrians at the bottom may be moving along the shortest path, they are likely to join the lane moving in the same direction to reduce conflicts with

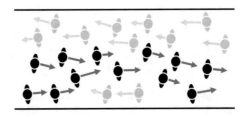

Fig. 5.9 Examples for interactions considered at the operational level. People usually have different walking speeds and the two gray pedestrians shown at the bottom will probably try to join the lane moving in their direction to reduce conflicts even if the route may get partially longer

opposite directed people. Also, people usually do not walk too close to the wall and tends to hug corners even if the shortest path would require them to touch them (as discussed in Chap. 2). This sort of low-level behavior is computed in the operational level.

5.4.3 Concluding Remarks

From the above examples, it should be now clear that crowd motion has to be modeled using the three levels of behavior: strategic, tactical, and operational. However, setting the scale for each level and defining the model that could better describe the behavior on each level largely depends on one's objectives and needs. Most of the commercial software available for crowd management has been originally developed for fire evacuation and has been later extended to implement transportation related mobility and leisure activities (such as visiting a shopping mall). Typically, both operational and tactical levels are implemented and inter-operating in modern commercial software, thus leaving to the user the task to define the conditions on the strategic level (in other words, the user needs to define scenarios that will be simulated).

In the following sections we are going to present more details on the various simulation models. However, when models are considered individually, there is often the tendency to closely look at their properties, neglecting the general picture provided by the three levels of behavior. It is therefore important to remind that even a good software could lead to inaccurate results when its conditions at its boundaries are not set keeping in mind a broader perspective. In short, also in simulation, a collaboration between stakeholders is necessary and the key of success. If simulations are performed for a stadium without knowing the capacity of the connecting station, results may look fine, but problems will arise in reality at the boundaries.

Finally, in light of what discussed above, one should consider that modern commercial software include several algorithms (route choice, individual motion, group motion, wheelchair navigation, etc.) whose combination determine the quality of a product. A specific software may be particularly accurate in considering mobility for people with disabilities, but may be less accurate in representing people's individual interactions. Software that works well on the operational level could perform good in evacuations, where route choice does not play a relevant role, but to model occupants behavior in a shopping mall or in a train stations in normal conditions, the capability to flexibly change routes on the tactical level could play a more important role. This means, again, that a simulation software has to be selected based on one's needs, regardless on it's overall evaluation.

5.5 Typical Models Employed in Crowd Simulation

Having illustrated general and common features of crowd simulation, the discussion will now continue considering the most relevant mathematical/behavioral models.

5.5.1 Cellular Automata

Considering historical development and easiness of understanding, Cellular Automata (CA) is being presented at first. CA is a popular microscopic model used to simulate pedestrian and crowd dynamics [25, 26]. Principles of CA are very simple, making it a very fast and flexible approach, allowing us to easily implement particular social behaviors observed in crowds.

CA was already introduced in the 1940s by mathematicians S. Ulam and J. von Neumann, and nowadays, it is used in a variety of fields, with traffic engineering being an application for which CA is particularly suited. A large number of variations of the model for pedestrians has been proposed over the years, and this section will only present the general concepts common among all variants. The notions gained through this section should allow grasping better strengths and limitations of pedestrian simulators based on CA.

Fundamental principles of CA are illustrated in Fig. 5.10. We will start by explaining the simple one-dimensional (1D) case, which should allow a better understanding of more complex bi-dimensional dynamics later on. Let us consider the case of people walking in a line, like the image represented in Fig. 5.10. For simplicity, in CA, people are represented as dots or "objects" filling a cell in a long grid. Since people cannot squeeze, and everyone has a particular volume given by her/his body size, we can assume each person can occupy only one cell at a time. People can move to the next cell (in the right direction for the case considered in Fig. 5.10) only if the next cell is empty. This emulates the congestion occurring in real crowds (which is somehow similar to vehicular traffic): If someone is standing in front of you on a

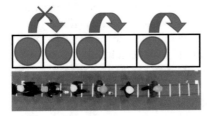

Fig. 5.10 Fundamental principles of Cellular Automata. Left: rules determining motion in a 1D case. People (indicated as circles) attempt to move from left to right, but motion is only possible when an adjacent cell is empty. Right: example for different time steps of CA simulation for pedestrians moving from left to right. People move with a given probability, which means motion does not occur all the time even if a cell is available

Fig. 5.11 Pedestrian space representation in CA. Moore neighborhood employs all surrounding cells (thus, eight positions), while Von Neumann only uses the four cells surrounding the central pedestrian (yellow arrows)

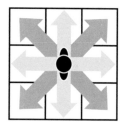

line, you cannot move forward. In addition, in CA, it is assumed that even if a cell is empty, people will not move all the times, but only with a given probability (which also occurs in reality when people are distracted, for example). The combination of both rules, move only when possible and not all the times, will generate a behavior like the one presented on the right side of Fig. 5.10.

While the 1D case presented in Fig. 5.10 is indeed used in crowd simulations, in particular, for the case of lanes formed at airports or in front of cash registers at supermarkets, people normally moves in a bi-dimensional space, turning left or right and choosing their preferred path depending on the surrounding environment.

As a consequence, a grid like the one presented in Fig. 5.11 is used for most of pedestrian simulators based on CA. Each pedestrian can move one cell at a time either using four directions (Von Neumann neighborhood) or eight directions (Moore neighborhood). The cell size is chosen to correspond to the average size of people, with most simulators using cells in the order of 40 to 50 cm.

Several methods are used to determine the cell that one pedestrian will chose when moving one step at a time, and we will not go into details because quite complex algorithms are employed on the purpose. However, it is important to know at least the so-called "static floor field" used to "guide" pedestrians to the destination.

The static floor field is a sort of map that allows us to determine which cell is closer to the exit or the destination. For example, when pedestrians attempt to exit a door (like in case of evacuations) maps similar to the ones represented on the left side of Fig. 5.12 are used. Regardless of where a pedestrian is located, if she/he choices the "whiter" cell in her/his neighborhood, she/he will be able to reach the destination as soon as possible.

Computing the static floor field is not an easy task [28], and quality of crowd simulators may depend largely on the way the static floor field is computed. As Fig. 5.12 shows, even for the simple case of a single door evacuation, the simulation result changes depending on the approach taken to compute the static floor field. As the environment grows in complexity, it becomes increasingly difficult to compute the static floor field, and simple crowd simulators may not be able to handle such situations.

In general, commercial crowd simulators have automatic tools that allow us to automatically compute those maps using CAD files or based on floor diagrams drawn in the user interface. It is also possible to set individual destinations for each pedestrian, thus defining several maps for each entity simulated (as required in the strategic level).

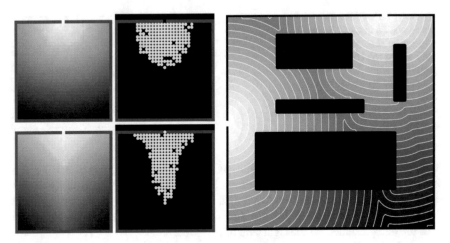

Fig. 5.12 Maps used to guide pedestrians to the exit. People will move one cell at a time trying to go to the neighboring "whiter" cell. Images on the right side show two different approaches to compute those maps in the case of single door evacuation, with results for those simulations given in the center. The right map represents a more complex scenario involving obstacles, walls and two separate exits (the white locations with openings). Reprinted figure with permission from [27]. Copyright © 2004 IEICE

The static floor field is only one of the many elements composing complex CA-based crowd simulators, and additional methods are used to account, for example, for following, anticipating [29], wall avoidance behaviors [30], pressure forces [31], or different walking speeds [32]. In CA models, it is also possible to account for groups [33] (e.g., couples or families), people with disabilities [34], elderlies, and infrastructural elements like escalators or stairs.

Listing all the special models that can be implemented in CA-simulators would be a difficult and an incomplete task because there is no agreement on the correct model to reproduce, for example, group behavior or wheelchair dynamics. Also, it is not always possible to know which algorithm is used in commercial software programs, as each company uses a different approach.

However, a common point of CA-simulators lies in their computational speed. Figure 5.13 compares results from a simulation performed using a CA model with video frames from a real experiment. To compute the complete egress (consisting of about 65 computational steps), a normal desktop computer took less than 0.1 s–much faster than the time it took to people to leave the room in the real case (about 18 s). The frames from the simulation also show a feature of CA models, namely their quite coarse visualization. As the scenarios get large (like the case of Fig. 5.4), a smoother motion is seen, but for small scenarios or when details are shown, a rather unnatural behavior is observed. In general, CA models tend to be accurate when the motion of people is considered on the crowd-level, but considerations are difficult on the individual level. For instance, the simple scenario considered in Fig. 5.13 correctly predicts the complete egress time (about 18 s), but the position of each person is

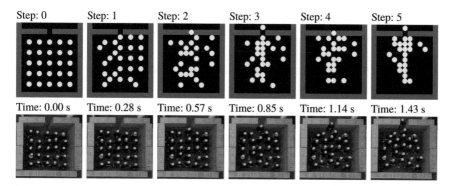

Fig. 5.13 Frames from a CA simulation and comparison with the related experimental case. Images of the simulation are shown every computational steps and experimental images are relative to the equivalent moment. In this case, a different static floor field could be used to better reproduce qualitative features (i.e., people's positions)

different from the real case (this also relates to the method used to set up the static floor field, as discussed earlier).

Further, CA-based simulators usually require multiple simulation runs to get accurate results. In the example above, the egress time of 18 s is correctly predicted when the average of many simulations is taken, but each simulation run leads to partially different results (the fastest one taking around 15 s, and the slowest more than 25 s). Finally, it is important to mention that CA simulators usually comprises a large number of parameters that adjust specific behavior of individuals, for example the "motivation" in hurrying up or how much people tend to follow each other or how strong is the group cohesion. While commercial software typically adjusts these parameters automatically, one should know that such parameters exist, and the results will change depending on the parameter set.

5.5.1.1 Advantages/Disadvantages

To summarize, the biggest advantage of CA-based crowd simulators lies in the simplicity of the model, which translates into very short computational times and ease of customization. It is also relatively easy to adapt CA models to work in a multi-CPU environment, thus allowing the use of supercomputers and further decrease computational time. Hence, CA models are well suited for applications where computational time is of primary importance, like real-time crowd prediction or large scenarios involving thousands (or even millions) of people. Also, CA models are generally very flexible, and although the degree of customization changes from product to product, it is easier to implement specific functions to existing CA models compared to other approaches.

Among the strongest disadvantages of CA models is the course representation of crowds. While this does not affect the results themselves, it may be an issue when animations of crowd moving need to be presented to customers or to people not familiar with these crowd simulators. People tend to trust simulation results if animations look real, and when experimental evidence is not provided, it is difficult to prove that results are indeed correct (which is usually true although people are moving in an apparently coarse fashion).

In addition, the large number of parameters [35–37] and the need to perform several simulations runs partially affect the excellent performances of CA simulators. Although computational time is very short, multiple simulation runs are required, slightly increasing the overall time needed to get the final (average) result.

Finally, CA models need a clear destination for each pedestrian and may not work correctly when people wander and/if people often stop without any particular reason (like to watch a shop's window).

5.5.1.2 Suitable applications/scenarios

CA models are well suited for slightly dense to very dense crowds and are often used for evacuations and simulations of extreme scenarios. CA models are suggested when a large number of people with very different characteristics are considered and when the destination/whereabouts are clearly defined. Also, CA models are very accurate when lanes or queues are considered.

Train stations, transportation hubs, and airports are a good targets for CA-based crowd simulations since people usually have a specific destination and need to reach it in the shortest time possible. Aircraft, building, or even city evacuation is also a typical scenario where CA models are used.

Finally, CA models are also well suited for real-time applications where predictions of crowd conditions need to be performed in a very short time. Using CA models, it is relatively easy to perform simulations based on pedestrian positions detected using sensors and predict possible risks occurring in the near future (more on this will be discussed in Chap. 7).

5.5.2 Social Force Model

The social force model (belonging to the more general family of force-based models) was proposed in the 1990s by Helbing and Molnar [38]. It has been widely used in academic research and commercial applications to simulate pedestrian behavior under various conditions [39–41]. The social force model belongs to the category of microscopic models, which means that each pedestrian is computed individually. However, in contrast to CA, a continuous space is used to simulate pedestrian behavior.

In the social force model, pedestrians' positions are computed using force potentials. In some way, pedestrians are considered like electric charges attracted toward

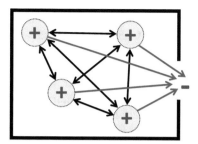

Fig. 5.14 Schematic representation of four people evacuating from a room with a single door under the social force model. People are modeled like positive electrical charge and their destination take a negative charge

their destination. To understand how the social force model works, the illustration in Fig. 5.14 may help.

In the approach used by the social force model, we may assume that people are like electric charges. Pedestrians, taking a positive charge, are attracted toward the destination, which takes a negative charge, but at the same time, they try to stay as far as possible from each other. In some way, it is considered that social relations generate repulsive forces among people who move toward their destinations. Hence, the model is referred as "social force."

An important aspect of the social force model is that since people are treated like electric potentials, they are not assigned a size but simply try to stay as far as possible from each other. Unlike the CA model, in the social force model, people may partially "overlap" each other if special considerations are not included in the computational algorithm.

How much the force between people change when they get close to each other and how fast people move toward the destination is computed using mathematical expressions, which may slightly depend on the variants of the social force model. However, although several modifications of the original model have been proposed over the years, the general nature of the model remains unchanged.

The main difference between CA and the social force model is clearly illustrated in Fig. 5.15. Since people are not constrained to cells, they can move to any position, resulting in a very smooth movement of the crowd. However, the cost for such a smooth motion lies in the computational efforts required to obtain the position during each step. Although each computational step was almost 0.3 s in CA, in the social force model, very small time-steps are used (0.01 s here). In other words, many calculations are required to calculate the motion of the crowd over a short time period. For instance, taking the example considered here, it took 33 s to compute the positions of all pedestrians during the complete egress (although computational time could have been reduced by taking larger time-steps, partially reducing accuracy), which was correctly predicted as 18 s long (in line with experimental data). In other words, it took almost twice the time it took to evacuate the room to predict how long it would take to evacuate it.

In addition, one should mention that simulations tend to get slower as the number of people is increased. In CA, the increase in computational time is proportional to the increase in the number of people: If a doubly large crowd is considered, the computational time will be doubled. In social force model, a doubly large crowd usually takes more than two times to be computed, although rapid improvements are being made to reduce this effect by employing more efficient algorithms.

On the other hand, the computational approach of the social force model does not require multiple simulations to get an accurate final result (or the number of repetitions required is much lower than CA simulators). Repeating the simulation shown in Fig. 5.15 will generate almost identical results. In addition, the number of parameters used in social force models is generally limited, thus making the model simpler than CA from this point of view.

5.5.2.1   Advantages/Disadvantages

To summarize, one of the biggest advantages of social force simulators is the smooth representation of collective crowd motion, thus making the results highly realistic and credible. However, with the improvements of visualization techniques, targeting in particular 3D visualization, also different approaches (including CA) can generate more or less realistic animations.

Since the social force model also belongs to the family of microscopic simulators, it is possible to set up properties of each pedestrian individually [42], thus making it suitable for diverse heterogeneous crowds and to consider more complex social interactions such as groups or families.

In addition, since a limited number of repetitions (if none at all) is sufficient and parameters are small in numbers, social force simulators are comparatively easy to use and calibrate [43]. Finally, it should be mentioned that a large number of commercial software are based on this approach, and therefore, it is possible to choose based on

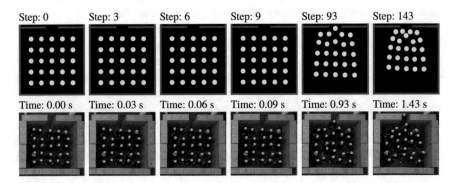

Fig. 5.15 Social force model simulation and comparison with the related experimental case. Images of the simulation are shown, and every computational step and experimental images are relative to the equivalent moment

more practical aspects such as ease-of-use, user interface, or price between solutions having a similar computational core.

The most evident among the disadvantages of social force models is the long computational time, although increasingly efficient algorithms are partially eclipsing this drawback. However, the relatively lower computational speed could limit the application of these models for real-time applications, unless supercomputers are used [6, 7]. In this regard, it should be also mentioned that given its particular nature, it is more difficult to have social force models working on multiprocessors and large computers, and smart solutions are required to cope with this problem (although commercial software products typically employs such solutions).

Also, it is generally more difficult to use social force model in complex environments compared to CA approaches. Internal walls, stairs, and escalators will need particular considerations. Again, commercial software products have features to automatically overcome those problems, but the complexity involved in the task make them less reliable.

Finally, like CA models, social force models require a clear destination to work efficiently. When people are not precisely aiming at a particular destination with time constraints, setting up proper conditions may be difficult.

5.5.2.2 Suitable applications/scenarios

Social force models are well suited to study facilities in the development phase, when computational time is not very relevant but quality in the presentation of the results is important. Typically, social force model is accurate for low to medium dense crowds and tend to be slightly unrealistic for highly dense crowds where "overlapping" of agents in simulation may become an issue (but this also depends on the specific product and parameters setting).

Given the considerations above, the social force model may be used to study everyday traffic in transportation facilities, where densities are usually never exceedingly high values and origin/destination is well defined. In general, scenarios that are good for CA are also adequate for social force models, though CA tend to be more accurate at high densities while social force model for sparse dense crowds (also considering that computational time tend to increase more rapidly with the number of people in the social force model).

5.5.3 Network Models

Network models (or similar approaches) are used in a variety of fields and are also the base for complex calculations related to the dynamics of human society [44, 45]. When the transportation network in a given area is well defined and timetables for trains, buses, and public services are available and reliable, then it is relatively easy to predict how people will move within that network and which area will be busier

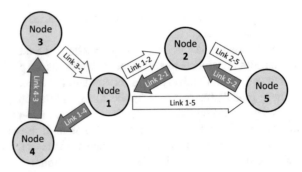

Fig. 5.16 Typical structure of a network model. Nodes are connected by links with different directions. Note that only links in one direction may exist between different nodes. Number for nodes are given with random order here, names for links refer to the connecting nodes. In real applications, each node correspond to a particular region/area and each link represents a set of transportation routes

at a particular time. However, network models rely on a very abstract representation of the space and results are reliable only when the abstract representation does not differ much from reality.

To better explain these concepts and further discuss the potential and issues related to network models, we should first explain the two fundamental principles of network models: nodes and links, both schematically represented in Fig. 5.16. A node represents a given area. Taking Fig. 5.3 as an example, a node may represent a neighborhood or a station within a city or a larger area such as a whole country. A link represents the set of routes between two nodes. If only one road connects two areas and there is no other way to go from one area to another, then that single route will be the link in the network model. If there are multiple routes and ways to go from one place to the another, then the link will need to consider the different ways of transportations and the different routes or, alternatively, multiple links with the different properties are to be created.

Defining the border or the region that a single node represents in reality is not an easy task. For example, an island in the middle of the sea with a single village of few houses around the harbor can be easily modeled as a single node. The daily ferry connecting the island with the closest city will summarize the link pointing to that node. However, it is difficult to define the node and links in large cities where areas are not clearly separated from each other and there are hundreds of ways to go from one point to another. For example, should the center of a city considered as a single node or is better to divide it in multiple small areas, considering that many people move inside it? Of course, this depends on the scale considered, but, again, creating the right network is not easy.

Even when the topology (or the shape) of a network model has been defined, there are still additional problems to solve. In particular, the properties of each node and link need to be accurately defined. Each node can have a maximum number of people (or population) depending on its size, and each link will have a maximum

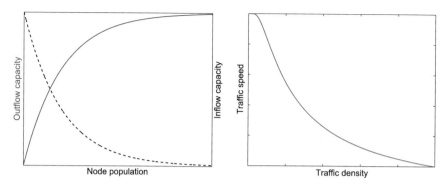

Fig. 5.17 Examples of typical expressions used to describe properties of nodes and links. When node population changes, the maximum in- and outflow is affected. Similarly, traffic speed (or transit time) in a link is affected by traffic density in the same link

flow (the number of people can pass through it in a given time) depending on the size and frequency of transportation means representing it.

To make things more complex, we should mention that in most of the cases, the dynamics of nodes and links is not simple and need to be defined according to mathematical descriptions. In fact, generally, the population of one node cannot increase at the same rate all the time. When an area (node) is completely empty, people can move in it very quickly, but when congestion build up, then it takes more time to accommodate the same number of people. Take the example of a large shopping mall: When parking lots are all empty and there is no car in the area, then a car can enter quickly and go straight to the parking spot closest to the entrance. Under these conditions, the number of customers will grow very quickly. But when the parking is close to capacity, people will have to drive around looking for an empty spot and the number of customers will grow slower. A similar dynamic is seen in nodes. When the flow is low, the time to go from one location (or node) to another is very short, but at high flow rates (when congestion occurs) it takes a much longer time. Some typical examples for the dynamics of nodes and links are given in Fig. 5.17.

To summarize, accuracy of network models therefore depends on how good is the representation of the space being studied and how much information we have on the system. In countries with a well-developed public transportation system, people use that public transport to move within cities. Mobility therefore depends on the transportation network, and modeling using the same network is rather accurate and effective. However, in developing countries and/or regions that largely depend on private forms of transportation, defining nodes and links is more difficult as there are several ways to move from origin to destination.

5.5.3.1   Advantages/Disadvantages

A clear advantage of network models is their simplicity and scalability. While micro-scopic models simulate each person individually, and geometrical details are required for the space people are moving in, network models consider a large group of people moving along combined transportation routes. Hence, network models can be built for any scale (as already described in Figs. 5.2 and 5.3). Since the simulated structure for a building is similar to the one for a city, which is in turn similar to the whole world, it does not matter how large is the scale, computational time will always be the same. Therefore, when large scales are considered (which is often the case), network models are much faster than any other approach (microscopic models in particular).

In addition, network models only require combined figures for capacity of nodes and links, so it is possible to perform simulations also when only estimates are available for road or rail infrastructure on a large scale. For instance, if a new train line is expected to transport 100,000 people per day, that information may be taken as it is to model its impact on the area without needing further details.

On the other hand, the biggest disadvantage of network models is the difficulty of making up the network and defining properties for nodes and links. In this sense, a large work is required in the preparation of the model, while calculations are very fast and efficient. Also, a small modification of the model may lead to rethinking a large part of it, since properties of neighboring nodes and links need to be redefined carefully. In brief, network models require knowledge and know-how to be built.

Also, results gained from network models are typically approximative, both on the spatial and temporal scales. Although it is always possible to adapt both scales, network models are generally used for large scales, and therefore, one cannot know which area is the most "dangerous," but only which area is more congested. To further study details, a microscopic model is required, but, linking network and microscopic models requires expertise and time (although it should be ideally done when all behavioral levels have to be combined).

5.5.3.2   Suitable applications/scenarios

Network models are appropriate to model existing transportation networks such as subways, local trains, or highways, in particular when a large proportion of the population use this infrastructure. It would be therefore possible to estimate the change over a subway stretch when for example a new train/road train line is being introduced. In general, because of the complexity involved in the construction of the network and its properties, network models are well suited for structures that do not physically change over time, but only usage change. For example, one can use a network model to simulate the effect of large events on the subway system. During large events like the Olympics or trade fairs, transportation network will not change much (possibly except for shuttle buses or similar temporary services), but time schedules need to be adapted and eventually supplementary buses introduced. Implementing those changes on an already existing network model is quite simple, and results are generated in a short time. Further studies on the local level (how people move inside the train station) can be performed using microscopic models based on the results from the network model.

5.5.4 Alternative Approaches

In the previous section, the models most commonly used in crowd simulators were presented in detail. Those models were chosen because they allow a quick understanding of some of the fundamental aspects of crowd modeling: representation of space, calculation of people's motion at each step and different degrees of detail (from individual to large uniform crowds). In this section, minor and trending alternatives are presented. The knowledge gained in the previous section should help in understanding each approach.

5.5.4.1 Velocity-based models

These kinds of models are somewhat similar to the approach by the social force model, but instead of trying to stay as far as possible from each other, in velocity-based model, people attempt to reduce the collision time [46].

In velocity-based models, people will therefore find the direction that allows reaching the destination while avoiding collisions with others. When collisions cannot be avoided, the walking speed is reduced eventually arriving almost to a full stop when density are too high to rule out the risk of collisions. A schematic illustration of the differences between social force and velocity-based models is given in Fig. 5.18.

Velocity-based models typically have similar advantages and disadvantages compared to the social force model but generally consider collision avoidance in a more

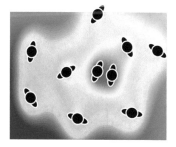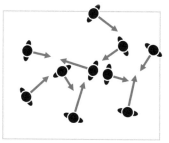

Fig. 5.18 Left: social force approach; people try to maximize their distance while moving toward the destination (undefined here). Right: velocity-based approach; people try to avoid collisions by adjusting speed and direction

natural way. They may therefore be more appropriate for situations where people move in very different directions and collisions would occur easily.

5.5.4.2 Behavioral (discrete-choice) models

In behavioral models, at each step, pedestrians choose their walking direction and speed from a limited number of possibilities [47]. Each pedestrian has a limited number of directions (as illustrated in Fig. 5.19) and may choose to slow down, maintain the current speed, or accelerate (also given in Fig. 5.19), forming a set of possible choices (33 in total in the case considered in Fig. 5.19).

The combination of stepping direction and speed change creates a sort of map representing all possible choices. Using experimental data gained from observations, it is possible to determine how people choose among the several possibilities and how the decision-making process changes depending on the location of the destination and the one of other pedestrians.

In simulations, each pedestrian performs a decision at every step (as schematically represented in Fig. 5.20), thus determining the overall motion of the crowd.

Behavioral models can be considered a trade-off between CA and social force approaches: motion dynamics is more fluid than CA models, but computational speed is faster then social force models. In general, a large number of parameters are required to correctly reproduce the decision-making progress, but, on the other hand, it is relatively simple to calibrate the model using experimental data. A remark-

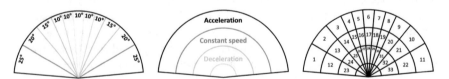

Fig. 5.19 Schematic representation of the motion strategies accounted for in behavioral models. Both future direction and change in velocity are considered. Reprinted from [48], Copyright (2009), with permission from Elsevier

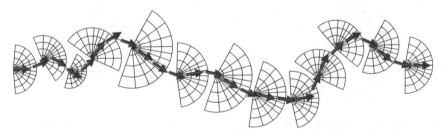

Fig. 5.20 Illustrative representation of a pedestrian trajectory determined using the behavioral model. Decisions are performed at every step thus resulting in the final trajectory represented here. Reprinted from [48], Copyright (2009), with permission from Elsevier

able drawback of behavioral models is that they are not widely used in commercial applications.

5.5.4.3 Continuum models

Continuum models adopt a macroscopic approach and assume people as fluids (or gases) with properties such as density and speed to be computed using complex mathematical equations [49–51]. Several continuum models have been proposed over the years, and the most important aspects have been already discussed in the introduction while presenting the macroscopic approach (see Fig. 5.1 in particular to get a better image of continuum models).

Continuum models are mainly used in research and practical applications are limited. They may become a potential candidate when extremely dense crowds are considered and they may be particularly fast and accurate under these very special conditions.

5.5.4.4 Data-driven prediction (model-free approach)

Recent developments in the field of machine learning and artificial intelligence have led to the emergence of a new approach for crowd simulation that is purely based on data [52, 53]. Basically, computers are "trained" using a large number of trajectories and, if training is performed well, are able to predict the walking pattern of one person considering the surrounding environment.

Given their purely statistical approach, data-driven systems can predict, for example, people stopping without any particular reason, if the data that have been used for training contained a similar behavior. In addition, data-driven solution can be successfully used to predict patterns of people entering the surveyed area (inflow). Machine learning is particularly powerful in reproducing patterns observed during different time periods and weekdays and can be therefore used to create the inflow of pedestrians in simulated areas (also for other models).

While limitations of typical pedestrian models lie in the nature of the model that is the heart of the system, the strengths and limitations of data-driven approaches lie in the data used for training. In other words, data-driven approaches are very good at predicting situations very similar to the scenario used for training. For example, if a shopping mall is used for training, data-driven solutions will be able to successfully reproduce the dynamics of people at low density and frequently stopping. When the same simulation is used for a congested train station, the results may be highly inaccurate, since the dynamics observed for hurrying crowds at high density is different from that for relaxed shoppers.

At the moment of writing, data-driven solutions are mostly limited to pioneering research, but an increasing number of studies is being published every year and we believe this approach may become one of the leading solutions in the near future.

Table 5.1 Important technical characteristics to be considered when choosing a crowd model

Computational requirements	Low … High
Individual pedestrians' properties	Completely heterogeneous crowds …
	… Completely homogeneous crowds
Special models available	Groups, stairs, escalators, elevators, combined traffic, wheelchair…
Route choice	Fixed … Adaptive/Automatic
Quality of animation/visualization	Rough … Smooth

5.6   Simulator Selection and Comparison

5.6.1   Selection Criteria and Relevance

After having discussed detailed aspects of the different models used in crowd simulators, it is now time to compare them and propose a methodology to select the approach that is better suited to one's needs. Like the previous chapter on sensors, we wish to consider the selection process from two perspectives: capabilities/technical aspects of simulators and environment/conditions relative to the envisaged employment. Although, for most of the users, the selection of a crowd simulator translates into choosing between different software products (or consulting firms using those products), in this section, we will only consider the major models discussed above (CA, social force, and network models) and added data-driven solutions considering the recent trends. We refrained from listing the various commercial software since their functionality, user interface, target usership, and price are changing rapidly and evaluation will need to be updated constantly. The criteria considered here for models can be also applied on specific software products, thus representing a universal approach in selecting crowd simulators. Nonetheless, at the end of this section, additional aspects that apply on commercial software are also listed.

Table 5.1 presents important aspects related to crowd simulators, and it can be seen as summarizing what a simulator can do. To start with, computational requirements is surely an important aspect to consider: Some simulators are able to generate results for thousands of people in a short time on laptop computers, while others require dedicated supercomputers. Next, one should consider the possibility to set individual properties for groups or individual pedestrians. This is important when modeling very heterogeneous crowds. In addition, the availability of special models within the crowd simulator has to be verified. In particular, group behavior or stairs may not be included in all simulators, and accuracy for those models may be very different between specific products. If, for example, stairs or escalators are present in large number in the area to be studied, one needs to play a particular attention on these aspects. Next, route choice capabilities are important. In some models, pedestrians have their origin, destination, and route fixed. However, in reality, people determine their path depending on the conditions along the route, if it gets congested alternative routes are considered. Some simulators may be better than others in considering these aspects and computing alternative routes depending on the conditions. The final point to consider is the quality of the animations and more generally the visualization of the results (this aspect will be discussed in the following section more in detail). Although it is generally possible to later post-process results depending on one's needs, simulators directly providing presentable results are generally preferred.

After having determined technical characteristics regarding the different solutions being considered, it is important to specify what are the constraints relative to the scenarios which will be studied and the environment where simulators will be used. Those constraints are listed in Table 5.2, which basically summarizes what the simulators are expected to do and under which conditions will have to work. At first, budget plays an important role in determining which products are accessible and which are not. Here, it is important to divide the costs on a yearly basis, as license and support generally need to be renewed. Next, the main scope for simulation needs to be clearly specified. Some simulators include many options and allow to go into details but require a long time to generate results: these are well suited for planning. Others are less detailed but very fast, thus being better for real-time applications. As already discussed in presenting the models, the scale of the studied scenario also contributes in limiting feasible products/solutions. Similarly, the motivation of the simulated pedestrians needs to be carefully considered. When origin-destination is clearly defined, then a large number of simulators are suited, but only few are able to deal with dynamics found in shopping centers or hospitals, where short-distance apparently unnecessary movements are frequently observed. The population being simulated also need to be surveyed, at least in a summarized way. Age and health condition affect walking speed, while unfamiliarity with the environment (for example foreigners) affects the way people navigate. Finally, the condition being simulated has to be defined since behavior in normal conditions is generally different from emergencies. To conclude the discussion on constraints relative to the use of crowd simulators, one needs to evaluate the expertise of future users. Some software is designed to be used by people without expertise on computational tools, while others may require advanced computer skills including some knowledge on programming.

Based on the criteria presented in Tables 5.1 and 5.2, each pedestrian model has been evaluated, and results are presented in Tables 5.3 and 5.4. These tables may help identify the best approach and later choice-specific products in a structured way.

It is, however, important to notice that, as individual products are evolving, differences between pedestrian models are getting smaller and differences between products larger. As a consequence, the content of Tables 5.3 and 5.4 may rapidly change. Nonetheless, we believe the criteria presented here will always be helpful in evaluating different models.

Table 5.2 Constraints relative to the environment where crowd simulators will be employed

Yearly license cost Hardware cost	Total cost required to buy and maintain the simulation software
Simulation scope	Design, planning, monitoring, real-time applications
Perspective scale	Region, city, neighborhood, architectural complex, building, floor, room
Simulated environment	Transit location, shopping area, sightseeing, music event, school, hospital…
Perspective crowd	Age, health conditions, locals/foreigners, gender, wheelchair users, children…
Simulated condition	Everyday situation … Emergency
Expected simulator's users	Beginners, entry users, crowd/simulator experts

5.6.2 Commercial Software, Code Development, or Outsourcing?

Although knowing about pedestrian models, understanding how they work and being able to select the right one is surely important to prevent potential issues in pedestrian projects, most often the biggest doubt for crowd managers lie on whether it would be more proper to buy a license for a commercial software, acquire or develop one (maybe based on freely available codes) or outsource the simulation task to a specialized company. Obviously each option has merits and demerits, and it often depends on the budget available, the complexity of the simulated scenario, technical experience of the crowd manager, and future needs. However, to help in case such a decision is needed, a few suggestions will be added as follows.

Commercial software products represent professional solutions that are often validated, trusted by several organizations and provided with extensive documentation.

Table 5.3 Classification of different pedestrian models based on technical characteristics

	CA	Social force	Network model	Data driven
Computational requirements	Medium	High	Low	Very high
Individual pedestrians' properties	Possible	Possible	Not possible	Not possible
Special models available	Several	Several	Limited	Not available
Route choice	Largely dependent on specific product/solution			
Quality of animation /visualization	Rough (typically)	Smooth	Rough in space	Smooth

Table 5.4 Classification of different pedestrian models based on potential applications and usability constraints

	CA	Social force	Network model	Data driven
Yearly license cost	Largely dependent on specific product			
Hardware cost	Low	Medium		High
Simulation scope	Design, real time	Design, planning		Prediction
Perspective scale	Building, region	Building	Region, city	Building
Simulated environment	Upon setup		Motion only	Relative to data
Perspective crowd	Upon setup		Homogeneous	Relative to data
Simulated condition	Normal or emergency conditions			Normal only
Expected simulator users	Entry user	Beginner	Entry user	Expert

This comes, however, with a cost, both in financial terms and in the time needed to learn how to use them and make sure simulation is correctly setup. Having a professional reliable software does not guarantee accurate results. Users also need to understand the product and be able to set up scenarios representative of the existing conditions. It should be also emphasized that modern commercial software can be highly automated, so users looking for a solution to be implemented into a more complex system could also benefit from them (e.g., if sensing and simulation have to be coupled as discussed later in Chap. 7).

If small simple infrastructures have be modeled (like a single floor) on a low budget, then opting for freely available programs could be an option. Nowadays, there are several open-source software [54–57] that can be used with some basic IT know-how and may be employed for simple scenarios (although most of them are limited to non-commercial use). Some also comes with an user interface, thus requiring little or no programming knowledge. However, validation is usually not strictly performed and users will need to setup several parameters with little or no documentation. While validation is somehow possible using some tips provided later and/or comparing with experimental data [58–60], a lack of documentation may impact results negatively. On the other side, it would be needless to say that users looking for complete control over a simulation model should either develop their own or use an available one as a starting point.

If, however, simulation is required for a specific purpose, and it will be a once in a lifetime task (or done quite rarely), then consulting a specialized firm could represent the best solution. In this case, choosing the best firm is important, and care should be taken in checking previous projects carried out by that firm (if possible). Companies specializing in fire engineering may have little experience in regular mass transportation. Also, it is fundamental to stress what is the expected outcome from simulation and what can be provided to that firm. Often, CAD data are required for accurate simulation, and alternative data may have to be prepared if those are confidential and cannot be shared with third parties.

To conclude, we should also remind that, if different types of simulation may have to be run for several contexts, then a diversification through several solutions is also possible and often the case for diverse projects [3].

5.6.3   Choosing a Commercial Software

If a commercial software is chosen to carry out simulations independently, then selection criteria slightly change toward more practical aspects.

Validation or verification should be the most important criterion in this case. Since commercial software usually do not allow modifications to the computational core (i.e., the model used and the related algorithms), it is imperative to select a product that produce valid and reliable results. If conditions observed in reality cannot be reproduced in simulation, people may be at danger even when risks are low and confidence among stakeholders may be lost.

Next, after validation, more practical aspects should be considered. Commercial software usually comes with a complex user interface and several functions (see for example Fig. 5.21). Even when an intuitive user interface is provided, it is usually difficult to understand all the functions without a proper documentation. For this reason, the availability of manuals, tutorials, and training videos will also play an important criterion in selection. Most users are typically self-taught [3], so, under this perspective the importance of documentation should be even more obvious.

Finally, capability to automatically import/export data is playing an increasingly relevant role as application program interface (API) are being commonly used to connect several software solutions. Most commercial simulators provide tools (or SDK) to programmatically read input conditions or export results to allow post-processing using third-party software. However, these capabilities largely depend from product to product. In this regard, the possibility to import CAD files can also play a relevant part in the selection. Software that automatically import and recognize pedestrian areas from complex geometries could reduce the amount of time needed to construct a simulation scenario.

5.7   Evaluation and Improvement of Simulation Results

So far, only preparation of scenarios and computational methods have been discussed, and nothing has been said on the final outcome of simulations: results. In discussing on methods to evaluate and improve results, we will, however, only focus on microscopic models as they are the ones more commonly used in crowd management and

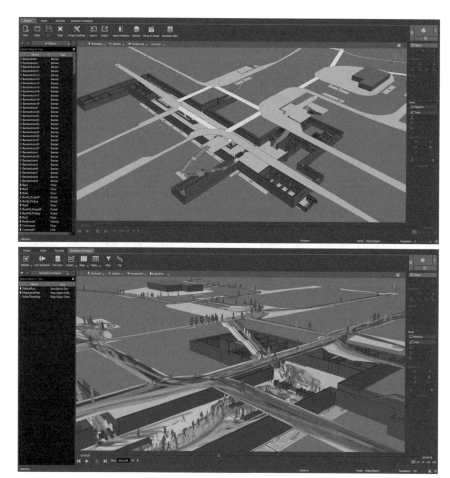

Fig. 5.21 Screenshots from a commercial software in which a transit hub is modeled. The image at the top shows the user interface for scenario setup, the image at the bottom the results (a heatmap showing more congested/busy routes)

they represent the majority of available products. Also, interpreting results is usually more difficult in microscopic models, and a few tips could help in this regard.

In the next section, we will present methods to summarize results in forms of maps and graphs, but, in microscopic models, usually the first outcome of a simulation is available in form of animation. It is therefore important to be able to assess results already from animation and grasp possible issues within the model/software chosen. Being able to assess animations can help to evaluate software, find issues in the built scenario, or determine whether a firm in charge to perform the simulation has correctly understood the conditions.

5.7.1   Evaluation of Simulated Motion

In evaluating simulated motion only qualitative aspects can be considered (we will discuss quantitative interpretation in the next section), and here, we will present some advices which may become useful on this purpose. Experienced users or people working daily with crowds should be able to "feel" whether an animation looks unreal, but sometimes the quality of the graphics could be misleading, whereas a realistic 3D representation could be seen as accurate despite the motion being different from a real crowd.

Therefore, systematically checking for specific features in animations is important. This aspect is particularly important if a simulation is commissioned, and therefore, it may not be possible to know details on the software used and the settings employed. Looking at the animation could help getting some clues on how the scenario was set up, which model was used and its accuracy and whether the scenario correspond to conditions at the facility.

Being able to assess crowd motion and its accuracy from animations is also important when evaluating a software. Very often commercial software developer allow to test their products for free in a limited time period (usually one month). Learning how to use a complex crowd simulator requires time, and therefore, it may be not possible to check all settings and functions during the trial period. However, tutorials or worked examples are often provided and could be used to get a feeling of what the software is capable to. Understanding the settings used for these worked tutorials can be very difficult for a new user, and therefore, evaluating the output could be a comprehensive solution to rate the software on overall.

Also, during the testing phase, it is clearly not possible to perform complex simulations such as the ones that will be performed during the envisaged applications. It is therefore important to create a simple scenario that may allow us to evaluate the capabilities and the user interface for situations close to expected future deployment. This testing scenario changes very much from customer to customer since expectations are very different depending on the application. Some organizations may be interested in egress (stadium/arena), while other on waiting time (airport, service counter). So, considering a microscopic scenario which better represents the macroscopic environment to be simulated is important during evaluation.

Considering what discussed above, there are few scenarios/locations that allow us to perform a first-hand evaluation of the capability of a crowd simulator without requiring to set up complex geometries or dig into advanced settings. From here on, we will present these simple check-points and explain which phenomena are expected and how does the quality of a simulator relate with the results.

In addition, inspection of simulated motion allows to grasp some important clues on the calculation methods employed. Since many products are provided as black-boxes, and it is not possible (or very difficult) to know how calculations are performed in core algorithms, test and result screening is the only way to gain information on this regard. With more clues on the methods used for calculation, it is easier to predict limitations of a given product and have more realistic expectations.

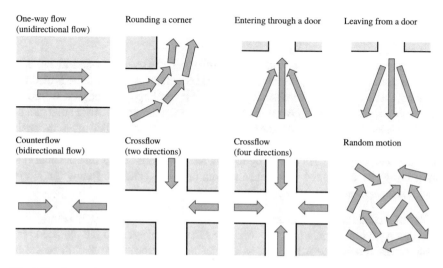

Fig. 5.22 Cases of pedestrian motion representing a set of scenarios to test crowd simulators [61]. Note: "crossflow" is used here instead of the general "intersection" term of Chap. 3 due to the perpendicular angle between both flows. Reprinted from D. C. Duives et al. [61], with permission from Elsevier

According to Duives et al. [61], pedestrian motion observed in most public spaces can be divided into eight cases, which are illustrated in Fig. 5.22. Most of these scenarios can be easily set up in most of the crowd simulators and given their geometrical simplicity little knowledge on the user interface of the product is required to generate some results. Also, each of those cases can be found in complex environments, which may be given as worked examples and may be also included in a simulation project assigned to an external firm. In each of these scenarios, a particular behavior is expected from the simulated crowd; failing to reproduce the expected behavior indicates a limitation of that product that may warn on potential limitations for more complex environments. Independently on the results, each scenario allows to evaluate some specific features of the simulator and to test if realistic settings can be used when preparing for a specific study.

Table 5.5 summarizes ideally expected results (assuming a virtually perfect simulator is used) and points to check for each of the cases considered in Fig. 5.22. After selecting the best computational approach and having tested different products with the criteria given in Table 5.5, you are ready to perform your final decision and start using your simulator for real applications or you can accept the results from an appointed firm. If you are not satisfied with the results, you may follow the advices given below to improve them.

5.7.2 Improving Simulation Results

Pretending to reproduce exactly crowd motion may be an over-expectation, but usually it is always possible to improve results and should be certainly done if discrepancy between simulated and observed behavior is too large. Although it would be impossible to list all modeling issues, there are some common mistakes that can be easily avoided. It should be mentioned that both beginners and skilled users are likely to make mistakes; the former ones because of their lack of experience and the latter ones because they may act driven by habits, often without taking into account that some things have changed over time and with product's updates. Below is a list of common mistakes with proposed solutions [62].

- **Use of default settings/parameters:** Simulators usually comes with settings targeting a general population, but conditions may be different in the modeled scenario. Important properties such as the desired walking speed should be set in line with expected conditions. If those properties are difficult to measure/predict, several simulation scenarios should be done to check how those settings will affect the results. Also, it is important to perform at least minimal site surveys for new scenarios to adapt conditions to reality.
- **Using a software/model for everything:** A software/model that has been successfully used in a specific context may not generate equally good results if that context is changed. Even when a software is validated or calibrated using experimental data, we should remind that accuracy will be lost if the simulated scenario differ from the one used in validation. Evacuation or egress is different from casual walking and software that worked well for a single floor may not be as good when a multistory building is simulated. While budget limitation may not allow to acquire several products, care is required for scenarios overly deviating from the suggested use. In those cases, it would be preferable to acquire some data on-site, if possible, in order to be able to judge the accuracy of the model in the new context.
- **Commercial simulators are not a single model:** The models discussed earlier only relates to pedestrian motion in flat surfaces. Simulating people on stairs or in escalator is a complex task as boarding and landing include non-trivial behaviors. Similarly, modern elevators include complex algorithms to judge on which floor to stop based on several factors, and those models may not be available in simulators. In this sense, commercial software is made of several algorithms, and if the final result is accurate for a complex structure, this does not mean that the achieved accuracy translates to each component. If, for example, a simulator is working well for a single floor, but elevators are poorly modeled, it would be better to work on each floor separately and perform hand-calculations for elevators separately.
- **Graphics and behavior:** If animation looks good, it does not mean behavior is correctly reproduced. Although this seems obvious, it is quite easy to get impressed by the graphics, neglecting the fact that a model is expected to reproduce the collective behavior and not the appearance. In some cases, it may be preferable to set each agent (the simulated person) using a default neutral object (i.e., single color, trivial shape, simple walking animation) rather then using too realistic represen-

Table 5.5 Expected phenomena and points to check when studying the scenarios presented in Fig. 5.22. It should be reminded that no software can exactly reproduce crowd motion as seen in reality, so the points listed here are to be seen as idealistic expectations

One-way flow (unidirectional flow)	
Expected phenomena	• The group speed decreases as the number of people increases. • When the density is two people per m², speed is about half of the free walking speed. • People sometimes deviate laterally and do not move "perfectly straight." • Some sort of waves may appear at high densities when people are almost at still.
Points to check	• If speed is different among people, the model may consider different walking speeds. • If some people move in group, the model may account for group behavior. • What is the maximum density of the model? Values above $10\,\text{m}^{-2}$ are unrealistic.
Rounding a corner	
Expected phenomena	• When crowd density is low, people perform a shortcut passing very close to the corner. • As the number of people increases some need to turn far from the corner. • Velocity is lower close to the corner.
Points to check	• By checking how trajectories change for repetitions with the same settings, it is possible to get a clue on the capacity of the model to generate similar random situations. • People should be able to turn also at high densities (speed will be lower). • Do people tend to stay away from the wall? If no, the model is slightly unrealistic.
Entering through a door	
Expected phenomena	• Total time required to have all people passing through the door is slightly less than double for a double large crowd. • At high densities, sometimes people obstruct themselves and flow through the door is not continuous (sometimes nobody cannot leave for one or more seconds due to congestion, this is also known as "clogging".)
Points to check	• Which shape is formed by the crowd in front of the door? This gives a hint on how people determine their destination and are guided to it. A round shape around the door suggests a very competitive model. • Are you able to get different shapes for the crowd in front of the door (by changing model settings for example)? When there is no hurry, regions close to the wall are not much occupied (check the experimental images of Fig. 5.12 and Fig. 5.13, the model considered there does not correctly reproduce this aspect). In emergencies, people are pushed toward the wall.
Leaving from a door	
Expected phenomena	• People spread out in different directions. • People do not get stuck after leaving the exit.
Points to check	• How large is the directions' spread? Can you set up individual destinations for people or groups or people? • Do groups split up and reform after leaving the door (if the model considers groups).
Counterflow (bidirectional flow)	
Expected phenomena	• People get organized in lanes to some degree. • A complete deadlock (people cannot reach the other side) almost never occurs.
Points to check	• Do lanes occur very easily? Imitation behavior may be too strong in the model. • Do people bump into each other? If so, model may not consider collision avoidance to a sufficient degree.

(continued)

Table 5.5 (continued)

Crossflow (two directions)	
Expected phenomena	• Stripes are formed under certain conditions and move in a direction 45 degrees relative to each flow (or in the angle formed by both flows). • At low densities, some people take a "long route" partially passing in the target corridor of the other group. • At high densities, flow after the cross is very intermittent. People from only one direction pass through the crossing, followed by only people from the other direction. People barely gets mixed in the middle.
Points to check	• Do you get a complete stop from both directions already at low densities? If so, the model may be too conservative.
Crossflow (four directions)	
Expected phenomena	• A sort of circular motion (like a roundabout) forms around the center. This sort of self-organization forms as people try to reduce collisions. • Lanes form in each corridor; the space taken by people leaving the cross is smaller compared to people entering it.
Points to check	• Also here, you can check the conservativeness and the limits of the model. Do people get stuck very easily? What is the maximum density your model can handle? By using large and dense crowds in all directions, the maximum density allowed by the model should appear. • Do you observe a different behavior at low and high densities? In general, macroscopic behavior observed in reality tends to be different depending on the density.
Random motion	-
Expected phenomena	• People may develop a form of self-organization over the long run, possibly moving in a circular way around the center of the "room."
Points to check	• How random is the movement of people? Can you set up simulations so that people will sometimes stop? This feature may be useful for commercial spaces. • Do you recognize a natural behavior when people try to avoid each other? This gives you a clue on how collision avoidance is managed by the simulator.

tations (i.e., different colors for each body part and complex stepping motion). Incongruities in collective behavior may be more apparent if simple graphics is used.

5.8   Result Visualization

Even when you are satisfied with the results, you must ensure that you will be able to efficiently present them to stakeholders, decision-makers or customers. Therefore, to conclude this chapter, we wish to briefly comment on the different ways to visualize results relative to crowd motion. Again, also in this section, we will mostly consider microscopic models, especially because they are the ones offering the largest range of visualization options. Macroscopic and network models usually have limited possibilities to visualize the results and selection of reporting methods is simpler and more logical.

As stated above, microscopic simulation programs usually allow to visualize results of simulations using 3D realistic animations (see Fig. 5.23 for example). 3D animations are a powerful way to present results to people not familiar with crowd simulation and pedestrian traffic. Using 3D animations, it is possible to get a realistic idea of the pedestrian traffic in a facility before it is actually built and people start moving it in. Latest developments in computer graphics now allow to create very diverse crowds with people having different cloth colors and faces representing several ethnic attributes. The way people move is also increasingly natural (legs and arms are animated), thus creating a sense of realism when animations are produced.

However, when results have to be analyzed and if a comparison with experimental values is needed, then animations become useless. From a simple animation, it is difficult to say which region is the most congested or how long people have to stay in line. Therefore, from here on, we will introduce some common quantities that are typically used to "measure" pedestrian crowds in simulation.

To avoid restricting the discussion on specific simulation methods or software products, we use a controlled experiment as an example showing the differences between different quantities and methods for visualization. For the scope of this section, we may assume that results are not relative to a controlled experiment but are obtained from a very accurate simulator able to reproduce with extremely good accuracy real situations.

Figure 5.24 presents the example considered here: 43 people need to leave a room (4 m × 7 m in size) from an 80 cm exit positioned along the longest side. The example considered here is somewhat similar to the case considered in Figs. 5.13 and 5.15, but the initial position and the number of people are different.

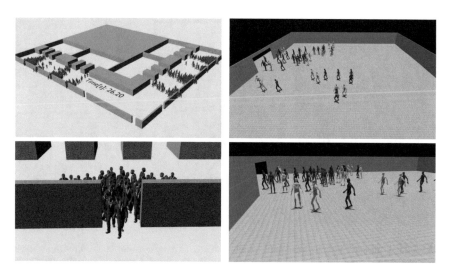

Fig. 5.23 Examples of 3D visualization of microscopic simulation results. Courtesy of Luca Crociani (left) and Satori Tsuzuki (right)

A very simple yet efficient way of visualizing the dynamics of people is by making use of their trajectories (as illustrated in the center of Fig. 5.24). Trajectories have the big advantage of providing a quite clear image of the way people move but still leave room for interpretation of the results. Where trajectories are closer to each other, it is possible to guess that densities were high. A lot of empty space suggest low densities. Sometimes different colors are also used to show speed on trajectories, giving a more detailed picture of how people move.

An alternative way for visualizing moving direction and speed is by making use of arrows (as shown on the right side of Fig. 5.24). Each arrow (also referred as vector in more technical terms) shows the average walking direction in different areas of the room, and the length of the arrow is relative to the walking speed. In this way, it is possible to understand that all people converge toward the exit and they have to slow down as they get close to the door. The use of arrows is very effective and generally simple to obtain, but depending on the simulation method used, results may look very rough (especially if CA models are used). Also, the use of arrows does not say much about the number of people present. A single person transiting in an area not walked by other people could fill that area, thus potentially resulting in a misleading interpretation.

Another way of visualizing results is to make use of "heatmaps" showing different quantities with a color scale. For example, speed (independently on the walking direction) can be visualized as shown in Fig. 5.25 (left image). Areas with a high speed appear darker compared to low speed areas that appear in light colors. As a reference, we should remember that typical walking speed when no obstacles are present is of 1.4 m/s.

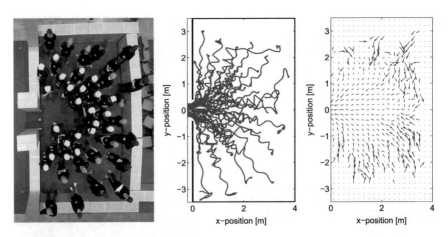

Fig. 5.24 Left: egress being considered in this section; 43 people gather in a room 4 m × 7 m in size. When the "start" signal is given they start leaving the room. Center: trajectories relative to people evacuating the room [63, 64]. Each line represents the path of one person in one experimental run. Right: direction and intensity of speed (this image has been generated considering multiple repetitions of this experiment). Reprinted from [66], Copyright (2018), with permissions from Elsevier

The representation using speed is simple, but the information provided could be misleading. For example, it is not possible to know if low speeds were relative to a dense crowd or people simply waiting. In general, speed is useful when the main purpose of people is to move and differences are large among moments of the day.

As already stressed in the previous chapters, density (measured, again, in people per square meter), is another quantity typically used in crowd simulators and real situations. Clearly, higher values for density are relative to more dangerous conditions although it is difficult to set thresholds defining typical values for density. Table 5.6 attempts to provide some examples of densities in typical situations, but those values need to be considered only for reference. LOS is also very commonly used in simulators, especially if non-critical every-day scenarios are to be modeled. However, it is important to remind that LOS is defined for specific structures, so it would be better to confirm whether areas such as staircases employ the corresponding definitions.

As the example of Fig. 5.25 shows, density is very practical in identifying the regions that are the most crowded and, for the specific case selected, the area close to the exit shows a particularly high density. Without going into details, we should add that estimating pedestrian density is not an easy task (as was already discussed in Chap. 2) and different solutions have been proposed to smoothly represent it. Therefore, the quality of a simulation program needs also to be tested considering these aspects. Also, timing chosen to represent density is important. Some areas may be crowded over a short time, so taking a long-term average may not be appropriate. Maximum density could be also used to make sure unacceptable levels are never reached within the premises.

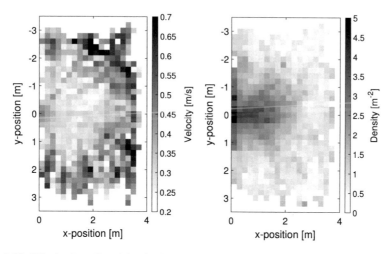

Fig. 5.25 Velocity (speed) and density in a controlled egress experiment. In this case, a grid of 0.2 m is used to present the results, but often smoothed profiles are employed to provide a visually more appealing representation. The results are the average of multiple experimental runs. Reprinted from [66], Copyright (2018), with permissions from Elsevier

Although density is surely one important (if not the most important) quantity used to evaluate pedestrian crowds, it has also some limitations. While speed considers only dynamics (how fast people move), density is static (how many people are in a specific area in a specific moment). None of them can give information on how smooth people move or how organized they are. Over the years, there have been many attempts to measure congestion or motion efficiency. Figure 5.26 show some special quantities that may be employed to study an egress scenario. The flow measures the "traffic amount," and crowd pressure and congestion index are both quantities trying to assess how smooth is the motion of groups of people.

Waiting time, which can be defined as the time when speed is below a given value (0.1 m/s for example), can also be used to evaluate, for example, conditions in areas with lanes (check-in areas in airports for example). In this case, rather than using a map, the waiting time for each pedestrian could be computed and an average for all people present in the region (i.e., how long people stay in that area) may be used to study changes in design of the facilities. Waiting time may be also useful to evaluate

Table 5.6 Typical crowd conditions at different levels of density (reproduced from Chap. 2 for convenience)

Density range	Crowd conditions
Less than $0.25\,\mathrm{m}^{-2}$	Complete freedom of motion, people can walk in the desired direction without having to consider other pedestrians. This condition is encountered for example in large uncongested public plazas or residential areas.
0.25–$1.0\,\mathrm{m}^{-2}$	Freedom to select individual walking speed and direction is restricted, and pedestrians need to consider others to avoid collisions. At this density, emergent behavior may form, for example lanes may spontaneously form in corridors.
1.0–$2.0\,\mathrm{m}^{-2}$	Walking at constant speed becomes difficult, and continuous speed adjustments are required. At this density, pedestrians may partially move in an intermittent way, but walking is still possible and there is no need to stop.
2.0–$3.0\,\mathrm{m}^{-2}$	Continuously walking is very difficult and progresses are made by shuffling. Visual field is restricted, and judgments are only possible based on neighboring pedestrians. Densities above this level should not be accepted during design, not even for short periods.
About $6.0\,\mathrm{m}^{-2}$	Maximum density sustainable for long time. Packed trains in congested cities usually reach this value during morning rush. Although this density represents a very unconformable level, it can be physically sustained for long periods of time. However, at this density, psychological tolerance may go beyond acceptable limits if the situation does not improve on the long run.
More than $10\,\mathrm{m}^{-2}$	Almost certainly causalities will occur. This value is not uniquely defined, but analysis of video footage from crowd accidents revealed that densities higher than $10\,\mathrm{m}^{-2}$ were reached when people started collapsing. Some reports also reported densities up to $15\,\mathrm{m}^{-2}$ during accidents.

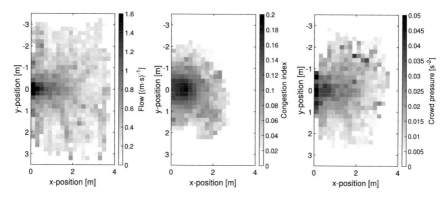

Fig. 5.26 Example of more complex quantities that may be used to analyze crowd dynamics during egress [65–69]. Congestion index measure "smoothness" of pedestrian motion, with 0 being a completely aligned arrangement and 1 being the most chaotic case likely leading to casualties. Crowd pressure attempts to measure a similar property although extrema are not specifically defined (the lowest the better). The results are the average of multiple experimental runs. Reprinted from [66], Copyright (2018), with permissions from Elsevier

the efficacy of advertisement. Locations where people wait for a long time are more attractive than locations where people walk at high speeds.

When testing one simulator, it is important to consider the means (tools) that are available to evaluate the results and how accurate they are. Most of the software allow to obtain speed and density, but quality of representation may be different from product to product. Simulators providing special indexes and build-in measures may help investigating each case more in depth, but validity (and openness) of the proposed measure needs to be checked using typical scenarios like the ones presented in the previous section. If one needs to post-process results using special indicators, it is also important to check whether the software allow to export results in an accessible format.

Table 5.7 presents the typical quantities used in crowd simulator providing a short description of what that quantity measures, how can be employed in real applications and what need to be checked when testing the ability of the simulator to display that quantity. Table 5.7 may be used as reference when evaluating visualization performances of crowd simulators.

Table 5.7 Typical quantities used in the visualization of crowd simulators. For each quantity, information gained, typical application, and important points to check in regard to its use are given as reference

Quantity	Information gained	Typical applications	Points to check
Speed	Fastness of motion *How fast is the crowd?*	Transportation hubs Crosswalks Corridors	Is it possible to see direction and magnitude? Is the vector (arrow) representation possible? Are sudden changes visible?
Density	Concentration "Crowdedness" *How much is it crowded?*	Useful in many situations	Is the representation smooth? Is it possible to see the maximum density? How is the grid defined?
LOS	Level of service *How "comfortable" is the area for the people?*	For non-critical every-day conditions	Is LOS known by those looking at the results? Is it based on the structure? Is the representation smooth? Which version of LOS is used?
Flow	Amount of "traffic" *How efficient is motion?*	Useful in many situations	Are alternative measures available? Is the definition given? Is it clear? Is the representation smooth?
Congestion	Smoothness of motion *How "smooth" is motion?*		
Waiting time	Time spent standing *How much time spent waiting?*	Counters, entrance Advertisement	Will the customers, stakeholders, etc. understand it?

References

1. Zheng, X., Zhong, T., Liu, M.: Modeling crowd evacuation of a building based on seven methodological approaches. Build. Environ. **44**(3), 437–445 (2009). https://doi.org/10.1016/j.buildenv.2008.04.002
2. Templeton, A., Drury, J., Philippides, A.: From mindless masses to small groups: conceptualizing collective behavior in crowd modeling. Rev. Gener. Psychol. **19**(3), 215–229 (2015). https://doi.org/10.1037/gpr0000032
3. Lovreglio, R., Ronchi, E., Kinsey, M.J.: An online survey of pedestrian evacuation model usage and users. Fire Technol. 1–21 (2019). https://doi.org/10.1007/s10694-019-00923-8
4. Xia, Y., Wong, S., Shu, C.W.: Dynamic continuum pedestrian flow model with memory effect. Phys. Rev. E **79**(6),(2009). https://doi.org/10.1103/PhysRevE.79.066113
5. Guo, R.Y.: Potential-based dynamic pedestrian flow assignment. Transp. Res. Part C Emerg. Technol. **91**, 263–275 (2018). https://doi.org/10.1016/j.trc.2018.04.011
6. Lohner, R., Baqui, M., Haug, E., Muhamad, B.: Real-time micro-modelling of a million pedestrians. Eng. Comput. (2016). https://doi.org/10.1108/EC-02-2015-0036
7. Makinoshima, F., Imamura, F., Abe, Y.: Enhancing a tsunami evacuation simulation for a multi-scenario analysis using parallel computing. Simul. Modell. Pract. Theor. **83**, 36–50 (2018). https://doi.org/10.1016/j.simpat.2017.12.016
8. Lohner, R., Muhamad, B., Dambalmath, P., Haug, E.: Fundamental diagrams for specific very high density crowds. Collect. Dyn. **2**, 1–15 (2018). https://doi.org/10.17815/CD.2017.13

9. Lopez-Carmona, M.A., Garcia, A.P.: Cellevac: an adaptive guidance system for crowd evacuation through behavioral optimization. Saf. Sci. **139** (2021). https://doi.org/10.1016/j.ssci.2021.105215

10. Hoogendoorn, S.P., Bovy, P.H.: Pedestrian route-choice and activity scheduling theory and models. Transp. Res. Part B Methodol. **38**(2), 169–190 (2004). https://doi.org/10.1016/S0191-2615(03)00007-9

11. Papadimitriou, E., Yannis, G., Golias, J.: A critical assessment of pedestrian behaviour models. Transp. Res. Part F Traff. Psychol. Behav. **12**(3), 242–255 (2009). https://doi.org/10.1016/j.trf.2008.12.004

12. Schadschneider, A., Klingsch, W., Klüpfel, H., Kretz, T., Rogsch, C., Seyfried, A.: Evacuation Dynamics: Empirical Results, Modeling and Applications, pp. 517–550. Springer New York (2011). https://doi.org/10.1007/978-1-4419-7695-6_29

13. Hensher, D.A., Rose, J.M., Rose, J.M., Greene, W.H.: Applied Choice Analysis: A Primer. Cambridge University Press (2005)

14. Wooldridge, J.M.: Introductory econometrics: a modern approach. Cengage Learning (2015)

15. de Dios Ortúzar, J., Willumsen, L.G.: Modelling transport. John wiley & sons (2011)

16. Ben-Akiva, M., Lerman, S.R.: Discrete choice analysis: theory and application to travel demand. Transportation Studies (2018)

17. Beale, L., Field, K., Briggs, D., Picton, P., Matthews, H.: Mapping for wheelchair users: route navigation in urban spaces. Cartograph. J. **43**(1), 68–81 (2006). https://doi.org/10.1179/000870406X93517

18. Church, R.L., Marston, J.R.: Measuring accessibility for people with a disability. Geograph. Anal. **35**(1), 83–96 (2003). https://doi.org/10.1111/j.1538-4632.2003.tb01102.x

19. Ding, D., Parmanto, B., Karimi, H.A., Roongpiboonsopit, D., Pramana, G., Conahan, T., Kasemsuppakorn, P.: Design considerations for a personalized wheelchair navigation system. In: 2007 29th Annual International Conference of the IEEE Engineering in Medicine and Biology Society, pp. 4790–4793. IEEE (2007). https://doi.org/10.1109/IEMBS.2007.4353411

20. Dzafic, D., Link, J.A.B., Baumeister, D., Kowalewski, S., Wehrle, K.: Requirements for dynamic route planning for wheelchair users. In: International Conference on Indoor Positioning and Indoor Navigation, vol. 27, pp. 1–4 (2014)

21. Kasemsuppakorn, P., Karimi, H.A., Ding, D., Ojeda, M.A.: Understanding route choices for wheelchair navigation. Disabil. Rehabil. Assistive Technol. **10**(3), 198–210 (2015). https://doi.org/10.1007/978-3-540-70540-6_164

22. Neis, P.: Measuring the reliability of wheelchair user route planning based on volunteered geographic information. Trans. GIS **19**(2), 188–201 (2015). https://doi.org/10.1111/tgis.12087

23. Crociani, L., Vizzari, G., Yanagisawa, D., Nishinari, K., Bandini, S.: Route choice in pedestrian simulation: design and evaluation of a model based on empirical observations. Intelligenza Artificiale **10**(2), 163–182 (2016). https://doi.org/10.3233/IA-160102

24. Li, M., Shu, P., Xiao, Y., Wang, P.: Modeling detour decision combined the tactical and operational layer based on perceived density. Phys. A Stat. Mech. Appl. **574** (2021). https://doi.org/10.1016/j.physa.2021.126021

25. Blue, V.J., Adler, J.L.: Cellular automata microsimulation for modeling bi-directional pedestrian walkways. Transp. Res. Part B Methodol. **35**(3), 293–312 (2001). https://doi.org/10.1016/S0191-2615(99)00052-1

26. Burstedde, C., Klauck, K., Schadschneider, A., Zittartz, J.: Simulation of pedestrian dynamics using a two-dimensional cellular automaton. Phys. A Stat. Mech. Appl. **295**(3–4), 507–525 (2001). https://doi.org/10.1016/S0378-4371(01)00141-8

27. Nishinari, K., Kirchner, A., Namazi, A., Schadschneider, A.: Extended floor field ca model for evacuation dynamics. IEICE Trans. Inf. Syst. **87**(3), 726–732 (2004)

28. Li, S., Li, X., Qu, Y., Jia, B.: Block-based floor field model for pedestrian's walking through corner. Phys. A Stat. Mech. Appl. **432**, 337–353 (2015). https://doi.org/10.1016/j.physa.2015.03.041

29. Suma, Y., Yanagisawa, D., Nishinari, K.: Anticipation effect in pedestrian dynamics: modeling and experiments. Phys. A Stat. Mech. Appl. **391**(1–2), 248–263 (2012). https://doi.org/10.1016/j.physa.2011.07.022

30. Kirchner, A., Nishinari, K., Schadschneider, A.: Friction effects and clogging in a cellular automaton model for pedestrian dynamics. Phys. Rev. E **67**(5) (2003). https://doi.org/10.1103/PhysRevE.67.056122

31. Henein, C.M., White, T.: Macroscopic effects of microscopic forces between agents in crowd models. Phys. A Stat. Mech. Appl. **373**, 694–712 (2007). https://doi.org/10.1016/j.physa.2006.06.023

32. Weng, W., Chen, T., Yuan, H., Fan, W.: Cellular automaton simulation of pedestrian counter flow with different walk velocities. Phys. Rev. E **74**(3) (2006). https://doi.org/10.1103/PhysRevE.74.036102

33. Vizzari, G., Manenti, L., Crociani, L.: Adaptive pedestrian behaviour for the preservation of group cohesion. Complex Adap. Syst. Model. **1**(1), 7 (2013). https://doi.org/10.1186/2194-3206-1-7

34. Feliciani, C., Murakami, H., Shimura, K., Nishinari, K.: Efficiently informing crowds-experiments and simulations on route choice and decision making in pedestrian crowds with wheelchair users. Transp. Res. Part C Emerg. Technol. **114**, 484–503 (2020). https://doi.org/10.1016/j.trc.2020.02.019

35. Nowak, S., Schadschneider, A.: Quantitative analysis of pedestrian counterflow in a cellular automaton model. Phys. Rev. E **85**(6) (2012). https://doi.org/10.1103/PhysRevE.85.066128

36. Feliciani, C., Nishinari, K.: An improved cellular automata model to simulate the behavior of high density crowd and validation by experimental data. Phys. A Stat. Mech. Appl. **451**, 135–148 (2016). https://doi.org/10.1016/j.physa.2016.01.057

37. Zeng, W., Chen, P., Yu, G., Wang, Y.: Specification and calibration of a microscopic model for pedestrian dynamic simulation at signalized intersections: a hybrid approach. Transp. Res. Part C Emerg. Technol. **80**, 37–70 (2017). https://doi.org/10.1016/j.trc.2017.04.009

38. Helbing, D., Molnar, P.: Social force model for pedestrian dynamics. Phys. Rev. E **51**(5), 4282 (1995). https://doi.org/10.1103/PhysRevE.51.4282

39. Zanlungo, F., Ikeda, T., Kanda, T.: Social force model with explicit collision prediction. EPL (Europhys. Lett.) **93**(6), 68005 (2011) https://doi.org/10.1209/0295-5075/93/68005

40. Friis, C., Svensson, L.: Pedestrian microsimulation. a comparative study between the software programs vissim and viswalk. Master's thesis, Chalmers University of Technology (2013)

41. Heydemans, E., Sumabrata, R.J.: The analysis of pedestrian's facility level of service at pondok cina rail station's platform using ptv viswalk. In: MATEC Web of Conferences, vol. 278, p. 05001. EDP Sciences (2019). https://doi.org/10.1051/matecconf/201927805001

42. Pan, X., Han, C.S., Dauber, K., Law, K.H.: A multi-agent based framework for the simulation of human and social behaviors during emergency evacuations. Ai & Soc. **22**(2), 113–132 (2007). https://doi.org/10.1007/s00146-007-0126-1

43. Shi, X., Xue, S., Feliciani, C., Shiwakoti, N., Lin, J., Li, D., Ye, Z.: Verifying the applicability of a pedestrian simulation model to reproduce the effect of exit design on egress flow under normal and emergency conditions. Phys. A Stat. Mech. Appl. **562** (2021). https://doi.org/10.1016/j.physa.2020

44. Ezaki, T., Nishinari, K.: Potential global jamming transition in aviation networks. Phys. Rev. E **90**(2) (2014). https://doi.org/10.1103/PhysRevE.90.022807

45. Ramezani, M., Haddad, J., Geroliminis, N.: Dynamics of heterogeneity in urban networks: aggregated traffic modeling and hierarchical control. Transp. Res. Part B Methodol. **74**, 1–19 (2015). https://doi.org/10.1016/j.trb.2014.12.010

46. Karamouzas, I., Skinner, B., Guy, S.J.: Universal power law governing pedestrian interactions. Phys. Rev. Lett. **113**(23) (2014). https://doi.org/10.1103/PhysRevLett.113.238701

47. Guo, R.Y., Wong, S., Huang, H.J., Zhang, P., Lam, W.H.: A microscopic pedestrian-simulation model and its application to intersecting flows. Physica A Stat. Mech. Appl. **389**(3), 515–526 (2010). https://doi.org/10.1016/j.physa.2009.10.008

48. Robin, T., Antonini, G., Bierlaire, M., Cruz, J.: Specification, estimation and validation of a pedestrian walking behavior model. Transp. Res. Part B Methodol. **43**(1), 36–56 (2009). https://doi.org/10.1016/j.trb.2008.06.010

49. Helbing, D.: A fluid dynamic model for the movement of pedestrians. arXiv preprint cond-mat/9805213 (1998). https://arxiv.org/abs/cond-mat/9805213
50. Hoogendoorn, S., Bovy, P.H.: Gas-kinetic modeling and simulation of pedestrian flows. Transp. Res. Record **1710**(1), 28–36 (2000). https://doi.org/10.3141/1710-04
51. Twarogowska, M., Goatin, P., Duvigneau, R.: Macroscopic modeling and simulations of room evacuation. Appl. Math. Modell. **38**(24), 5781–5795 (2014). https://doi.org/10.1016/j.apm.2014.03.027
52. Kouskoulis, G., Spyropoulou, I., Antoniou, C.: Pedestrian simulation: Theoretical models vs. data driven techniques. Int. J. Transp. Sci. Technol. **7**(4), 241–253 (2018). https://doi.org/10.1016/j.ijtst.2018.09.001
53. Duives, D.C., Wang, G., Kim, J.: Forecasting pedestrian movements using recurrent neural networks: An application of crowd monitoring data. Sensors **19**(2), 382 (2019). https://doi.org/10.3390/s19020382
54. Korhonen, T., Hostikka, S.: Fire dynamics simulator with evacuation: Fds+ evac: Technical reference and user's guide. Tech. Rep, VTT Technical Research Centre of Finland (2009)
55. Horni, A., Nagel, K., Axhausen, K.W.: The multi-agent transport simulation MATSim. Ubiquity Press (2016)
56. Chraibi, M., Zhang, J.: Jupedsim: an open framework for simulating and analyzing the dynamics of pedestrians. In: SUMO Conference 2016, FZJ-2016-02717. Jülich Supercomputing Center (2016)
57. Zönnchen, B., Kleinmeier, B., Köster, G.: Vadere—a simulation framework to compare loco-motion models. In: Traffic and Granular Flow 2019, pp. 331–337. Springer (2020). https://doi.org/10.1007/978-3-030-55973-1_41
58. Feliciani, C., Murakami, H., Nishinari, K.: A universal function for capacity of bidirectional pedestrian streams: filling the gaps in the literature. PloS one **13**(12) (2018). https://doi.org/10.1371/journal.pone.0208496
59. Boltes, M., Holl, S., Seyfried, A.: Data archive for exploring pedestrian dynamics and its application in dimensioning of facilities for multidirectional streams. Collect. Dyn. **5**, 17–24 (2020) https://doi.org/10.17815/CD.2020.28
60. Murakami, H., Feliciani, C., Nishiyama, Y., Nishinari, K.: Mutual anticipation can contribute to self-organization in human crowds. Sci. Adv. **7**(12), eabe7758 (2021). https://doi.org/10.1126/sciadv.abe7758
61. Duives, D.C., Daamen, W., Hoogendoorn, S.P.: State-of-the-art crowd motion simulation models. Transp. Res. Part C Emerg. Technol. **37**, 193–209 (2013). https://doi.org/10.1016/j.trc.2013.02.005
62. Kinsey, M., Gwynne, S., Kinateder, M.: Evacuation modelling biases—research, development, and application. In: Fire and Evacuation Modeling Technical Conference (FEMTC), pp. 1–11 (2020)
63. Boltes, M., Seyfried, A., Steffen, B., Schadschneider, A.: Automatic extraction of pedestrian trajectories from video recordings. In: Pedestrian and Evacuation Dynamics 2008, pp. 43–54. Springer (2010). https://doi.org/10.1007/978-3-642-04504-2_3
64. Boltes, M., Seyfried, A.: Collecting pedestrian trajectories. Neurocomputing **100**, 127–133 (2013). https://doi.org/10.1016/j.neucom.2012.01.036
65. Helbing, D., Johansson, A., Al-Abideen, H.Z.: Dynamics of crowd disasters: an empirical study. Phys. Rev. E **75**(4) (2007). https://doi.org/10.1103/PhysRevE.75.046109
66. Feliciani, C., Nishinari, K.: Measurement of congestion and intrinsic risk in pedestrian crowds. Transp. Res. Part C Emerg. Technol. **91**, 124–155 (2018). https://doi.org/10.1016/j.trc.2018.03.027
67. Feliciani, C., Zuriguel, I., Garcimartín, A., Maza, D., Nishinari, K.: Systematic experimental investigation of the obstacle effect during non-competitive and extremely competitive evacuations. Sci. Rep. **10**(1), 1–20 (2020). https://doi.org/10.1038/s41598-020-72733-w
68. Hosseini, O., Maghrebi, M., Maghrebi, M.F.: Determining optimum staged-evacuation schedule considering total evacuation time, congestion severity and fire threats. Saf. Sci. **139** (2021). https://doi.org/10.1016/j.ssci.2021.105211

69. Zanlungo, F., Feliciani, C., Yucel, Z., Nishinari, K., Kanda, T.: A pure number to assess congestion in pedestrian crowds

Chapter 6
Crowd Control Methods: Established and Future Practices

Abstract Behavior of crowds may change any time and methods to control their motion and ensure safety are required. Crowd control needs a progressive approach in which static solutions simply relying on information provision represent the base on which gradually restrictive measures physically limiting crowd motion are implemented upon necessity. To successfully control crowds, it is important planning a strategy in advance and knowing which methods are available. In this chapter, a five-stage approach using different strategies at each stage will be presented and discussed. Generally speaking, crowd density determines which solution is the most appropriate at each stage. For sparse crowds, information provided by signage, direction indicators, and maps is sufficient to ensure an efficient motion of people. As density increases, intervention by trained personnel will be needed, first in form of advices and later by more restrictive guidance. For dense crowds, steering by physical means such as barricades or dedicated queuing lanes becomes necessary. In extreme cases, police or even the army may be called to enforce discipline to the crowd. Each of these stages (with the partial exception of extreme situations) will be covered in detail by highlighting which factors are relevant to ensure an effective control. At the end, emerging trends in the frame of crowd control will be also discussed. Throughout the chapter, practical advices and examples will be given to better explain each strategy.

6.1 Introduction

Understanding, measuring, and predicting crowd behavior is important, but in most of the cases, the goal is to influence people's dynamics and improve their comfort and safety. In other words, crowd control is necessary to ensure that people move smoothly without creating congestion or dangerous motion patterns. In general, there are various strategies to control crowds, and methods typically depend on the crowd density and the criticality of the situation. The biggest differences between various strategies are summarized in Fig. 6.1 and will be discussed below in detail.

However, before interpreting Fig. 6.1, it is important to remark that each control strategy (each stage) does not have to be considered as a separate set of actions that can be used to keep people under control. Instead, each stage is built upon the pre-

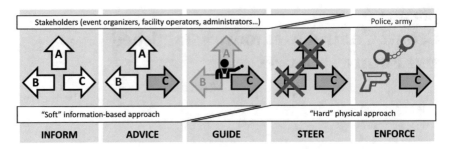

Fig. 6.1 Schematic representation of different stages of crowd control [1, 2]

vious one, and a control strategy can be effective only if it is conceived as a gradual approach. In general, information is the principal way to control people, and any strategy needs to be conceived based on this fundamental mean. However, as the crowd density increases, information alone may not be sufficient to control people, it may become necessary to employ physical measures. As a last resort, when even "peaceful" control strategies are not effective, force may have to be used through police or army involvement. The responsibility of stakeholders is to do everything possible in order to avoid this situation, but should it happen because of unpredictable circumstances (e.g., in the case of a terrorist attack, or an infiltration of violent individuals into a peaceful event); it is important to be prepared for this scenario. However, since this book focuses on crowd management for general stakeholders, strategies related to crisis management and law enforcement by force will not be covered. In the following introduction, we will present the principal characteristics of each stage, and more specific aspects will be covered in the dedicated sections of this chapter.

When crowds are sparse, information is sufficient to influence their motion. In this context, the way in which information is presented has a drastic effect on decision-making among pedestrians. While information is the predominant strategy in the "inform" and "advice" stage, the way in which it is presented is the main difference between both stages. In the "inform" stage, all information necessary for people to make decisions is provided in a neutral, informative manner. Signs, maps, and colored paths are some typical examples of the methods used in the "inform" stage. People moving within a space therefore can choose their path based on the information they have. In Fig.6.1, directions A, B, and C are presented in the same way, allowing the pedestrians to decide the direction they wish to take. In the "inform" stage, information is neutral, and typically static, meaning that it is prepared to address a general and universal usership. Some degree of customization is possible depending on the characteristic of the location (the signs used in a hospital differ from those used in an amusement park), but information will be uniform inside the area considered. Also, in the "inform" stage, it is not possible to reach in different ways particular subjects within the crowd; everyone will receive the same information. Therefore, in the "inform" stage, crowds are considered as a uniform element, and strategies are prepared accordingly.

In contrast to the "inform" stage, in the "advice" stage, information is prepared to influence the decisions of people. Information channels used in the "advice" stage can be the same as those employed in the "inform" stage, but tricks will be employed to have people choose a particular option rather than others. In the example shown in Fig. 6.1, route C is given in green, thus suggesting (without being explicitly given) that the particular direction is beneficial compared to others. In this regard, the so-called nudge approach (which will be discussed more in detail at the end of the chapter) is particularly suited in the "advice" stage. An important characteristic of the "advice" stage is that people are influenced without being aware of it (or without noticing it too much). As a representative example, one may also think on the products' sales ranking in a shop: Informing the customers on which product sell the most will influence them in making their purchase but does not imply that one product is better than the others. The ranking has an informative nature (showing which product sells the most), but the aim is obviously to influence customers' decisions. The same strategy is employed in the "advice" stage of crowd control. The methods and strategies used in the "advice" stage are typically more dynamic than those of the "inform" stage since messages have to be changed to reflect changing conditions. Audio messages (via loudspeakers, megaphone, etc.), information monitors, or light signs are some of the means employed at this stage. In the "advice" stage, it is also possible to adapt information to the specifics of the crowd and/or to deal with only a part of it. For example, it is possible to advice passengers boarding a given flight to move to the security inspection by using only specific loudspeakers located in an area where passengers are waiting and streaming the message in a specific moment. The announcement may be repeated if many passengers are still not showing up in the gate. On the other hand, the time table showing the scheduled flights will not change from the first appearance until departure (information is static and neutral), thus leaving the decision to move to security screening for the passenger to make.

The "guide" stage represents a transition from a soft, information-oriented control strategy, to a hard, physically oriented method. In this stage, people still have all information and options available but are strongly influenced into choosing a particular one. At this level, it is clear to users that they are being directed toward a particular option. In the example shown in Fig. 6.1, this time, directions A and B are given in red to prevent people from using them, and the guidance staff indicates the suggested direction. Differences between the "advice" and "guide" stages are not always evident, and there is sometimes an overlap between both strategies. However, the most remarkable difference between the "guide" and "advice" stages is the fact that in the "guide" stage, people are aware that are being guided, and although they may still choice a different alternative, they will have to take the moral responsibility in regard to their choices (other people may look at them in a "bad" way). In the "guide" stage, stakeholders usually tend to take a more active role, for example, by appointing supervisors inside the crowd to provide guidance (staff and/or volunteers). Loudspeakers or visual messages may also be used to guide people, but the language and expressions used will have a much stronger weight (compared to the "advice" stage). One may for example consider the difference between the announcement advising passengers to move to the boarding gate and the final call for a flight.

Passengers can still ignore the last call message and spend time shopping, but they will be aware of the risk and consequences (it will be harder for them to pretend that they did not notice/hear the call). Information in the "guide" stage tends to be more specific and targeted as it is usually intended to reach a specific group of people or a delimited area. For example, the name of the passenger may be announced in the final call message, and the audio message may be streamed in a specific area (departure only for instance). As already mentioned, physical means may be also used to a limited degree, for example, security personnel may be located in specific locations during a firework event to guide people thorough a junction. By using loudspeakers, personnel may urge people to keep to the right/left side of the walkway. People may still disobey the indications, but they will certainly be aware they are not acting in the proper way.

The "steer" stage marks a clear passage between the information-based and the physical approach. For example, the above-mentioned right/left-walking behavior will now be imposed by separating the walkway into two lanes and forcing people to walk on the right/left side. Further, as shown in Fig. 6.1, now only direction C is open, and people are refrained from using path A or B. Examples of the means used in the "steer" stage are fences, waiting lines, and turnstiles. People's freedom of choice is now very limited, and decision-making is almost completely entrusted to the stakeholders, who need to constantly monitor the crowd and take rapid decisions to maintain safety. A limited number of individuals may still be able to go against the rules imposed by organizers, but they will do it at their own risk and will be generally responsible in case their actions lead to dangerous consequences. On the other hand, stakeholders need to be aware that should a problem arise during crowd control in the "steer" stage, and their strategy will be very likely investigated straight away for possible negligence. The "steer" stage is based on physical measures, but it is important to remind that the overall control approach is based on a gradual build-up of strategies, and therefore, information is still provided, and this information provision is fundamental to ensure that people are efficiently steered. For instance, when a route is closed (A or B in Fig. 6.1), it is important that people are advised and guided toward route C and that information present in the area is updated to ensure people know about the layout change. In addition to informing people, during the "steer" stage, it is important that there is an efficient exchange of information among the staff involved in the event and/or supervising the area. Although the exchange of information is also important in the "guide" stage, people in the crowd can typically act locally, but in the "steer" stage, a global picture of the situation is necessary, and everybody on the stakeholder's side need to be aware of the situation.

The "enforce" stage is the most extreme scenario. Like in the "steer" stage, people have no freedom (or very little) with regard to their actions, but the main difference is that when the "enforce" stage comes into action, police is involved, and people creating troubles may get arrested or be subjected to force. In this stage arrests, water cannons, tear gas, or simply brute force may be used to get the crowd under control. To conclude the explanation on the events shown in Fig. 6.1, the main difference between the "steer" and "enforce" stages is that routes A and B are still closed and inaccessible, but careless individuals trying to go through A or B anyway may be

Table 6.1 Relevant aspects related to each stage of crowd control

Stage	Inform	Advice	Guide	Steer	Enforce
Crowd density	Very low	Low	Medium	Medium to high	Generally high
Approach	"Soft" (information)	"Soft" (information)	Combination	"Hard" (physical)	"Hard" (physical)
Competence	Designer, architect and administrator	Administrator	Administrator and crowd supervisor	Crowd supervisor	Police/army
Control time scale	Very long	Medium	Short	Short	Very short
Feedback from the crowd	Very limited	Limited	Substantial	Substantial	Safety level only
Target	Universal	Universal	Specific	Specific	Very specific
User freedom	Complete freedom of choice	Unconsciously influenced	Consciously influenced	Little freedom of choice	No freedom (or very limited)
Decision-making	Users completely	Users (influenced)	Administrator (users can disobey)	Administrator	Police/Army
Required knowledge	Wayfinding and design	Wayfinding, communication, and marketing	Communication skills	Crowd motion and behavior	Legal code, crisis management

arrested or tackled by the police who is now responsible to ensure crowd safety. Actions in the "enforce" stage may be directed toward single individuals or small groups and are therefore precisely targeted. In addition, decisions at this level are taken very rapidly in line with the latest updates on crowd conditions.

The main aspects of crowd control relative to each stage discussed above are summarized in Table 6.1. The following sections will deal with the elements that are relative and common to all the stages of crowd control, namely: information management and physical measures. While there is no clear division between the different stages, each one is characterized by a different balance of these two elements.

6.2 Objectives of This Chapter

This chapter aims at explaining the methods that can be used to influence the way people move by using both information and physical measures, both in a static and a dynamic way. At the end of this chapter, readers should be able to understand which approach is necessary depending on the situation and what solutions are available to control crowds under different conditions. Also, readers will need to understand what are the steps involved in setting up effective systems for crowd control and what are the inputs and outputs necessary in each step.

There are clearly some limitations on the suggestions that can be made for good practices on crowd control since it is a discipline that mostly relies on experience and the capabilities of an individual or organization. On the other hand, it is also possible to prepare a good crowd control strategy to avoid relying solely on experience and know-how. A reliable system of crowd analysis based on appropriate sensors and planning or preparation using simulators that can recreate what-if scenarios surely help in effective crowd control and reduce the burden on the personnel, thus providing a margin for critical situations that are beyond any possible prediction. Therefore, we would like readers to go through this chapter by recalling the different technologies and tools that have been presented in the previous chapters and what they learned about crowd characteristics (and theories).

We would also like to remind the readers that each level in crowd control involves complex aspects of several disciplines where the point of view changes greatly from expert to expert, depending on their background. Psychologists will provide suggestions different from lawyers with regard to important points while controlling crowds. Designers and architects may also have different viewpoints on the same topic. In this chapter, we attempt to provide a general perspective focusing on the most important aspects of each component of crowd control. For instance, design and architecture play a very important role in wayfinding, which is one of the most important elements of the "inform" stage. Mass psychology and social science are important for communication, which is the central part of the "advice" and upper stages. Understanding crowd motion is, on the other hand, relevant in the "guide" and "steer" stages, and experts on crowd dynamics are probably the most experienced persons for this purpose. Readers interested in specific aspects of each topic are addressed to the references provided at the end of this chapter.

Finally, we would like also to mention that the "enforce" stage will not be covered in detail in this chapter. In extreme situations when even planned crowd control methods are not effective, there may be the need to enforce specific measures by police and/or military personnel. In this context, preparation plays a marginal role and good practices almost completely rely on experience and know-how (in fact, this book aims at never getting to this point). Enforcing decisions on people is legally restricted to law enforcement personnel, and crowd managers are not required to know details regarding this (except remembering that this solution has to be a part of a plan as the most extreme scenario). Also, to conclude, what can be done and what cannot be done with regard to enforcement is strictly bound by the local laws, and it is not possible to provide a general overview for all national and local variations. People seeking advice on how to deal with extreme situations should consult with the local law enforcement authorities.

6.3   Information Management—Laying the Fundamentals for an Effective Crowd Control

Information is essential to ensure that crowds move in an ordered way and to guarantee a satisfactory and pleasant experience to the people visiting a public space. Information management represents the basis of crowd control in the "inform" and "advice" stages and also plays a fundamental role in the upper stages as people need to be aware of situational changes. Since it is through information that people are moved to specific directions under noncritical conditions, it is important to understand the methods that are available to influence them and the effect that these methods have on overall crowd motion.

In particular, we will distinguish between three methods that can be used to deliver information to crowds: static and dynamic information provision and communication. As indicated in Fig. 6.2, the differences between these approaches basically lie in the amount of feedback from the crowd and the capacity to change information content based on the situation.

When there is no feedback from the crowd, we can define the information provision as static. Examples are signs and maps that are merely informative and will not change depending on the amount of people looking at them or the time of the day. Of course, it will be possible to change a sign or map if layout changes, but this will happen very rarely and will require a substantial amount of work and preparation. Static information provision generally falls into the concept of "wayfinding," which is a multidisciplinary approach covering design, architecture, psychology, and traffic engineering, with the aim of navigating into complex structures easier and more intuitively. Static information provision plays an important role in the "inform" stage and represents the basis for every crowd control strategy. Small events or crowds limited in size may be simply managed using loudspeakers and oral messages, but generally, a reliable system of wayfinding providing information in a static manner is required for larger facilities or events. Although wayfinding is important and effective

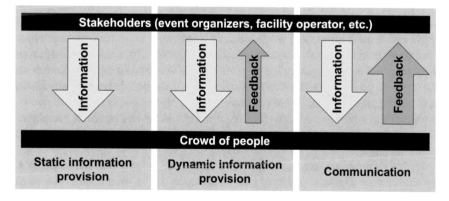

Fig. 6.2 Differences between static and dynamic information provision and communication

in achieving a balanced use of public spaces, it has its own limitations. For instance, the information provided is not based on the real-time context, and therefore, static information provision is sufficient only for the "inform" stage, where crowds are sparse and areas to be controlled very large.

It is, however, possible to dynamically change the information delivered. For example, flight timetables are updated based on the time and air traffic conditions. In train stations, changes in platforms are also communicated using screens and announcements. Also, information on the waiting time at different service windows is updated based on the real-time conditions. This type of information provision requires a variable amount of feedback, and we will define these systems as "dynamic." In some cases, the dynamic nature is simply limited to the time of the day, but more complex systems may combine feedback from several sensors to provide the best information. Dynamic information provision is mostly used in the "inform" and "advice" stages. Preprogrammed information systems (such as train or flight schedules) are usually intended to provide neutral information that is simply updated, but advices may be given considering several feedback variables (e.g., the "please move to gate" message, which is intended to advice people to hurry up). Information design and management for dynamic systems is based on principles similar to those for wayfinding, but the time variable needs to be taken into account. The biggest challenge in dynamic systems is of a technical nature since the system should be robust to unpredicted changes and failures. Dynamic information provision can be performed in a fully automated manner (where information management is all embedded in a computerized system) or in manually (where information is all prepared by humans evaluating the situation based on their intuition or experience). Semiautomatic information provision is typically preferred, where people choose between different options based on the preprocessed options provided by automatic systems.

In this section, we will define "communication" as the most dynamic type of information provision, where an equal exchange of information is performed between the crowd and stakeholders. Consider for example an information point. The staff need to listen carefully to the questions of the customers to provide a satisfactory answer and to advice or guide them. In this sense, there is a substantial amount of feedback from the crowd. Usually, communication cannot be planned in advance since it changes greatly with the context (and the feedback). However, it is possible to prepare and train the staff on the manner of communicating efficiently with a crowd and to prepare them for possible situations by sharing information relative to the event/location and the expected profile of guests/customers. Although some people are naturally skilled in communicating with large crowds, training and preparation surely help in making communication better and more efficient. Briefing and debriefing are also important elements that make communication more efficient and ensure constant improvement over long term.

In this section, we will cover the three aspects of information management to provide readers a general image of how information can be used to control crowds. Again, we should mention that each method needs to be considered gradually and good crowd control practices need to start from the bottom level, adding elements as the situation gets critical. Also, since there is no perfect division between the three approaches, one should read this section as a gradual approach toward an increasingly crowded scene.

6.3.1 Static Information Provision: Wayfinding and Its Role in Crowd Control

Wayfinding is an important element in the design of complex pedestrian environments since it allows people to move seamlessly without becoming disoriented or lost [3–5]. In the case of very large projects, wayfinding experts will usually take up the task of designing a range of signs, maps, and landmarks so that people will find their way naturally, but for small buildings and/or in case of limited budget, this important task may be dealt internally within the managing organization. While there is no recipe to success for a wayfinding project, some general guidelines can be followed to ensure that at least the minimum requirements are met.

Finding the best solution for wayfinding is not always easy because the expectations and perspectives differ greatly depending on the person involved. According to Carpman and Grant [6], three types of people are directly influenced by the good or bad outcome of a wayfinding project: users, staff, and administrators. From the users' perspective, wayfinding is important mainly because of the following reasons:

- **Being lost is a waste of time**: You may have many things to do, and you cannot lose your time wandering, for example, in a hospital searching for the right place to go.
- **Being lost is stressful**: If you are in a hospital, you are usually not there for a nice reason. You might be nervous, and getting to the right place could become a difficult task. For some people, the mere idea of having to transfer in a large airport is stressful because they assume that they will get lost.
- **Being lost is frustrating**: Getting back to the same place after 15 min can be very frustrating and may let people down with regard to their ability to get to the right place.
- **Although organizations are supposed to help us, they seem less informed than us**: If information provided by the staff is not clear and accurate, you might feel even more helpless.

On the other hand, staff working in large buildings such as hospitals [7], train stations, and airports are also affected by wayfinding. This includes both the people directly involved in providing information to users (this will be also considered in the following parts) and the normal staff working there (doctors, train conductors, flight attendants, cleaning staff, etc.). In particular, from the staff point of view, wayfinding is important because of the following reasons [6]:

- **You want to appear competent**: Imagine that somebody asks you for directions in the office you work. You decide to help that person to get to the desired place but you get lost on the way. Such an experience can be very embarrassing and can undermine the image of the organization.

- **Everybody wants to be able to do their job (efficiently)**: If patients get lost in a hospital and arrive late to their appointments, doctors will find it hard working on schedule. Similarly, if people get lost in the airport, flight attendants may have to call them, thus creating unnecessary stress and making the airport noisy.

Finally, administrators too have an interest in having a good wayfinding design. From their viewpoint, wayfinding is important because of the following reasons [6]:

- **Wayfinding ease is a part of caring for users**: Users clearly perceive when information provision is carefully studied and when it is approximately sketched.
- **Wayfinding ease helps organization market their facilities and services**: An airport with a clear and yet artistic wayfinding approach may become a landmark destination for travelers and could get attention from newspapers and magazines, which may eventually feature it as an example.
- **Customer disorientation results in specific problems**: For example, delivery is strongly affected by wayfinding. If deliveries are made difficult because couriers get lost, management is also affected (in the worst case, deliveries may also arrive to the wrong place).

We should also remember that disorientation does not discriminate by age, gender, profession, degree, or fame. Most people become lost or disoriented at one time or another. However, there are some people who are directionally challenged, and face more problems finding their way compared to others. While there is no solution to make sure that nobody gets lost, there are designs that make sure most of the people get promptly to their destination.

In the following sections, we will explain how a wayfinding system is conceived, maintained, and updated by covering the most important elements used to inform people in public spaces [4]. Specific examples and case studies will be used to show problems caused by ineffective wayfinding designs and present possible solutions.

6.3.1.1 Wayfinding Design Process

Wayfinding is not a once-in-a-time task, but a continuous process by which pedestrian traffic is analyzed to identify locations where information is needed, and the efficacy of the proposed solutions is evaluated later to eventually perform modifications. During the development of a new system, it is, therefore, important to leave some room for later modifications as places do change and the habits of people too do so. Similarly to what suggested by Gibson [4], in general, the development of wayfinding solutions can be divided into three stages with different requirements and involving different people. The three stages along with substages are described in details in the following sections.

Fig. 6.3 Map for a hypothetical university campus

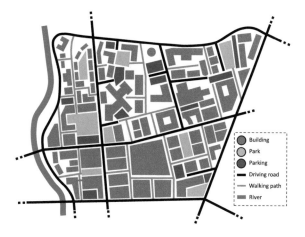

Planning

The planning phase is probably the most important one in the creation of a wayfinding system since it lays the basis for the next stages. To better explain the concepts introduced from now on, we will use a hypothetical university campus as a continuous example. A map representing the layout of buildings, parks, parking, and all connecting driving and walking roads is presented in Fig. 6.3.

The planning stage is further divided into three different phases to be executed in order:

- **Research and analysis**: The target site for the wayfinding project is examined, and preliminary meetings are carried out with all institutions/organizations involved to understand the objectives and limitations. For improvements and/or wayfinding projects to be built on already existing structures, site visit is important. In this context, the expert point of view is surely important but interviews of randomly selected people are also necessary to understand the requirements from the user's perspective. For new constructions, all considerations have to be done based on architectural plans. Patterns for vehicular and pedestrian traffic are to be identified. These will form the basis for the design program. Figure 6.4 shows the results of the research and analysis task for the example considered here. The layout of buildings, entrances, exits, and gates is plotted on a map to predict the way vehicles and people will move inside and around the campus. The wayfinding designer examines these diagrams and creates recommendations and a strategy to place signs and their content.
- **Strategy**: Based on the results of the previous phase, a strategy for the wayfinding system will be proposed. This should contain concrete ways to provide information and directions for a place and to address user requirements. Design goals and schematic outlines are defined in this stage. Figure 6.5 presents an example showing different strategies inspired from urban models in cities: connector model (e.g., Yamanote line, Tokyo, Japan; or The Forbidden City, Beijing, China), district

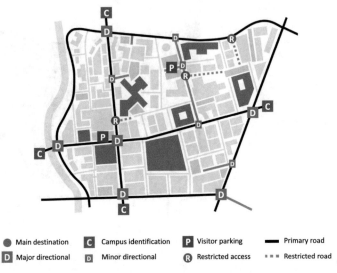

Vehicular traffic analysis

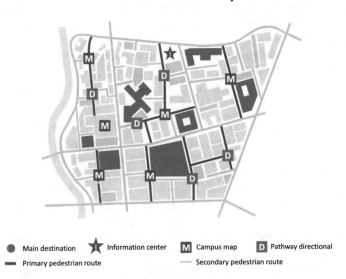

Pedestrian traffic analysis

Fig. 6.4 Site analysis for pedestrian and vehicular traffic for the example considered in Fig. 6.3. In this case, we are assuming that a wayfinding system (or something similar to it) already exists, and planners are analyzing the site to create recommendations for an improved system. For new buildings, the same analysis will have to be done based on intuition or simulations and expected user behavior

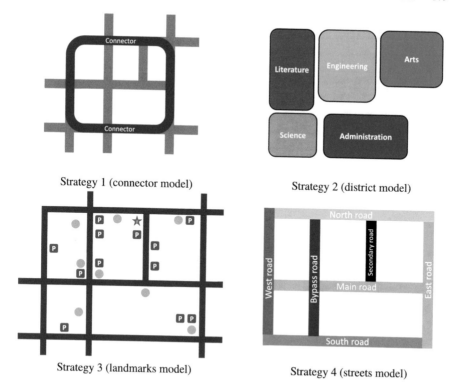

Fig. 6.5 Different strategies to guide people through the campus shown in Fig. 6.3

model (e.g., University of Cambridge, UK), landmark model (e.g., Rome, Italy; or Paris, France), and the street model (e.g., New York, USA; or Sapporo, Japan).

- **Programming**: Having studied traffic paths and defined the strategy, it is now time to determine the location and type of each sign. The cost of the wayfinding project is determined during the programming phase, and it is therefore important to determine in detail the number and types of signs needed. A schedule database containing each sign can help scaling the costs by adapting to the needs of the client (the database will help complete this task quickly by changing the cost of each element). Table 6.2 lists some of the signs that may be considered in the programming phase, with the corresponding illustration provided in Fig. 6.6. Figure 6.7 presents the results of sign programming, and the schedule database is given in Table 6.3.

Design, construction, and implementation

The design stage is the key stage where all signs are designed and minor details determined. This stage is based on the previous planning stage, and now, the focus is

Table 6.2 Types of signs, corresponding codes, and brief descriptions

A1 Station ID	Signs identifying a location; freedom of design
A2 Building ID	
B1 Directional–strap mount	Signs providing directions; design is free
B2 Directional–overhead ceiling	
C1 Regulatory–wall mount	Signs regulated by law; design is fixed and determined by codes
C2 Regulatory–strap mount	

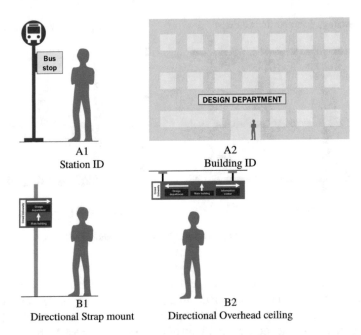

A1
Station ID

A2
Building ID

B1
Directional Strap mount

B2
Directional Overhead ceiling

Fig. 6.6 Illustrative example for the type of signs contained in Table 6.2. In this stage, the specific design is not determined yet, but general illustrations showing the main differences can help

only on the single signs and wayfinding elements. The locations and types of signs are not important anymore. Here, each element should look beautiful, be clear, and be produced using the right material keeping in mind the initial budget. The design, construction, and implementation phase can be further subdivided:

- **Schematic design**: In this task, different designs are tested, and the general branding strategy is defined. Although the details are still not defined for each sign, it is important to define the approach for the whole system. The color palette, suggested fonts, language, and approximate sizes will be defined in this task. It is important to maintain continuous dialog between the parties involved because the wayfinding system should be not only effective, but also respectful of the image of the institution where it is used. An opera concert hall will need a different, more

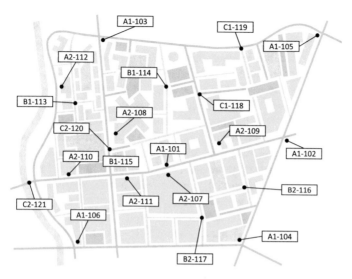

Fig. 6.7 Sign programming for the example of the university campus. Details are provided in Table 6.3

Table 6.3 Sign message schedule for the example university campus

Type	No.	Arrow	Messages
A1	101		Crowd University—Administrative building bus station
A1	102		Crowd University—East gate bus station
A2	107		Administrative building
A2	109		Design department
B1	113	↑	West park
			Administrative building
		←	Engineering department
			Visitor information center
			[Braille]
B1	114	←	Visitor parking
			Art department
		↑	Administrative building
B2	116	↑	Administrative building
		→	Design department
C1	118		Access restricted
C2	120		(Identification message TBD)
C2	121		Speed limit inside the campus 30 km/h

Not all signs provided in Fig. 6.7 are listed here since this information is only for illustrative purposes

classic, and traditional approach compared to a sports center where administrators would probably like to give an energetic and dynamic image to their facilities. Multipurpose exhibition halls or transportation hubs need to adopt a simple, clear, and neutral approach given the very wide range of users.

- **Final design development**: This is the task where all signs, maps, and wayfinding elements are determined in detail. Every aspect of each sign is determined: color, font, size, material, and finishes to be used during construction is defined. The previously discussed schedule is completed by determining exactly which design will have a specific sign, which text will be shown, and where and how will the sign be fixed to the architectural elements. This is also the time when more engineering aspects are resolved, considering, for example, how to power the elements that need electricity. Once the design is decided, only extraordinary modifications are possible, and these should be extremely limited to avoid increasing the costs.
- **Construction**: This is the moment when the elements of wayfinding are actually physically manufactured. Although there is no exact time schedule for determining the manufacturing firm, selection from among different potential candidates should start as soon as the engineering requirements of the project are clarified. Although the designer needs to create a documentation to be submitted to the manufacturer who will produce the elements based on her/his documents, it is important that continuous dialog is maintained to ensure that final parts correspond to the requests from the client. During the construction, aspects related to demolition need to be considered. Recyclable materials are preferred, and nondestructive fixing methods might have to be considered to avoid damaging structures that have important cultural or historical significance.
- **Implementation, administration, and staff training**: This is the moment when the constructed wayfinding elements will be actually installed at the appointed locations. It is important that the implementation is prepared in advance to minimize the transition period from the old to the new wayfinding system (for existing structures). It is also important to define the administration of the wayfinding system: Who is responsible for changes; to which area is the responsibility limited; and how to address eventual modifications. Staff training is also an important part of this last task. The people who are directly involved with guidance need to understand the wayfinding system to be able to efficiently provide assistance to users. These people need to know about navigation changes in the wayfinding strategy as their (old) way of providing guidance may not be consistent with the new system.

Post-implementation evaluation

Although the creation of a new wayfinding system is considered finished when the elements are laid down, it is important to adopt a critical stance to eventually address deficiencies or improve the approach adopted. This post-implementation phase is divided into the following tasks:

- **Analysis and evaluation**: In the initial phases of the implementation, it may be necessary to survey users to understand if the new system is fully understood and appreciated. Accustomed users may find the new system less effective than new users, but one should focus on the problematic elements rather than paying too much attention on the overall evaluation. People who have been involved in the wayfinding project (the designer in particular) may be also interested in the post-implementation feedback. They could also make use of this knowledge to eventually plan improvements.

- **Modifications and continuous staff training**: Although it is not easy to make substantial changes to the wayfinding system, some elements can be modified in a relatively short time. Booklets or handout material could provide guidance through alternative routes that are not sufficiently considered in the wayfinding system. Also, the staff needs to be continuously educated on the peculiarities of the wayfinding system (this will also be discussed more in detail in the following parts) to ensure a satisfactory user experience. Certain places may get popular over time (consider for example a shopping mall with several shops) thus requiring a different guidance strategy and it is important that the information is provided in a consistent way among staff members.

- **Maintenance**: It is not uncommon to see unlighted signs or missing letters also in places where wayfinding plays an important role such at airports or transportation hubs. Maintenance aims at avoiding these problems by taking quick action. In this regard, people working in a place should be aware of the consequences that a crumbling wayfinding system can have on the whole organization (remember also the introduction provided earlier) and should know who to report malfunctions or deficiencies.

6.3.1.2   Elements of Wayfinding and Design Variations

In the previous section, we discussed how a wayfinding project is carried out and what are the relevant stages. Now, we delve into the specifics and consider the elements that compose a wayfinding system and the important points for creating variations that successfully represent the branding strategy of a specific place while providing effective guidance to the users. We will start by presenting different categories of signs as proposed by Gibson [4] and later consider more design-specific aspects.

Categories of signs

In general, the signs used in wayfinding can be divided into four categories (some of them were already briefly presented in the previous example): identification, directional, orientation, and regulatory signs. Specifics and examples for each category are presented in Table 6.4.

Table 6.4   Categories of signs used in wayfinding, their characteristics, and representative examples

Identification	Directional
These signs are used to display the name and the function of a place or a space. They may be used for a room, a single building, or a gateway. They usually appear at entrances and exits and/or at the beginning and end of roads. While their purpose is mainly functional, their design can be also used to impose the character, personality, identity, and historical context of a place.	Directional signs are the backbone of the circulatory system of wayfinding because they offer important cues needed by users to move within a space. These signs can be used for both vehicular and pedestrian traffic. The design should be chosen to integrate well with the environment, but they also need to be easy to recognize and interpret. The messages of single signs needs to be simple but consistent with other signs available in the same space.
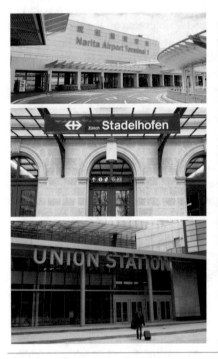	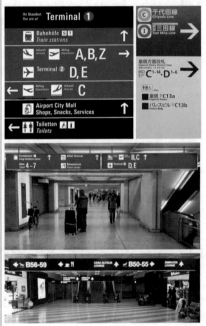

(continued)

Table 6.4 (continued)

Orientation	Regulatory
Orientation signs allow people to navigate within complex environments; they are typically represented by maps usually containing the "you are here" indication. It is important that these signs are consistent with other wayfinding elements: building and road names must be consistent. For facilities where occupancy changes are likely, a digital electronic sign may be more convenient as indications can be changed easily.	Regulatory signs describe what can be done and what cannot be done. While some of them are simple (e.g., "no smoking"), some may include a list of rules to be followed. In some cases, regulatory signs have to comply with legal codes, especially the ones regarding vehicles. Regulatory signs should not undermine user experience, but they still have to be large enough and clearly visible to be effective.
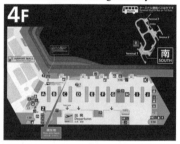 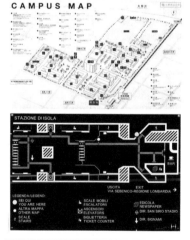	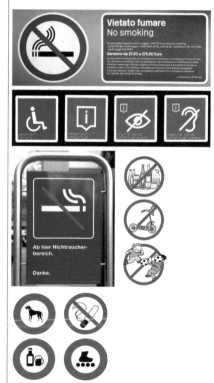

"Narita Airport Terminal 1" photo courtesy of Narita International Airport Corporation and "Union Station" photo by Sean Thoman on Unsplash

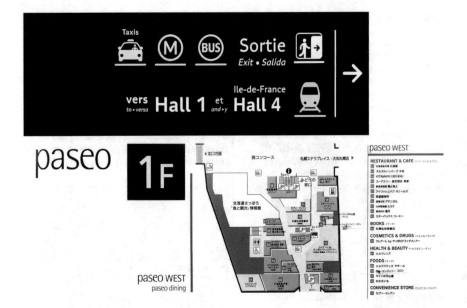

Fig. 6.8 Examples of fonts use and the font size. In the figure in the upper panel, different sizes are used in the different languages with the local language (French) having the largest font. Font size and style is also used to highlight the most important information. In the lower panel, a stylized, personalized font is used to increase branding identity of the location. Large size is used to attract the attention of passersby, while a smaller font is used to provide details to users who carefully read the map

Typography, color, and layout

Regardless of the type of signs used, there are some ways to change their perception and enhance the message being delivered. Typography, layout, and color have a strong influence on the nature of a sign and should be adapted to the environment while considering the branding strategy of the specific infrastructure where they are placed.

Typography refers to the used font and its size. It is important that the same type of font is used throughout the wayfinding system and that the font chosen is representative of the environment where it is located but still is easy to read and identify (some examples are provided in Fig. 6.8).

In addition to the font chosen, the color and color combination play a relevant role in making a wayfinding system efficient as well as elegant. In this context, it is important to remember that colors have psychological effects that are mostly common for all people (e.g., blue is better for studying compared to red [8]) as well as of a more individual nature that is related to cultural or ethnic membership. Hence, colors should be carefully selected with regard to the desired function and usership.

Since colors are usually used in combination (text and background being a very common case), contrast and visibility are also important. To increase readability,

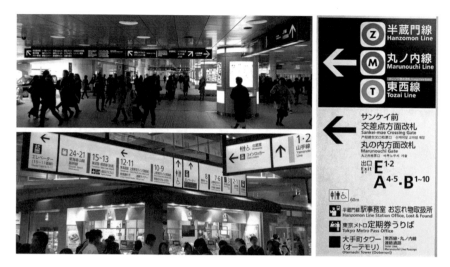

Fig. 6.9 Choice of colors in directional signs. Left: the use of strong contrasts makes the text easy to read, though the combination of different colors further improves readability (bottom left). Right: color combinations are used to create a clear distinction between the upper and lower sides of the sign

there should be a strong contrast between the text and background (see for example the signs in Fig. 6.9).

Finally, the manner in which different elements are arranged together also contributes to the overall harmony of a wayfinding sign. Elements of similar importance should occupy similar spaces, and details should be accessible only from a close distance and should not cause a disturbance when seen from further away.

Symbols and maps

Symbols represent the unspoken language used in wayfinding. They can be found in all wayfinding systems and should be understandable without explanation. Universal symbols should be clear to everyone, regardless of cultural membership, gender, or age (e.g., the symbols for the toilet, wheelchair, escalator/elevator, and WiFi). Although variations are possible, they should be limited to the minimum to avoid creating confusion. Original symbols may be also used, for example, to indicate a train line or to mark a particular building inside a campus. The use of those symbols can minimize the need of text to describe each element.

Maps are also an important element of wayfinding and are particularly relevant for large infrastructural complexes. There are different ways to improve the readability of maps, and the choice depends on the characteristics of the site. In places where there is a clear division among areas, grouping several buildings into sectors may be the best choice. In complexes formed by characteristic buildings (e.g., historical ones),

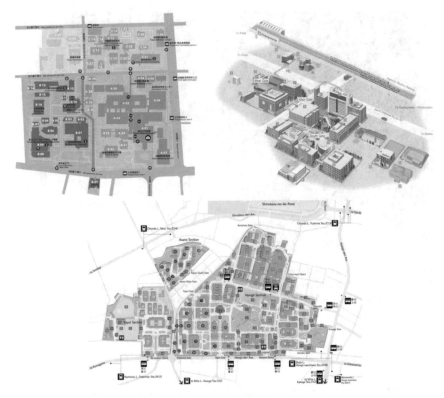

Fig. 6.10 Examples of maps used for university campuses. Left: a division of the surface into different sectors is clearly performed using colors (Tohoku University, Seiryo Campus, courtesy of Tohoku University). Bottom: surrounding streets and train stations are depicted to provide orientation (The University of Tokyo, Hongo Campus, courtesy of The University of Tokyo). Right: the specifics of the various building are used to distinguish each element (courtesy of Mukogawa Women's University)

reproducing the buildings on the map may help navigation. Refer also to Fig. 6.10 for a few examples on the different approaches.

Forms, materials, and media

Finally, we present a small remark on forms, material, and media. It is especially important to consider whether illumination or waterproofing is needed. If so, one may have to reconsider the design as lighted signs or waterproof signs are more difficult to design and construct. For nonlighted signs, it is important to take into account the fact that the wayfinding strategy may be different during day and night.

Further, with the ubiquitous presence of smartphones, a digital wayfinding approach too may be considered. In this case, connectivity is a major issue. Foreigners may not be able to access the content, and alternatives need to be provided if they represent a large portion of the users. In this regard, it is also important to check whether the wayfinding strategy is consistent with navigation apps. If the two approaches are in contradiction, users may get lost. In extreme cases, it may be necessary to notify the mapping authority or modify the wayfinding strategy.

Wayfinding for people with disabilities

Although in the discussion above, visual means have been presented as the main element of wayfinding, it is essential to remember that users may be visually impaired and/or may have restricted or impaired movements. Hence, alternatives to printed text (e.g., Braille) in maps and at crucial locations are necessary for visually impaired people. It is also essential that the navigation is consistent with the type of disability. For example, indicating stairs is not very important for wheelchair navigation, but visually impaired people will still need this information.

Hence, during the development of a wayfinding strategy, it is necessary to take advice from people with disabilities and/or experts as understanding their perspective is usually challenging for people without disabilities and without any personal experience regarding a specific disability.

Further, the guidance staff too should be familiar with the wayfinding alternatives for people with disabilities. For example, if a visually impaired person asks for directions to a place where access is difficult to her/him, the guidance staff should recognize the issue and assist the person until she/he reaches the destination.

6.3.1.3 Examples of Wayfinding Issues

Here, we shall delve into some typical challenges that are often encountered in wayfinding systems. The previous paragraphs should have made the problems and their relevance clearer. In this section, we present case studies. They are summarized in Table 6.5, which presents issues and possible solutions.

6.3.2 Dynamic Information Provision: Adding the Time Variable to Wayfinding

Pedestrian environment is a dynamic place where users strongly contribute to changes in the environment. Even the best wayfinding system cannot take into account variations over the long term, and commercial spaces or transportation hubs are likely to assist changes in pedestrian traffic caused by changes in tenancy or timetables. When a layout change becomes the new definitive standard, and further changes are not likely, then modifications to the wayfinding system may be necessary. However,

Table 6.5 Examples of issues related to wayfinding systems and possible solutions

Map inconsistency

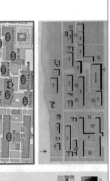

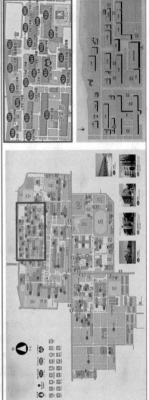

Issue: A university campus makes use of several maps to guide visitors and staff. A large map is located at the main entrance to show all buildings and connecting streets, while other maps are located inside the campus to provide guidance inside the areas corresponding to each department. However, the full campus map and the department map are not fully consistent with alternative names being used and details presented in one map not appearing in the other. The issues possibly originated from the fact that one map is older than the other and employs a partially different naming scheme. Visitors receiving indications with the new names may not find the buildings in the old map.

Possible solution: Completely remove the old map or substitute it with the same full map appearing in the main entrance having a correctly located "you are here" sign. A temporary solution (to be used only while waiting for a definitive solution) may also include to add a legend showing the correspondence between the old naming and the new (added) naming schemes.

(continued)

Table 6.5 (continued)

Directional sign inconsistency	Sign interpretation
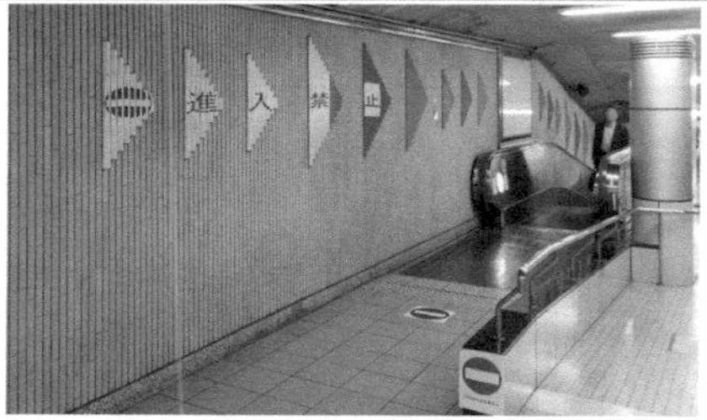	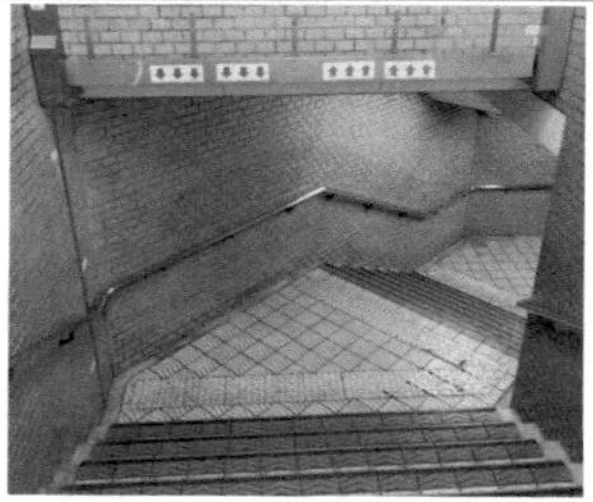
Issue: Arrows indicate a direction which is not allowed.	Issue: Arrows do not make it clear which side should be taken; following the arrows in the walking direction lead to the right, but left is suggested in the text (not shown here).
Possible solution: Completely cover the arrows or paint them with a color close to the background.	Possible solution: Use only one set of arrows, and change color or size of the walking direction to make it clear that it is the suggested direction.

(continued)

Table 6.5 (continued)

Information board illumination/contrast	Identification sign location / size
Issue: In the upper image, the train timetable cannot be read because of poor illumination and the strong light coming from the surroundings. Clock and current time are however clearly seen in the background.	Issue: Identification relative to the building is clearly recognizable only when the entrance is reached, thus nullifying its principal function.
Possible solution: A backlighted board such as the one shown in the lower picture presents clearer text, even when under strong sunlight. See also the next section for topics relative to dynamic signage.	Possible solution: Placing a bigger sign on the external side of the roof may make it more easily recognizable without interfering with the overall design.

if changes occur on a daily basis or are limited to a specific place and moment, then a dynamic way to address people may be required.

Consider for example an airport or a train station. Number of gates and platforms are determined and hardcoded to the signs and will be changed only on rare occasions if the building is modified or expanded. However, the time and destination of trains or planes leaving from each platform or gate will change many times during the day. Most importantly, changes beyond the schedule will have to be communicated promptly, considering verbal communication has now become an additional and important element of information provision and should be added to the underlying wayfinding strategy. Besides using a larger number of channels to provide information, the timing is the most important issue to be considered in dynamic information provision.

For all dynamic systems, in the case of a manual or semiautomatic approach, it is important that the people managing it are the ones who have the best overall image of the situation. This kind of feedback is possible only if the staff within the organization share information efficiently; in addition, nonrelevant information should be filtered to avoid putting too much pressure on operators who have to create the messages to be delivered to the crowd.

Finally, since timing is the most important aspect of dynamic systems, it is fundamental to provide the right type of information at the right moment. As a general rule, when something unexpected (e.g., an accident or a service interruption caused by technical problems) occurs, the initial communication regarding the event should arrive to the crowd within 3 min of the event's occurrence. An additional communication with more details (e.g., how long it will take before the service resumes) should arrive no later than 5 min after the first communication (therefore, within 8 min of the event's occurrence). Conservative estimates are suggested when giving information in regard to service suspensions or delays.

6.3.2.1 Dynamic Visual Messages

Dynamic visual communication aimed at advising crowds of people can be generally analyzed by using considerations valid for wayfinding, since the design and the locations of the signs play an equally important role for both static and dynamic content. However, the temporal component should be considered closely in the dynamic approach. A dynamic approach should be preferred only when there is an adequate system ensuring that information is correctly updated. In short, feedback is required, and countermeasures must be taken should the feedback not work. Consider, for example, the case of a dynamic train schedule that is updated only based on the time. Travelers looking at the board will assume that information is updated based on real conditions, and if a train is delayed, the time and order of departures will change. However, if there is a disagreement between the displayed information and real conditions, people are very likely to get anxious and create a burden to the guidance personnel who will have to deal with their requests. Therefore, if a dynamic system cannot reflect real conditions, a static, less complex approach is preferred. People looking a printed train schedule are clearly aware that delays cannot be displayed and therefore are prepared for inconveniences.

Another important element related to dynamic visual communication is the possibility of switching to the manual mode in the case of technical issues or to completely turn off the system if it becomes unreliable. In this regard, it is important that people dealing with information provision are aware of who is allowed/responsible for manual changes. It is not uncommon to see papers with handwritten messages put in front of displays because people do not know who can change the content of the displayed message.

Another issue related to dynamic visual messages is related to the integration into the wayfinding system. Since it is simpler to change the design of the dynamic content, sometimes the design adopted in dynamic systems becomes gradually different from that in the static wayfinding system, which has not changed at all. Therefore, it is important that upgrades in the dynamic system are limited to the technical aspects and the design is in line with the existing static elements. Two design approaches with similar objectives may only create confusion to users who may wonder if it is the same organization that is delivering information.

6.3.2.2   Internet Pages

With the widespread use of internet and mobile connectivity, it may be useful to consider putting online the content of visual messages or preparing dedicated pages to inform users. Although putting information online seems rather simple, internet traffic should be considered. Internet traffic can dramatically increase depending on the gravity of the situation. Although a simple server may be sufficient to provide information during normal operation, it may become overloaded in the event of emergencies when users outside the facility may start accessing the dedicated page. For example, when an airport is closed because of adverse weather conditions, family and friends of passengers may want to know the current situation, and passengers to fly in the following days will be interested in being updated on the situation. When external sources (such as media) start reporting on the case, people get different sorts of information and will want to double check the official content. Then, not only the number of users but also the frequency of access increases, thereby putting a lot of pressure on dedicated servers.

Social networks (Twitter, etc.) and external services can be a useful alternative, since these systems are typically accustomed to large internet traffic and can deal with rapid changes. However, note that in most cases, users are allowed to comment on pages, creating a sort of communication that may be difficult to control. Therefore, while internet traffic is clearly an issue, user interaction also needs to be considered closely when internet services are used to deliver information.

Another important aspect to be considered when preparing internet pages to deliver information is that most of the users may not be on the site when checking the page. While dynamic visual messages can be interpreted from the context of people being inside the facilities and some content can be implicit, internet pages

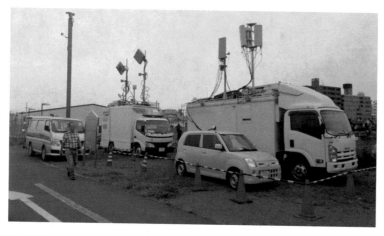

Fig. 6.11 Mobile antennas used to increase connectivity during crowd events

also need to provide access to more detailed information that can help understand the content provided. In this sense, internet pages complement visual messages, allowing people to access more detailed information without having to put too much information on monitors.

Finally, a fundamental aspect related to internet content is the connectivity. Setting an announcement saying "for more information, check our internet page" implies that users should be provided with connectivity to access the internet. In places with many international users, this would mean creating dedicated WiFi spots, and in remote locations, it may be necessary to increase the number of antennas to reduce network congestion (see Fig. 6.11 showing a mobile antenna).

6.3.2.3 Dynamic Audio Messages

Audio messages are a form of information provision that can only (or mostly) be used in a dynamic context (Fig. 6.12). There is no meaning in having the same message being repeated all the time (except for advertisement purposes, but this is beyond the scope of this book). Audio messages are used in airports to inform regarding the closing of a gate or in train stations to announce the arrival of a train. The content and goal of audio messages can be very different. They might be used to announce an earthquake or a fire or to provide less critical information such as the imminent closure of a shopping mall. Audio messages can be easily automatized, and it is also possible to create a large range of messages by recoding only parts of messages and later join them depending on the situation. Latest technologies also allow creating messages directly by using a computerized system that reads prepared texts. Thus, while it is now possible to create any sort of message and having it read aloud at the desired moment, it is important that the content and the timing are chosen accurately.

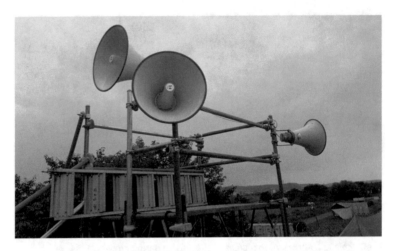

Fig. 6.12 Loudspeakers placed outdoor during a firework event used to deliver audio messages

According to Zuliani [9], in general, several aspects need to be considered when preparing audio messages, and the most important ones are listed below.

- **Constant update**: Audio messages need to be updated if there is any change in the layout of the building and/or if the names of exits/landmarks change. If the content changes very often (e.g., in exhibition or multipurpose halls), it may be more practical to have members of the staff reading the most variable parts and have the system read out only the service messages. To give an idea on the importance of updating audio messages, we can remember the 1996 Düsseldorf airport (Germany) fire, which claimed the lives of 17 people [10]; during this accident, the prerecorded massages broadcast during the first 10 min had not been updated after a layout change, and as a result, passengers were led to the most dangerous area of the airport [11].
- **Importance of words**: In preparing the messages, it is crucial to use simple language that everyone can understand; there is a widespread tendency to use overly technical language. This tendency sometimes arises because the people creating these messages are experts with good knowledge of the location and the procedures, but customers (many of whom may be first-time users) do not necessarily understand the language employed. Further, complex and technical expressions may be used to minimize the gravity of the situation. This should be avoided as people usually perceive that something is happening, and if the difference between the message content and their perception grows too large, they may start worrying about the worst. Moreover, the use of even a single complex word may undermine the comprehension of the whole sentence as people tend to get stuck on the word that they cannot completely understand. In this regard, the Keep It Short and Simple (KISS-rule) may summarize what detailed above. Finally, it is important to recognize the intrinsic valence of each word. In fact, words are never neutral.

Examples of positive words are "earning," "comfortable," "modern," "new," "simple," "useful," and "advantage." In contrast, "complicated," "expensive," "fear," "difficult," "disturbing," "must," "loss," "danger," and "risk" are some negative words. Choosing the right word is important because it influences how people feel or perceive the message, and therefore, valence should be considered along with the content.

- **Length and repetition of messages**: The length of the message should be accurately calibrated. People may not be able to assimilate the full content of long messages, but short messages may not contain enough information. This occurs because in most of the situations where messages are delivered to crowds (and especially in emergencies), the short-term memory will act as the most relevant form of information storage. Typically, the first message can only attract people's attention, and only the later repetitions can provide information. Therefore, the maximum effect is obtained by repeating a message 3–5 times. Another important aspect is the possibility of announcing upcoming information and the timing of their communication (which should be in line with the initial announcement). This helps reducing the anxiety of people and keeps them focused on official announcements, giving less attention to external sources.
- **Intonation modality**: The tone used in the audio message should be consistent with the message delivered and should also avoid any emotional connotation. In the case of messages about emergencies or critical issues, it is essential that the tone urge promptness without creating fear or anxiety.
- **Necessity to repeat it in several languages**: If the crowd is expected of being composed of people from several countries/regions, it is necessary to provide a multi-language message. This makes the message longer and the part spoken in a particular language may come later in time. If the message is overly long, people may try picking up words from the previous announcements coming before the announcement is made in their own language, likely causing misunderstanding arising from the small knowledge of that language.
- **Check if the message is audible**: Finally, the audibility of the message should be checked—whether a message can be heard in the all areas considering the background noise. Alarms or sounds may be easily heard even under noisy conditions, but it is more difficult to understand verbal communications completely. Even a well-prepared message is useless if it cannot be heard correctly.

In short, the advantage of audio messages is that they can be prepared without urgency when there is enough time to consider in detail all the aforementioned delicate aspects. In addition, three other important aspects too need to be considered:

- Messages should be prepared by an expert who has knowledge of the communication language as well as the cognitive and emotional effects on the people listening to them.
- The message must correspond to what people feel about the situation occurring in order to be credible.
- Finally, the person responsible for activating the message and eventually also choosing between the available options must be selected. In some cases, an auto-

matic system (a train arrival, the end of a match or a fire alarm) may be employed, but in other cases, it should be activated by a human operator.

6.3.2.4   Combination of Different Methods

Different channels of information provision can be combined to reach a very large usership. Technological improvements now allow use of multiple channels simultaneously: A visual text message may be read aloud using an electronic voice and be put online at the same time. However, the priority should be to provide reliable information rather than having multiple channels. There is no meaning in putting online wrong or unreliable communications. In this context, it is also necessary to remember that creating an effective and reliable dynamic information provision system involves a rather large amount of work, and including additional channels will be an easy step if a solid platform is already available.

6.3.3   Communicating with the Crowd: Efficiently Adapting Style and Content

In some ways, communication capabilities should be regarded as a skill that some people have and some do not. In this sense, rather than focusing on methods and approaches, it is more important to focus on "who." Although communication can be learned and unskilled people can improve their abilities over time, skilled and experienced people will be able to instinctively cope with new situations. In contrast to dynamic information provision, where the content is prepared in advance and only selection is performed considering the condition of the crowd, in the case of communication, everything is done in real time. This situation puts a lot of pressure on the staff, who needs to act in appropriately even when the crowd reaction is not positive. Hence, the selection and training of the people who will deal with direct communication is of utmost importance.

Staff dealing with communication should able to control their emotions, but at the same time, understand the situation and carefully listen to internal communications. Therefore, it is important that people having foremost roles in communication should have sufficient experience or at least adequate training. Further, training and education strongly depend on the role (e.g., police communication with a crowd will be different compared to the answers provided at an information desk), and therefore, people should be chosen for their roles and trained accordingly.

Lastly, the physical appearance of appointed staff is important too. In general, for any kind of communication, it is preferable to have people wear clothes that make them clearly distinguishable from the rest of the crowd but still makes them seem as part of the crowd. Creating a sort of gap between the staff delivering messages

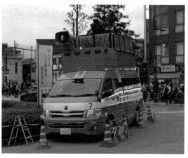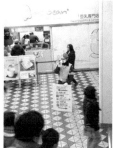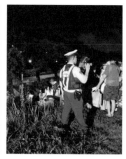

Fig. 6.13 Example of verbal communication with the crowd in different contexts

and the crowd receiving them may undermine the confidence of the people in the organization managing the event or facility.

6.3.3.1 Spoken Audio Communication

When something unexpected happens or when dynamic audio systems are not available, the only method to address crowds is by using loudspeakers or audio systems and speaking directly to them. Although the means of delivering information is the same as that for dynamic audio messages, the real-time condition makes it very different in terms of employment. Sufficient time is available to prepare recorded messages, and people reading them will be relaxed; the tone and the content can be adjusted for the situation. However, when operators speak to a crowd directly in front of them, their emotions may create contradictions between the message and the content. A trembling, loud voice telling people there is no danger and to stay calm may create more confusion rather than comforting the crowd as intended, because people will feel the urgency through the tone of the voice. On the other hand, if the message and voice are properly balanced, a positive effect may be created. For instance, the Landing Signal Officer (LSO) on aircraft carriers is trained to adapt their voice to the content. If a pilot is slightly below the flying path, the LSO will quietly ask "a little bit more engine," but if a pilot is dangerously below the flying path, the LSO will scream "engine!" [12].

Since oral communication requires a substantial feedback from the crowd, it is important that the staff dealing with it has direct contact with the people receiving the message. Supervisors should be so located that they are close enough to the crowd but do not obstruct the movement of people. Ideally, a location slightly above the crowd is preferred as it allows the staff to grasp the situation with a quick glance (see for example Fig. 6.13).

In addition to the selection of the message content, the manner and location of its delivery too are important; constant communication with organizers/stakeholders is also fundamental to ensure that no conflict occurs between what is communicated elsewhere. Hence, the people dealing with direct communication have multiple responsibilities: listening to internal communications, observing the crowd, reporting the local situation to organizers, and ultimately speaking to people using their voice or loudspeakers.

6.3.3.2   Information Desk and Walking/Mobile Information Staff

In vast complex buildings (such as airports, shopping centers, and exhibition venues) with a large usership, it may be appropriate to have an information desk or information point to provide information on demand (see Fig. 6.14). An essential skill for people working at these points is their capacity to understand requests from customers. Although many typical requests (e.g., "Where is the closest toilet?") could be answered in a routine way using material prepared in advance, the staff has to keep in mind that people asking for advice usually have little knowledge of the place. So, many requests will sound vague or difficult to understand (e.g., "I am looking for something to buy for my husband/wife." or "I am looking for the shop that a friend of mine suggested me but I don't know the name."). Therefore, sometimes, rather than providing the correct answer straightaway, asking the right question to the customer may lead to the best response, thus satisfying users (e.g., "Is your husband/wife a regular visitor of this facility?" or "Which kind of product does your friend usually buy here?").

Other important aspects of information desk are information sharing between colleagues and staff training. If there are multiple information desks in a facility, it is important that at least common requests are dealt uniformly. If somebody is looking for a particular place, it is possible that she/he will ask at multiple locations, and the information provided must be consistent at all times. Therefore, there should be a protocol to respond to common requests (we.g., "Where is the toilet?") but also adequate training on how to provide information for more complex situations. Although advice for more personal requests may change depending on the staff in charge, it is important that at least the style and the way of delivering information is consistent within the organization.

Finally, the people involved with information provision should be the first to be informed in case of any layout change or any kind of change within the facility (renovation work, temporary closure, service stop, etc.) as well as (to the maximum extent possible) in case of any changes in the services such as trains or bus lines or even weather forecasts (of course important changes in layout must be also shared with external stakeholders like the fire department).

In addition to information desks, it may be also useful to assign walking/mobile information staff either inside the crowd helping people or at locations where it is expected that people may need help. Since this type of staff will move around just like normal people, it is important that they can be recognized and distinguished easily. Clothes and style may be also adapted to best match with the requirements of the stakeholders. People standing in the lobby of a hotel have to be recognizable without interfering with the harmony of the area, while people giving information in

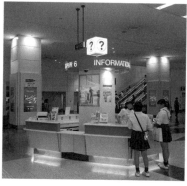
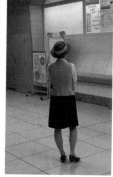
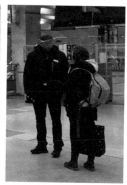

Fig. 6.14 Information desk (left), stand-by information staff (center), and staff providing information (right)

open air music festivals need to stand out from the crowd by wearing, for example, yellow cloths or some fluorescent items of clothing that are recognizable in darkness. As in the case of the information desk, mobile information staff too need to provide guidance consistently and uniformly.

6.3.3.3   Traditional and Social Media

Media are an ambiguous means of communication. While to some extent, some form of media communication may be considered as dynamic information provision (e.g., newspapers' internet pages that provide real-time news coverage), user interaction is increasingly playing a dominant role in the communication style of media agencies.

In the era of internet, social networks are also emerging as a new method to communicate with the crowd. In fact, in many social media (e.g., Twitter and Facebook), users are allowed commenting on news/communications and reposting them with added opinions. Hence, caution should be exercised when using these channels. It is possible that influential people reposting an official communication may gain more attention than the organization originally posting it. While in some cases, this could help spreading the information, in other situations, it may also lead to disinformation as the original message could be manipulated.

Timing is also an important factor. If an official communication concerning, for example, a critical situation during a crowd event is delayed, it is likely that participants will inform the public first. On the other hand, a hasty official communication may lead to unwanted consequences. Therefore, there should be a balance between being quick and providing a reliable and trustable message that could rapidly become the reference for people looking for information on the ongoing situation. A gradual approach is to provide essential information as quickly as possible and later add details [9].

In this sense, traditional media (newspapers, televisions, etc.) can play a central role as they represent an additional channel of official communication that can be used by stakeholders. Hence, it is important that media organizations be contacted as soon as an event is being organized and that large facilities have a point of contact should it be necessary to inform the media during crisis or critical situations. Even when dealing with (traditional) media, timing is relevant. If updates on the situation are delayed, representatives of the media will start investigating by themselves, potentially creating an alarming picture of the situation.

When dealing with any sort of media, it is important to provide updates on the current situation even when there is nothing new to report. Having a press conference scheduled and informing the media that nothing new has happened or that everything is fine is much better than creating an empty hole in the communication process as such gaps will be filled by media representatives and social media by collecting opinions from the crowd [9].

Finally, with regard to internet media, the possibility of using images is an additional aspect. Images too have not only a descriptive nature but also an emotional one. Therefore, care should be taken when using images as a part of the messages delivered through social media and/or provided to traditional media outlets.

6.4 Physical Methods to Safely Steer Crowds—Potentials and Limitations

When information is not effective to guide crowds in a safely manner, physical methods may be the only means to bring the situation under control or to avoid dangerous escalation. However, it is impossible or very difficult to dislocate physical elements when crowd density has already reached a moderate level. Also, actually moving structures around may worsen pedestrian traffic and hence should be avoided. Therefore, the strategy to employ physical means should be planned, and elements should be placed in advance. In short, only whether or not to use them and if so, the manner of using them will be decided by judging the condition of the crowd on site.

For this task, crowd simulators are a useful tool as they allow predicting locations that may need physical modifications to the architectural environment. However, since their accuracy is still limited and since prediction is also limited by the expected attendance and external factors, which are difficult to simulate, in most of the cases, considerations for physical methods are based on experience.

In general, the best approach is to identify locations that may need some intervention through physical modifications and prepare accordingly. It is much better to implement physical measures even if they are found to not be necessary later rather than be stuck in the opposite situation. In some cases, physical methods are already a part of the construction or are implemented as a mobile element that can readily change the layout of pedestrian traffic. An example is barriers used to line up people buying tickets or food at the entrance of stadiums. Since people usually come in large number shortly before matches or events, a similar situation is repeated on a regular basis. Hence, making these physical elements a part of the constructional environment is an appropriate choice. Airports use a slightly more flexible approach by lining up passengers using partitions that can be modified depending on the number of staff members available and other conditions. In this situation, fixing partitions to the ground would represent a too drastic solution, limiting their efficacy.

While the positions and functions of physical elements can be discussed well in advance of an event, their operation is limited to the duration of the event itself. It is, therefore, crucial to prepare and discuss the protocol with members of the staff to ensure that everybody knows who is responsible for implementing a physical change. For example, let us assume that the gates have been set up to control the inflow during a mass event. The gates themselves are useless if the staff responsible for their actuation do not know the protocol and when to open/close them. As discussed in Chap. 3 several accidents occurred because gates were not opened when necessary.

This means that physical methods have to be planned as part of a wider protocol where human resources and hierarchical organization play a fundamental and central role. Considering the example of the gates discussed earlier, the following points need to be clarified during the preparation of a mass event: who takes the decision to open/close the gates, how is this decision communicated to the person responsible to open/close the gates; and who will be that responsible person. Even structures that are supposed to be immobile (such as fences) need to be assigned to a member of the staff in case some trouble occurs (e.g., if a fence collapses because of a constructional defect).

Finally, we wish to remind the readers again that physical measures too are to be implemented considering information provision. A physical modification of the layout that results in changes in pedestrian traffic and circulation should be communicated to be effective, and the message will be more effective if people can predict or guess that such a modification may occur. For example, indicating the sections that permit one-way traffic on a map of a large crowd event will help people navigate inside the facilities, thus avoiding congestion created by people trying to enter a one-way path. Similarly, showing the location of the entrance (control) gates will help people predict possible long waiting times and consequently arrive psychologically prepared for the situation.

Now we will present some of the most classical approaches to physical measures. For most of the methods, the common goal is to reduce congestion in a single place. In large crowd events, it is unavoidable to have a large number of people, and congestion cannot be ruled out at all. However, if the crowd is spread out and light congestion is omnipresent but never excessive, then the risks for people are low. It is preferable to have many relatively small entrances rather than a single large one (assuming information is clear on entrance's locations). This principle is generally valid for all physical elements that aim at spreading out the crowd and partially limiting the creation of mass movements leading to a build-up of forces.

6.4.1 Crowd Control Barriers (Barricades)

Barriers are probably the most common method used to create physical divisions within a crowd or with external portions. Barriers, with some examples provided in Fig. 6.15, have multiple functions depending on where and how they are employed. Some of their functions are as follows:

- **Create a division between the accessible and inaccessible areas and/or areas with different characteristics:** The role of barriers is not only physical, but also psychological, and it aims to clearly set a mental division between the accessible and inaccessible areas. For example, barriers are used during parades to prevent people from entering the road. Higher and typically insuperable barriers are also used to distinguish and delimit areas that require a ticket purchased from open-access areas where everyone may be allowed in. Barriers may be also used to protect private properties if there is the possibility that people will enter them.
- **Protect people from a hazard or prevent occurrence of disorders:** Barriers can be used to avoid people from falling into a river or entering a rail track. In other cases, the crowd itself may be the hazard, for example when hooligans may try to invade the area of the opponent team. In this sense, fences also have a psychological function, and as such, in this particular circumstance (i.e., hooligans invading the area of the opponent team), it may be better that the opponents are not able to see each other (or at least not directly) to prevent provocation.
- **Avoiding the build-up of large pressure inside the crowd:** Under high crowd densities, so-called pressure waves may form with people being pushed in several directions in a short time. Under these conditions, the collapse of a single individual may create a dangerous avalanche potentially leading to death. Barriers may be used to split up the crowd into smaller groups and to ensure that if such a situation arises, the pressure build-up will not be overly high.
- **Canalize pedestrian streams:** Barriers may be used to divide two flows of people moving in opposite directions in a corridor (or a similar structure), thus avoiding the creation of the counterflow, which could lead to dangerous situations and accidents. Waiting lines (queues) may be also created by canalizing people into single lanes (this will be discussed in detail later on).

In all the cases, it is extremely important to ensure that barriers can withstand the pressure from the crowd also in the worst case. Accidents have often occurred because of collapse of barriers. Consequently, in order to perform their function, barriers should be sufficiently strong enough, hooked together if possible, and set at the right place in the right number.

Maintaining a balance between the flexible and safe employment of barriers is also not an easy task. Using too many barriers and hooking them together will limit pedestrian motion, and the barricade may also become an obstacle; for example, if it becomes necessary to allow access to emergency operators (medical assistance or firefighters). On the other hand, not using enough barriers may limit the control on the crowd and affect the safety of the people. A solution that allows to dynamically

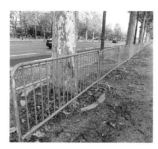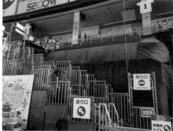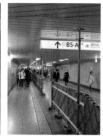

Fig. 6.15 Examples of use of barriers for pedestrian control. Left: barriers used to delimit pedestrian access during a military parade, center: flow separation on stairs (going up and going down use different sections), and right: flow separation in a corridor; an opening is left in the center of the barricade to provide some flexibility for crossing pedestrian traffic

change the level of connectiveness of the barriers is surely the most appropriate. This can be achieved by creating from the beginning some points where passages may be opened/closed and some of the barriers added/removed without interfering with the crowd movements.

6.4.2 Waiting Lines/Queuing Systems

Waiting lines are often employed to discipline pedestrian access to service windows. When crowd density is limited and there is little competition in accessing to a service, lines may form naturally (Fig. 6.16, right panel). However, when a large number of people have to be managed, there are numerous service windows, and/or there is a big competition to arrive first at the service window, chaos may easily occur, making crowd control difficult. Under such conditions, setting up waiting lines may be appropriate (see Fig. 6.16 for a few examples). Waiting lines too have a secondary psychological function as they make it clear to the people arriving that there is the need to line up and that shortcuts are not allowed.

Another advantage of waiting lines is that they make it simpler to estimate the waiting time. Since the number of people lining up until a given position is known or can be at least approximated well, the waiting time can be computed by knowing the average time it takes for one person to complete the operations at the service window. In short, the expected waiting time will be simply the product of the average service time and the number of people waiting (the left panel of Fig. 6.17).

Although waiting lines are simple to setup and manage, the way in which they are configured can affect their efficiency and ultimately the waiting time of the people. It is therefore important to understand which type of configuration fits best given the characteristic of the service provided.

Typically, two types of waiting lines are used: the fork type and the parallel type (a combination may be also used, see Fig. 6.17, right panel). In the fork type, a single line (that may be twisted to occupy less space as in the left panel in Fig. 6.17) is formed, and people are called to each service window as soon as it becomes accessible. In the parallel type, different lines are created in front of each service window.

The advantage of the fork type is that the waiting line is typically always filled with people and therefore each service window can work efficiently calling people when someone has finished. However, in this configuration, the distance between the end of the waiting line and the service window may be quite large, and for service windows far from the waiting point, the people waiting will have to be called out aloud.

On the other hand, in the parallel type, people are waiting right in front of the service window. So, transition time from one person to the next one is typically small. However, an uneven distribution of people in waiting lines and different service times for various windows may create empty lines, thus reducing the overall efficiency.

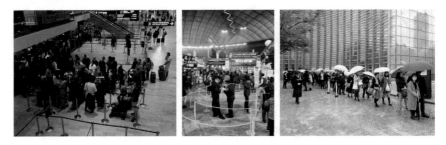

Fig. 6.16 Examples of different waiting lines. Left: fork-type waiting line set up in an airport, center: empty waiting line prepared during a mass event, and right: people naturally lining up in front of a ticket corner of a museum

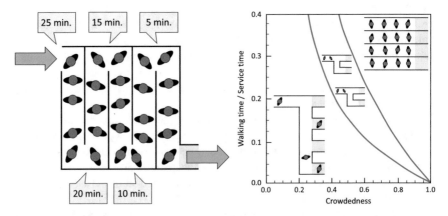

Fig. 6.17 Left: example of waiting time estimation in a waiting line. In this example, the average service time is supposed to be 1 min, and the waiting times are computed by counting the number of people. Right: diagram showing the optimal waiting line configuration given the amount of people waiting and the relative distance to the service window (shown in yellow) [13]. This case assumes four service windows, optimal configuration changes depending on the number of service windows, and additional parameters. Reprinted from Yanagisawa et al. [13], with permission from Elsevier

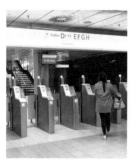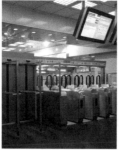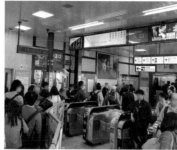

Fig. 6.18 Examples of one-way check gates used at an airport (left) and a metro station (center). Gates used in a train station (right, partially two ways and partially one-way). In both cases, entrance is restricted to people with a valid ticket, but a simple counting gate is also sometimes used to control the total number of people inside a facility

Using the diagram shown in Fig. 6.17 (right panel), it is possible to determine the best configuration given the crowdedness and the relative distance between the end of the waiting line and the service window [13]. Under congested conditions and short service times, the parallel configuration is preferred, while for uncongested situations where a long service time is expected, the fork configuration is more efficient.

Again, also considering the relative technical ease in counting people at service windows, creating adequate information with regard to waiting times in waiting lines is of utmost importance and will have a positive effect on overall crowd control. If possible, not only real-time waiting times but also expected waiting times for given period of the day and the week should be provided to help people schedule their visits and harmonize congestion.

6.4.3 Access Gates and Ticket Control

For facilities with a maximum capacity, the number of people entering and exiting has to be computed with extreme accuracy to ensure that the maximum capacity is never exceeded. Therefore, it may be necessary to setup check gates for people to pass through (see Fig. 6.18). Depending on the need, people may need to provide a valid ticket to open an automated door or may simply transit through the gate one by one.

Obviously, control gates are effective to count people only when a facility is completely closed, and flows are controlled at every access point. If data on access are available in real time or in a short time, access gates may be also used to control pedestrian flows (more will be discussed later). For example, when a facility is close to capacity, inflow may have to be reduced.

In general, an important point with regard to access gates is their direction. Gates that can be used only in one direction may not be able to act both as entrance and exit (or may need reconfiguration). On the other hand, gates that work in both directions may not be practical when people are simultaneously coming from both sides. Selecting the right type of gate for the right location is necessary. For both types, it is important that in the case of emergency or electrical failures, people can pass through without interference. It is not uncommon that emergency exits which are supposed to be open all the time are found to be closed during emergencies as the stakeholder prioritized preventing unauthorized entrance over safety.

In addition, a backup solution should be part of a protocol in the event that any kind of technical problem prevents the use of automated gates. Staff need to be ready on place and perform ticket control manually. If the number of tickets is not limited and entrance is free, the number of occupants cannot be maintained in case of technical failures. In this condition, an additional caution should be set to constantly checking crowd density and internal crowd conditions.

6.4.4   Flow Control and Bottleneck Effect

In many situations, it may be necessary to control the flow of people through specific locations. The gates presented above represent one solution, but they usually require significant investments and complex technical setup and are therefore typically used only in locations where large crowds are common. However, it is also possible to reduce pedestrian flow using architectural elements, and in this regard, bottlenecks are particularly useful.

As already discussed, in general, bottlenecks are simply restrictions along pedestrian routes. Every time a path becomes narrower, we speak of a bottleneck. For instance, doors or exits are also a bottleneck as people are forced to pass through limiting the flow. Although bottlenecks are a convenient way to reduce pedestrian flow, a failure in their use may be potentially dangerous and lead to unwanted consequences. Consequently, setting up the right size and selecting the right location of bottlenecks is of utmost importance.

In general, it is preferable having many small bottlenecks reducing the flow at several locations with a limited number of people, rather than a single large bottleneck where many people are packed. People far away from a bottleneck cannot understand the reason for their slowing down and may want to push slightly (maybe not on purpose). However, since pressure is transmitted from person to person, pressures easily build up in large crowds. This is why small bottlenecks are better: people can understand the reason for their slowing down and the pressure build-up is partially sustained by the surrounding structure.

Another reason justifying the use of relatively small bottlenecks is that the flow through them grows slower in comparison to their size. For instance, consider two doors—a 1.2-m-wide door and another 0.8-m-wide door. Despite being 50% larger in width, the flow through the former door is only roughly 15% higher that through the latter door [16]. As width increases, the differences in flow become less remarkable, but doubling the door width will probably never lead to a double pedestrian flow (except for extremely large widths).

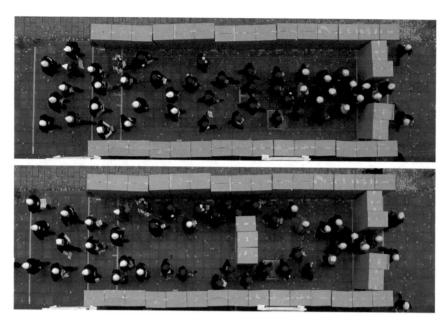

Fig. 6.19 Depending on their use, bottlenecks may allow to canalize people and spread out congestion over a larger area. Top: a single bottleneck (exit) is used to reduce flow; bottom: a double bottleneck is used before the final destination, thus allowing the reduction of congestion in the area before the exit [14, 15]. Courtesy of Xiaolu Jia

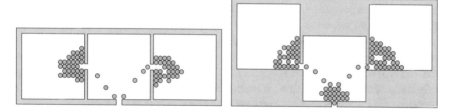

Fig. 6.20 Comparison of a triple room configuration where the location of the exit is different in the two external rooms. Since the flow is higher for exits located at the corner, the right configuration result in a higher flow of people moving to the central room. However, as a consequence, congestion occurs in the central room, limiting global evacuation efficiency. In fact, the overall evacuation time is lower for the left configuration since people arrive from the external rooms at a lower rate, but can leave the central room straight away [17]. Reprinted figure with permission from Ezaki et al. [17]. Copyright (2012) by the American Physical Society

An optimal use of bottlenecks may also allow spreading out congestion among several locations and finally increase overall mobility. Figure 6.19 shows that the use of a double bottleneck before an exit allows reducing pressure close to the door and promotes the formation of lanes [14, 15].

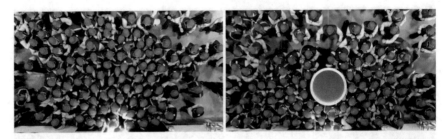

Fig. 6.21 Frames obtained during a controlled experiment designed to investigate the effect of an obstacle placed in front of the exit. Left: normal condition (no obstacle), right: a cylindrical obstacle is placed in front of the exit. In this specific case, it was found that the obstacle was somehow beneficial in noncompetitive scenarios but ineffective (or even detrimental) under highly competitive conditions [18]. Reprinted under Creative Commons CC BY license from [18]

Figure 6.20 presents a paradigmatic case in which the slowing down created by multiple bottlenecks allows speeding up the evacuation time of the whole complex. In Fig. 6.20, the left room configuration results in a lower total evacuation time because congestion is balanced among the different bottlenecks. In the right configuration, people from the external room reach the center too fast, thus limiting the overall system efficiency.

The example of Fig. 6.20 shows the importance of planning on the global scale with regard to the use of bottlenecks for spreading out congestion. If a complex pedestrian space is too optimized in a particular place, it is likely that congestion will occur when people leave that particular region and enter a less optimized area. It is therefore important to ensure that when optimization is performed, the system is conceived as a whole, and stakeholders being a part of the connecting system, are invited to the discussions. For example, if a stadium is well conceived and people are able to leave it in a short time, it is likely that congestion will occur in the connecting train stations or roads. Therefore, if pedestrian traffic is optimized inside the stadium, improvements in the connecting infrastructures are necessary as well.

Quite surprisingly, some research has also shown that the flow through bottlenecks can be improved by placing a cylindrical obstacle right in front of the exit (usually at a similar distance compared to the width of the exit, see also Fig. 6.21 for an example). The presence of the obstacle limits the conflicts among pedestrians, partially avoiding the formation of an arch among people obstructing the motion of the crowd [19, 20]. In general, depending on their design and location, obstacles may also act as elements guiding and canalizing the crowd. Figure 6.22 illustrates how a change in obstacle design will affect pedestrian motion, allowing the formation of organized lanes.

However, research is still ongoing to determine the conditions under which the presence of obstacles can be useful for increasing the flow through a bottleneck. While some evidence suggests an obstacle has benefits, some other studies did not find a significant difference from the situation without an obstacle [18, 21].

Finally, with regard to bottlenecks, note that no important information should be placed close to bottlenecks. People tend to stop to read information and having

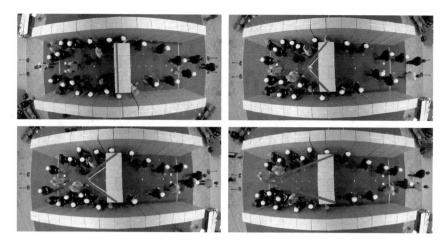

Fig. 6.22 Example of different employment possibilities in relation to obstacles. Obstacles may be useful to guide and canalize pedestrian flow in certain circumstances. In this case, a triangular shape is used to avoid the formation of nonaligned crowds at the sides of the obstacle. Courtesy of Xiaolu Jia

people stopping right in front of a bottleneck can dramatically reduce the flow in a location that is already quite critical with regard to traffic management. It this therefore preferred to place relevant information in large areas where stopping people do not pose an obstacle to the moving crowd.

6.4.5 Dynamic Routing and Guidance Staff

Physical measures are generally intended to force people in specific directions and to prevent them from entering places forbidden to the general public. However, it is preferred to consider alternative routes to be used in case of emergencies or in specific situations. For example, if the density along the most direct route from the main access station and a stadium reaches dangerous levels, it may be appropriate to divert people to a route with the same origin and destination but taking longer time (remember that stopping a moving crowd is never a good idea, most accidents occurred at dead ends). This kind of approach is generally referred as dynamic routing.

Dynamic routing cannot be improvised; it has to be carefully planned in advance as it requires physical elements (typically barriers), adequate information provision, and trained guidance staff. Guidance staff is particularly important because dynamic routing is typically used in situations with high density, and it implies a change in layout that can create problems for both first-time and frequent users. First-time users are likely to get lost in a new place, and frequent users may not notice the change and/or may neglect information provided as they move based on their habit.

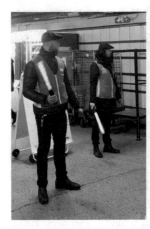 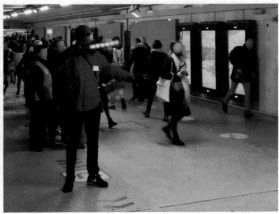

Fig. 6.23 Guidance staff on stand-by (left) and asking people to move to the right side in a narrow corridor (right)

Guidance staff therefore should ensure that everybody understands which direction to take and to discipline users who may be going against the rules.

Guidance staff is also important in the case of dynamic routing because they oversee a safe transition from a configuration to another. When a direction is changed, confusion may occur, and guidance staff is supposed to clarify to everyone where to go and eventually answer questions.

Even when dynamic routing is not in force, guidance staff may be employed in dangerous locations, for example if there are crosswalks with traffic light along a route, and people are likely to take risks. As for information staff, it is important that guidance staff is clearly recognizable (see for example Fig. 6.23) and has been sufficiently trained regarding what to do. An instruction such as "please control pedestrian traffic here." is not clear and may lead to individual interpretations of the correct control approach.

6.5   The "Nudge" Approach in Crowd Control

In addition to information provision and physical measures, an emerging potential method to efficiently control crowds is the so-called nudge approach. The "nudge" approach has gradually attracted the attention in several fields after the publication of a book describing its underlying principles in 2008 by Richard Thaler (who eventually got the Nobel prize in economics in 2017) and Cass Sunstein.

The "nudge" approach is best understood by considering an example often taken as a success story. Spillage around the toilet is a problem encountered in all male bathrooms around the globe. In an effort to tackle this problem, in 1999, Schiphol Airport in Amsterdam (Netherlands) added the image of a fly in the center of men urinals. As a natural unconditioned reaction, men were more likely to aim at the fly while urinating, thus reducing the spillage, which eventually dropped by 80% leading to a 8%-reduction in cleaning costs [22]. An important component in the nudge approach is that people are not forced toward a particular action, but there is an unconscious appeal that induces a person's autonomous behavior. In that sense, "advice" is given but the information is "invisible."

More generally, the nudge approach can be considered as a kind of invisible method to deliver information (as we already discussed while presenting the "advice" stage). When considered in the frame of crowd control, the concept of nudge is related to any architectural or environmental choice that alters people's behavior in a predictable way without forbidding any options or significantly changing their economic incentives. In other words, when a "nudge" is effective, people are unconsciously driven toward a particular action without noticing it and without having no particular or evident benefit from it.

In the case of pedestrian traffic, music is an example of an effective "nudge" approach [23]. It is known that walking speed can be increased by streaming music with a particular BPM (beat per minute). When the BPM of a song is close and slightly higher than the rhythm at which people move their legs, their walking speed increases naturally. People are naturally driven by the music without noticing it and without having a direct (personal) benefit from it. Since the efficacy of this approach is related to the stepping frequency, the music rhythm should be adapted to the speed of people and typically their density. For low density, a BPM of about 90–100 should be adequate, but higher densities require a lower BPM of typically about 70–80 [24].

Another example concerns light. Some evidence suggests that people can be driven using light [25]. In general, people tend to prefer bright areas over darker ones. As a consequence, a contrast in illumination can be used to steer people toward a particular place without directly telling them to move there.

From this point of view, the "nudge" approach can be considered a very soft way of providing information. Music, lights, colors, and the surrounding environment can be designed to have people moving in a desired direction without having to explicitly write signs or give orders to them. Although the "nudge" approach is still in an experimental phase and organizations are now starting considering applications, benefits from its successful implementation are big. User experience/satisfaction is among the biggest benefit in regard to this approach. Under the "nudge" approach, users are influenced but not directly guided. Hence, they tend to be not aware of being steered and enjoy the place they are in. Since satisfied users are also one of the goals of operators, the "nudge" approach represents one of the best solutions, providing benefits to both usership and stakeholders.

6.6 The "Self-Regulation" Approach

An invisible way to control crowds is the so-called self-regulation approach. Although this approach is still partially in a test phase and traditional methods are very likely to represent the standard also in upcoming years, it may be useful to know the general principle and consider "self-regulation" as an alternative with potential benefits [26, 27]. "Self-regulation" (sometimes also called "self-policing"), has been principally developed in the frame of police involvement during protests or potentially escalating events. In some ways, it is beyond the scope of this text. However, since we believe there are positive elements that can be learned from this approach of crowd control, we wish to briefly present its fundamental principles.

The concept of "self-regulation" originates from the so-called self-categorization theory (presented earlier in Chap. 2), which states that when forming a crowd, individuals do not lose their sense of identity, but simply shift from an individual identity to a shared social identity. Hence, individuals do not lose control over their behaviors, but shift from behaving in terms of their individual identity to behaving in terms of the norms and values exposed by their shared social identity.

In the "self-regulation" approach, the crowd is not controlled by stakeholders, but appropriate conditions are created so that people can control by themselves. Here, it is important that this does not mean that stakeholders have no role in crowd control; in fact, they may play an even more fundamental role compared to the traditional approach, but that stakeholders facilitate decisions taken collectively by the crowd instead of imposing their policy.

Although the methods making use of this approach are multiple, the general idea is to have members of the staff within the crowd interacting with them and at the same time reporting the situation to the control center using in part open channels like social media. In this regard, social media and/or public information channels play a central role as they are employed to (1) show to the public/usership the role of the policing staff, (2) inform the general public inside and outside the event location, while also (3) communicating with other staff members. Thus, a sort of shared knowledge is created in which both the stakeholders and the general public depend on the reliable information collected by the staff of the supervising organization. This context is important to create the conditions in which the crowd itself can take informed decisions ultimately leading to the "self-regulation." Such an approach has been made possible only recently due to increase of information channels and the possibility to inform a large audience with simple means (e.g., a smartphone may be sufficient).

Under the "self-regulation" approach, for example, instead of blocking disrupting actions in a forced way, they are documented as part of the event, allowing the rest of the crowd to know that somebody is trying to create troubles in a peaceful context and keep distance from those members. Obviously, examples of good habits need also to be documented to provide a clear picture of what is happening and to avoid a misunderstanding on the role of the stewards acting for the supervising organization.

Throughout the process, it is therefore important that there is continuous dialog with the crowd, both to show the role of the staff and to get clear information of the mood and motivation of participants. In fact, the goal is to achieve crowd control through consent and facilitate peaceful events through dialog and communication. From this perspective, it should be clear that learnings from the previous sections may also become useful in the context discussed here.

To conclude, it is necessary to remember that in order to reach successful "self-regulation," discussions with relevant organizations should start well before the organization of an event. Dialog between the organizers of an event and stakeholders involved in safety and crowd control is essential to guarantee that staff present on site is well received and their presence understood and tolerated from the crowd.

References

1. Tertoolen, G., Grotenhuis, J.W., Lankhuijzen, R.: Human factors en dynamisch verkeersmanagement: waar psychologie en techniek samenkomen. In: Colloquium Vervoersplanologisch Speurwerk (2012). (in Dutch)
2. Zomer, L.B., Daamen, W., Meijer, S., Hoogendoorn, S.P.: Managing crowds: The possibilities and limitations of crowd information during urban mass events. In: Planning Support Systems and Smart Cities, pp. 77–97. Springer (2015). https://doi.org/10.1007/978-3-319-18368-8_5
3. Mollerup, P.: Wayshowing: a guide to environmental signage. Lars Muller Publishers (2005)
4. Gibson, D.: The Wayfinding Handbook: Information Design for Public Places. Princeton Architectural Press (2009)
5. Carpman, J.R., Grant, M.A.: Design that Cares: Planning Health Facilities for Patients and Visitors, vol. 142. Wiley (2016)
6. Carpman, J.R., Grant, M.A.: Wayfinding: A Broad View, chap. 28, pp. 427–442. Wiley (2002)
7. Carpman, J.R., Grant, M., Simmons, D.: Wayfinding in the hospital environment: the impact of various floor numbering alternatives. J. Environ. Syst. 13(4), 353–364 (1983). https://doi.org/10.2190/590Y-QCBR-TBVN-B9PW
8. Costa, M., Frumento, S., Nese, M., Predieri, I.: Interior color and psychological functioning in a university residence hall. Front. Psychol. 9, 1580 (2018). https://doi.org/10.3389/fpsyg.2018.01580
9. Zuliani, A.: Azioni e reazioni nell'emergenza. EPC (2017). (in Italian)
10. National Fire Protection Association: Fire investigation summary – Düsseldorf airport terminal fire (1998)
11. Proulx, G.: How to initiate evacuation movement in public buildings. Facilities (1999). https://doi.org/10.1108/02632779910278764
12. Flin, R., O connor, P., Crichton, M.: Safety at the Sharp End: A Guide to Non-technical Skills. CRC Press (2017). https://doi.org/10.1201/9781315607467
13. Yanagisawa, D., Suma, Y., Tomoeda, A., Miura, A., Ohtsuka, K., Nishinari, K.: Walking-distance introduced queueing model for pedestrian queueing system: theoretical analysis and experimental verification. Transp Res Part C: Emerg Technol 37, 238–259 (2013). https://doi.org/10.1016/j.trc.2013.04.008
14. Jia, X., Feliciani, C., Yanagisawa, D., Nishinari, K.: Experimental study on the evading behavior of individual pedestrians when confronting with an obstacle in a corridor. Phys. A: Statist. Mech. Appl. 531, 121735 (2019). https://doi.org/10.1016/j.physa.2019.121735
15. Jia, X., Murakami, H., Feliciani, C., Yanagisawa, D., Nishinari, K.: Pedestrian lane formation and its influence on egress efficiency in the presence of an obstacle. Safety Sci. 144, 105455 (2021). https://doi.org/10.1016/j.ssci.2021.105455
16. Seyfried, A., Passon, O., Steffen, B., Boltes, M., Rupprecht, T., Klingsch, W.: New insights into pedestrian flow through bottlenecks. Transp. Sci. 43(3), 395–406 (2009). https://doi.org/10.1287/trsc.1090.0263
17. Ezaki, T., Yanagisawa, D., Nishinari, K.: Pedestrian flow through multiple bottlenecks. Phys. Rev. E 86(2), 026118 (2012). https://doi.org/10.1103/PhysRevE.86.026118
18. Feliciani, C., Zuriguel, I., Garcimartín, A., Maza, D., Nishinari, K.: Systematic experimental investigation of the obstacle effect during non-competitive and extremely competitive evacuations. Sci. Rep. 10(1), 1–20 (2020). https://doi.org/10.1038/s41598-020-72733-w

19. Helbing, D., Buzna, L., Johansson, A., Werner, T.: Self-organized pedestrian crowd dynamics: experiments, simulations, and design solutions. Transp. Sci. **39**(1), 1–24 (2005). https://doi.org/10.1287/trsc.1040.0108
20. Yanagisawa, D., Kimura, A., Tomoeda, A., Nishi, R., Suma, Y., Ohtsuka, K., Nishinari, K.: Introduction of frictional and turning function for pedestrian outflow with an obstacle. Phys. Rev. E **80**(3), 036110 (2009). https://doi.org/10.1103/PhysRevE.80.036110
21. Shiwakoti, N., Shi, X., Ye, Z.: A review on the performance of an obstacle near an exit on pedestrian crowd evacuation. Safety Sci. **113**, 54–67 (2019). https://doi.org/10.1016/j.ssci.2018.11.016
22. Halpern, D.: Inside the nudge unit: how small changes can make a big difference. Random House (2015)
23. Meng, Q., Zhao, T., Kang, J.: Influence of music on the behaviors of crowd in urban open public spaces. Front. Psychol. **9**, 596 (2018). https://doi.org/10.3389/fpsyg.2018.00596
24. Yanagisawa, D., Tomoeda, A., Nishinari, K.: Improvement of pedestrian flow by slow rhythm. Phys. Rev. E **85**(1), 016111 (2012). https://doi.org/10.1103/PhysRevE.85.016111
25. Corbetta, A., Kroneman, W., Donners, M., Haans, A., Ross, P., Trouwborst, M., Van de Wijdeven, S., Hultermans, M., Sekulovski, D., van der Heijden, F., et al.: A large-scale real-life crowd steering experiment via arrow-like stimuli. Collect. Dynam. **5**, 61–68 (2020). https://doi.org/10.17815/CD.2020.34
26. Reicher, S., Stott, C., Drury, J., Adang, O., Cronin, P., Livingstone, A.: Knowledge-based public order policing: principles and practice. Policing: J. Pol. Pract. **1**(4), 403–415 (2007). https://doi.org/10.1093/police/pam067
27. Gorringe, H., Stott, C., Rosie, M.: Dialogue police, decision making, and the management of public order during protest crowd events. J. Invest. Psychol. Offender Profiling **9**(2), 111–125 (2012). https://doi.org/10.1002/jip.1359

Chapter 7
Risk Management: From Situational Awareness to Crowd Control

Abstract A successful crowd management strategy is based on a correct risk assessment. Although a growing number of tools and technologies are available to crowd managers and it is increasingly easier obtaining information on previous events or accessing reports on crowd accidents, risks are sometimes difficult to be quantified without a structured methodology. In particular, it is important to link consequence and likelihood associated to a particular risk to judge its relevance in relation to various scenarios. Also, the dynamic nature of crowds makes it difficult to reach a good balance between a focus on short-term risky events, possibly leading to accidents, and long-term safety goals. This chapter will introduce a framework based on international standards to be used specifically for crowd management and its applications and limitations will be discussed in detail.

7.1 Introduction

After having discussed qualitative and quantitative characteristics of crowds and presented methods to detect and simulate them while also control their behavior, it is now time to make use of all this knowledge gained so far to quantify and analyze risks involved in crowd management. As already introduced in the beginning of this book, the final scope of the tools, methods, and technologies presented earlier is to guarantee safety and comfort of people inside a crowd. While this principle is easy to understand in conceptual terms, quantifying risks, and understanding when and how much comfort need to be sacrificed to ensure safety is not always straightforward. Mass gatherings, big events, or transportation facilities often see rapid changes in crowd density and other quantities (speed and flow in particular) and deciding whether safety should be maximized only during peaks or has to be considered on a much longer timescale is not an easy decision. Should security personnel be dispatched in large number only in critical moments such as before/after a game in stadia or in peak hours in train stations or a sufficient number has to be kept all the time in case of unpredicted events (e.g., a terrorist attack)? Of course a balance is needed, but defining that balance in terms of human resources is not straightforward. Another issue that is also not easy to answer could be: How is it possible to quantify risks for an event or a location that is new to the organizers? In this and the following chapter, we will try to answer these questions by also providing some practical solutions that may help quantifying risks involved with crowd management. As we will see, prevention is the key to ensure safety, and a constant feedback from people working closely to the crowd is necessary to identify possible shortcomings and continuously update safety protocols.

However, in this chapter, we will not discuss in details on the different types of risks to which crowd are exposed (e.g., fire, high densities, traffic accident, crime, etc.) as this largely depends on location, time, and the characteristics of the crowd. Here, we will focus on the methodology to analyze and quantify risks, particularly relating to the risks induced by the crowd itself (as we have seen in Chap. 3 when crowd is poorly managed and risk not adequately estimated a simple change in collective motion can lead to catastrophes). A framework for automatic risk estimation using sensing technology will become a key element of this chapter. Nonetheless, a more detailed discussion on common risks typically involved in the organization of large events and some possible countermeasures to prevent them will be given in the next chapter.

7.2   Objectives of This Chapter

Through this chapter readers should become familiar with the international standards used to define, classify and analyze risks and the implications in the frame of crowd management. The difference between on-site and off-site risk assessment should be clear, also considering the different tools and data available for both scenarios. Readers should also understand and get used to the methods used to quantify risks, in particular the relation between consequence and likelihood associated to a particular scenario. It is also necessary to fully understand the limitations imposed by the method presented here and remember that risk management is a teamwork performed involving all stakeholders and by employing different and alternative approaches. By the end of this chapter, readers should be able to assess more systematically risks involved in crowd management, plan how to use available technologies and when/how dispatch their human resources accordingly.

7.3   Risk Definition and Approach

Before entering into a detailed discussion on risk assessment in the frame of crowd management, it may be necessary adding a few words in regard to its context and definition. The latest international standards for risk management, ISO31000 [1], were drawn up in 2018. According to the ISO standards, risk is defined as "the effect of uncertainty on objectives." In other words, it is only possible to identify risks after objectives have been set. In addition, a particularity of the latest ISO standards lies in the great emphasis set on preventive risk management, which takes place before people get actually exposed to a particular risk (in the case of this book, the risk that a crowd accident resulting in injuries or death may occur).

Considering the points introduced above, it should be noted that, in terms of deviation from established objectives, both positive and negative effects are generally considered to be elements of risk that require management. However, for risk assessment for the purposes of crowd management, also considering the importance on preventive safety, this means that measures to reduce the risk of negative effects should be prioritized. Crowd management is, of course, intended to increase the level of both safety and comfort of the people who make up the crowd, but when risk level rises as described in Chap. 1, safety is more important than comfort from the perspective of human lives. In short, safety should always be the top priority, and the reduction or elimination of risk is a fundamental part of crowd management and control. It may nonetheless useful to remind that, in some sense, prioritize safety does not necessarily contrast with organizer's or operator's objectives. For instance, organizer has the added goal of making the planned event a success and operator will need to make a location enjoyable by its users. In this sense, safety usually correlates positively with the satisfaction of the people who attend an event or visit a facility and the two goals (safety and visitors' satisfaction) are usually aligned. But, when everything goes smoothly, safety may be underestimated in favor of comfort, and it is therefore important that care is taken to ensure that service is never given priority over safety in crowd management.

To align with ISO standards and taking into consideration the nature of crowds, in this chapter (as we also generally did in this book), we will focus on preventive safety, and we will not deal directly with evacuation safety and its associated risks. In short, we will consider how to minimize the likelihood that an evacuation is needed and reduce the consequences in that case. However, we assume that locations hosting large crowds are already prepared and designed to evacuate people, should it necessary due to unavoidable circumstances. For example, keeping in mind what learned in Chap. 2, the width of entrances and exits to a building should be carefully considered in terms of the building's purpose and capacity and according to local laws to ensure that everyone who is in the building can safely escape as quickly as possible in the event of a fire. In this chapter, we will follow the same principle, i.e., identify and quantify the risk related to weak points (e.g., exits) and potentially dangerous scenarios (e.g., fire). However, when preventive risk management is considered, a more macroscopic perspective need to be adopted, where not a single exit, but a large building or a festival ground as a whole are considered. If the same safety principles used to reduce risks *after* an emergency evacuation has been already started are also employed to minimize the risk of crowd incidents under normal conditions, then countermeasures against risk put in place during normal operations will have the effect of mitigating the danger of a more serious disaster in the event that an emergency occurs (and evacuation is needed).

To conclude, we should remind, that it is obviously difficult to completely prevent accidents, and we must therefore assume that emergencies may occur also when preparing policies or measures aimed at preventing risks. Accordingly, we should thoroughly eliminate risk factors during normal operation but also prepare in case the worst-case scenario may happen. Accidents occurring in normal conditions without external intervention and/or related to inappropriate evacuation design for predictable and common causes (e.g., fire or power failure) cannot be forgiven.

7.4   A Framework for Risk Management in Crowds

The descriptions which follow use a framework that refers to the ISO standards in terms of preventive safety, and the positioning of risk assessment and its input/output for crowd management within that framework is shown in Fig. 7.1 (more details on this diagram will be presented later on).

In general, risk management has to be seen as the task that includes both the assessment of a risk and its mitigation. The goal of risk assessment is to determine the so-called risk level through a systematic analysis focusing on where and when problems can occur, and the scale and likelihood of their occurrence. Risk assessment should always be performed before, during and after an event. Although the general procedure is similar for each case and the framework presented in Fig. 7.1 will always represent the central reference, data available before, during, and after an event are largely different. As a consequence, a different approach is also needed. In this book, we distinguish between on-site risk assessment, which is performed on real-time during an event, and off-site risk assessment, which is performed while preparing (or planning) for an event and when examining a completed one. This chapter will focus on on-site risk assessment, with off-site risk assessment covered in detail in the next chapter, but, to understand the differences between the two approaches a brief description covering both will be given as follows.

Fig. 7.1 Risk management in the case of crowds. Crowd control and strategies (summarizing what will be defined as "conditions" and "operating modes" in the next chapter discussing off-risk risk management in detail) could be directly defined based on information obtained by crowd sensing or related data, but a systematic approach through risk assessment is generally preferred and strongly suggested

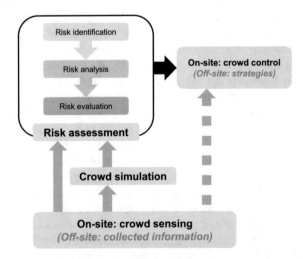

7.4.1 Off-Site Risk Management

When preparing for an event, it is fundamental to systematically predict any possible risk in advance and, if risk is judged too high, reconsider conditions and operating modes (summarized as "strategies" in Fig. 7.1) under which the event will be hold (both "conditions" and "operating modes" will be explained in detail in the next chapter). In addition, strategies to be used during crowd control should be defined, communicated, and understood by all stakeholders. For events hold on a regular basis risk assessment for a scheduled event may correspond to the risk assessment of the previous event, i.e., risks that may occur in the future may be predicted by examining potentially dangerous situations which already occurred in the past. However, for completely new events, risk assessment should start well before the event (usually months or years in advance) and the only mean to predict crowd behavior is by simulation or through the collection of information for similar events. As such, off-site risk assessment relies on the creation of scenarios that are used to estimate risks. Realistic and what-if or worst-case scenarios have to be created to assess both risks occurring during normal and abnormal operation.

The goal of off-site risk management is to reduce or completely eliminate risks by finding optimal conditions and operating modes for an event. This will also result in the definition of crowd control strategies, which will be employed should one of the predicted scenario occur. For instance, if while planning it is predicted that density could be high in a particular place at a particular time, flow lines and/or schedule need to be changed and reiterated until the risk is reduced to a sufficient level. On the other side, countermeasures should be put in practice to avoid a power outage during the event. However, at the same time, strategies to ensure safety of the crowd need to be also defined should this occur due to unpredictable circumstances.

7.4.2 On-Site Risk Management

On-site risk management should make sure that limit conditions set up during off-site risk management (which was performed earlier while planning) do not appear and therefore crowd needs to be constantly monitored and accordingly controlled. During on-site risk management, data are abundant and highly representative for crowd condition, and therefore, sensing data is the most important source of primary information. As already described in Chap. 4, this information can be gathered from cameras that are installed in various locations, sensors that count the number of people passing through gates or check points, the number of tickets sold, and/or location information gathered from mobile phones or electronic devices.

In general, there are two methods that can be employed to perform a risk assessment based on sensing data. One approach relies on chronological data to assess the risk based on crowd condition measured in the past. Data for, say, the last 10 min are collected, and based on this, data risk assessment over the last 10 min is performed. This method has the disadvantage to be relatively late in the evaluation since it relies on past data and, even if trends can be computed, they will always be based on past conditions. However, such an approach requires only data from sensors and is therefore relatively easy to implement.

In addition to this "simple" approach relying on chronological data, in recent years, a second method is rapidly emerging as an alternative to also take future conditions into account. Recently, there have been a number of cases in which risk has been assessed by inputting real-time crowd data into a computational system so that short-term predictions can be made about risk using simulated crowd behavior [2–4] (note that a prediction based on a model is different from a simple trend). Such scientific methods have become possible because crowd simulators have become more accurate, because it is easier to couple them with sensing systems and due to the rise in computational capabilities (as discussed in Chap. 5). Longer-term (but often less accurate) predictions are also possible by machine learning techniques for simple information such as the number of attendants or crowd density in a particular location [5]. However, in the case of machine learning, the capability to correctly predict future behavior depends on availability of training data relative to previous events or similar conditions. Thus (as already discussed), predictions tend to be inaccurate if observed behavior deviate from data collected in the past.

Although the two methods described above can be used to make automated risk assessments based on current or predicted crowd behavior, skilled staff often need to be present on site so they can judge the available information more comprehensively by also adding the precious value of their experience when making the final assessment. Having the best type of sensing techniques or the most experienced personnel does not guarantee a perfect risk assessment and a combination of reliable and abundant data evaluated by skilled professionals is always the best choice.

In the case of on-site risk management, crowd control is the direct result of risk assessment. For instance, if a high risk level is detected in a particular location actions are to be taken straightaway to reduce the risk level and consequently diminish the likelihood that something adverse may occur or the consequences in case of accident (or, even better, both at the same time). However, it is important to remind that strategies for crowd control are defined while planning an event, so the availability of on-site risk assessment does not eliminate the need for off-site risk management.

7.5   Risk Assessment

As already said, in this chapter, we focus on on-site risk assessment and, as such, from here on we will assume that a sensing system or a form of feedback is available to constantly monitor crowd conditions. Once those sensing data have been collected on the past, current and possibly also on the simulated (predicted) state of the crowd, the next step is using these results to identify, analyze, and evaluate risks as presented in Fig. 7.1. The three stages of risk assessment, i.e., identification, analysis, and evaluation will be described in this section by also introducing useful techniques to be used in each stage.

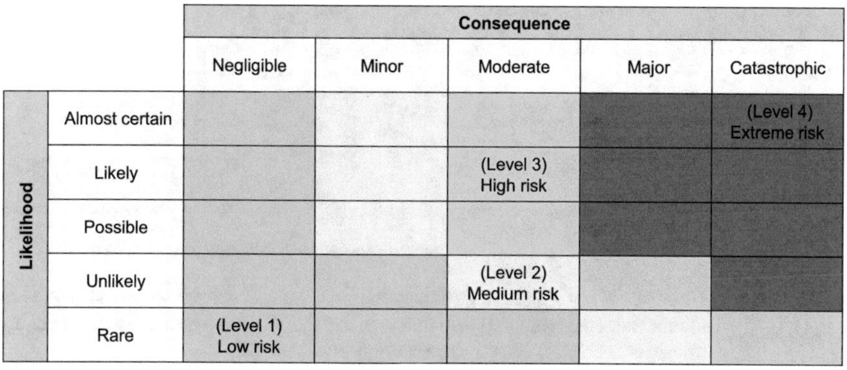

Fig. 7.2 Example for a matrix determining risk level

7.5.1 General Principles

With the overall image of risk assessment in mind, let us first describe the principles behind the determination of the so-called risk level. Although there are many potential ways to do so, in this book, we use a standard definition that combines the consequences of an event occurring and its likelihood. The risk level can be defined as the product between its consequence and likelihood, or in simple terms:

> Risk level = Consequence × Likelihood

To make the evaluation of the risk level more practical, consequence and likelihood may be both ranked on a scale from 1 to 5 to create a matrix with 25 combinations, as shown in Fig. 7.2. Four risk levels are set as shown in Fig. 7.2, with risk increasing from the bottom left of the diagram, where it is negligible and it will rarely occur, to the top right, where the consequences are catastrophic and the considered scenario will almost certainly occur. Furthermore, the boundaries between the four levels are arbitrary and may be adjusted as necessary to suit the circumstances of any given event (although, obviously, should always form some kind of oblique stripes from bottom left to top right) [6]. Generally speaking, crowd management uses level 1 for low-risk situations, level 2 for medium risk, level 3 for high risk, and level 4 for extreme risk. However, this scale can be adjusted so that it only uses three levels or modified in other ways as necessary.

Figure 7.2 shows the general theory behind determining risk level, and its application in the specific context of crowd management is discussed in detail later. In the following discussion, we will focus on crowd intrinsic risk assessment based on data from sensors (possibly combined with simulations) because it represents the most complex approach and also because it is, generally speaking, the only way to perform it automatically. However, risk assessment for events affecting the crowd as

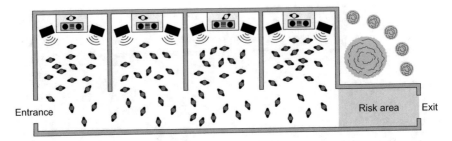

Fig. 7.3 Schematic example for a multistage dance floor in which people are schematically reproduced in small number (adapted from [7]). We may assume that the red region close to the exit is judged being the most risky area for which close monitoring is needed

a whole in a rather unpredictable manner can be also performed by solely relying on the matrix from Fig. 7.2. More will be discussed in the following section.

7.5.2   Risk Identification

When crowd motion is intrinsically concerned, the first step that is needed is to determine the risk level in a given crowd is by quantifying its properties as already described in Chap. 2. Although this should be already clear at this point, the three most important crowd properties that are considered in this process are:

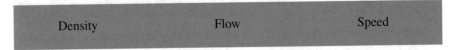

| Density | Flow | Speed |

As stated earlier, this sort of data need to be provided by a sensing system monitoring crowd conditions. However, as we have seen through this book, it is not always easy to uniquely estimate each value since they generally change by location to location and over time. Accordingly, the area for which risk assessment is required is divided up into sections as necessary, and the crowd density, speed and other variables are measured in each section. If the crowd is moving in a fixed direction, the flow rate can also be measured and used to calculate the number of people who will pass through the section within a given period of time.

The selected sections need to be representative of a particular region of the venue/infrastructure with the crowd within them behaving in a fairly uniform way. The scenarios presented in Chap. 5 to test crowd simulators, or the typical locations where accidents occur as given in Chap. 3 may constitute an example for these sections, although, upon necessity, larger or smaller areas may be used. Ideally, the selected regions should cover the whole area where the crowd move, but, when this is difficult, regions where accidents are more likely (and therefore risk high) need to be identified to allow the installation of cameras and/or sensors collecting real-time data or, when not possible, dispatch staff to constantly report on the conditions. These risky areas are typically identified during off-site risk assessment, thus limiting the aim of on-site risk assessment to monitor those areas and make sure that risks are never exceed or are not likely to be exceeded in the future.

To explain the following principles in an easier manner, we may assume that a multistage dance floor has an internal configuration as presented in Fig. 7.3. During off-site risk assessment, organizers will need to run a number of simulations or perform estimates taking into account the schedule of the events and adding additional variables such as the timetable of public transportation serving the location. In this context, both realistic and worst-case conditions need to be taken into account. We could further assume that after this preliminary analysis of the various scenarios, organizers assume that stages themselves represent low-risk areas (e.g., people are not expected to get overly excited and high densities may not form), but the region close to the exit could get easily packed, when, for example, late-night trains are about to leave. Since, in our example, this area may potentially lead to accidents, organizers therefore plan to set sensors closely monitoring the number of people around the exit and dispatch the best trained staff there. Again, to reduce the risk at minimum, the full surface should be covered, but, in our example we assume that only the red "risk area" is automatically analyzed and a sufficient number of staff will be nonetheless dispatched over the whole venue to make sure that even the low-risk stages are constantly monitored.

7.5.3 Risk Analysis

Next, we will explain how to calculate the values for "consequence" and "likelihood" that are needed to use the matrix of Fig. 7.2. Consequence is often calculated by using the density of the crowd. As density becomes higher, there is increasing pressure between the bodies in the crowd, and the risk of a snowballing crowd incident becomes greater. As such, the density of a crowd is directly proportional to the consequences of any incident that may occur. As discussed in Chap. 2, this concept was already used to define the level of service (LOS), and it is therefore meaningful to apply the same categories proposed by Fruin in his approach to define five levels of consequence, as shown in Table 7.1.

For the purposes of this table, LOS A and B, in which crowds have plenty of available space, have been combined into the "negligible" consequence, but it should be noted that acceptable density varies according to the situation, and these categories should be set according to the requirements of the event under consideration. Here, density has been considered since it is usually the most important crowd quantity, but it has a static nature, so if a crowd has a density corresponding to LOS B but is running (e.g., in a marathon) the consequences of an accident may be not completely negligible, although, very likely, not catastrophic. More on this aspect will be also discussed later on.

Table 7.1 Example of the relationship between LOS, corresponding density, and consequence in case of accident. Threshold values for density are indicated using Greek letters, which will be used later on (ρ is typically used to indicate density in physics and therefore also often used for crowds). Refer also to Fig. 7.4 for a visual representation

Consequence	Density range	Threshold density
Negligible (LOS A,B)	Below $0.43\,\mathrm{m}^{-2}$	$\rho_0 = 0.00\,\mathrm{m}^{-2}$
Minor (LOS C)	Between $0.43\,\mathrm{m}^{-2}$ and $0.72\,\mathrm{m}^{-2}$	$\rho_1 = 0.43\,\mathrm{m}^{-2}$
Moderate (LOS D)	Between $0.72\,\mathrm{m}^{-2}$ and $1.08\,\mathrm{m}^{-2}$	$\rho_2 = 0.72\,\mathrm{m}^{-2}$
Major (LOS E)	Between $1.08\,\mathrm{m}^{-2}$ and $2.15\,\mathrm{m}^{-2}$	$\rho_3 = 1.08\,\mathrm{m}^{-2}$
Catastrophic (LOS F)	Above $2.15\,\mathrm{m}^{-2}$	$\rho_4 = 2.15\,\mathrm{m}^{-2}$

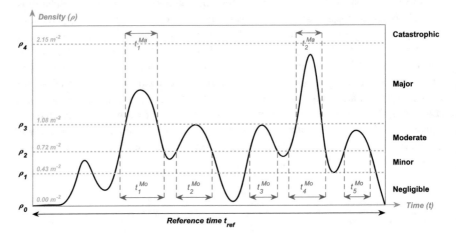

Fig. 7.4 Example on how to determine level of risk from density time series

So far, we have considered the spatial component of crowds, but, as mentioned, density does not only change over space, but over time too. Figure 7.4 shows an example of chronological data relative to crowd density that is gathered for a given section, for example, the area covered by the sensor considered in the example of Fig. 7.3.

We will now present a method that may be employed to use this data and calculate the likelihood of a specific risk scenario. The horizontal dotted lines have been added in Fig. 7.4 as a reference to indicate the different thresholds previously considered in Table 7.1. Next, time interval t_{ref} is defined as the reference time, i.e., the time interval for which crowd management is required. A detailed discussion will follow about the selection of this reference time, but, for now, let us assume that a time of 10 min is used, which, in general, could be a reasonable choice for most of the cases (but, again, selection depends on several considerations and details will follow).

Depending on the approach used, data within the reference time may be relative to the past conditions, could be a combination of past and predicted conditions or could be completely generated from a simulator assessing future conditions. If, for instance, data relative to the previous (predicted) 10 min are used, risk assessment will be relative to the past (future) conditions. If, for example, the historical data from the previous 5 min are combined with a simulation predicting the next 5 min an estimation of the current risk is possible.

Within this reference time, the total interval for which the crowd density exceeds each threshold line is calculated. As an example, the probability that consequences in case of accident are equal to or higher than moderate is calculated by looking at how long density exceeds ρ_2 as a proportion of reference time t_{ref}, by using the following equation:

$$P(\rho \geq \rho_2) = \frac{t_1^{Mo} + t_2^{Mo} + t_3^{Mo} + t_4^{Mo} + t_5^{Mo}}{t_{ref}} \tag{7.1}$$

in which "Mo" refers to "Moderate." By using a reference time of 10 min and setting numeric values to the example considered in Fig. 7.4, we have:

$$P(\rho \geq \rho_2) = \frac{1.25 \text{ min} + 1.00 \text{ min} + 0.78 \text{ min} + 1.04 \text{ min} + 0.74 \text{ min}}{10 \text{ min}} = 0.48 \tag{7.2}$$

The closer this value gets to 1, the more likely it is that an event with moderate consequences will occur.

In a similar fashion, the probability for an accident to occur and resulting in major consequences can be computed by considering the crowd density in the interval relative to "Ma" (standing for "Major"). If the same reference time used earlier is assumed, we have:

$$P(\rho \geq \rho_3) = \frac{t_1^{Ma} + t_2^{Ma}}{t_{ref}} = \frac{0.91 \text{ min} + 0.73 \text{ min}}{10 \text{ min}} = \frac{1.64 \text{ min}}{10 \text{ min}} = 0.16 \tag{7.3}$$

Obviously, the likelihood for an accident having major consequences is smaller than one having moderate consequences. Probability relative to any other given consequence can also be calculated in the same way.

It should be pointed out here that the duration of an incident is also an important factor when assessing risk. Even if density becomes high, there is little risk if the problem can be resolved instantly, while even medium density crowds can become high risk if they are allowed to remain so for a long period of time. This is properly reflected in the above calculations of probability. However, even though serious accidents rarely occurs, they can be underestimated if the reference time is set at too large a value. Consequently, the reference time should be kept short when sudden changes in density are expected to occur (e.g., if light rain is approaching during an open-air event and people are likely to move around more rapidly). If it is set at a long interval, countermeasures cannot be deployed in a timely manner, which also means that areas in which there are unexpected density fluctuations, such as connecting

Table 7.2 Likelihood and probability

Likelihood	Probability
Rare	Lower than 20%
Unlikely	Between 20% and 40%
Possible	Between 40% and 60%
Likely	Between 60% and 80%
Almost certain	Higher than 80%

routes between two sections, should be carefully monitored for any changes with shorter reference times.

Once the probability has been calculated using the methods above, the five-level likelihood considered here can be set according to the resulting probability. An example of this is shown in Table 7.2. Again, the boundaries proposed here are for reference, and actual values assigned to each level of likelihood will likely differ according to the nature of the event being assessed, so the levels should be given careful consideration before they are set.

Coming back to the example of Fig. 7.4 and employing Table 7.2, we can say that an event with moderate consequences is possible during the reference time (probability was 0.48, i.e., 48%) and an event with major consequences is rare (probability was 0.16, i.e., 16%). To simplify this example we did not explicitly compute the probability of events with minor and negligible consequences but we present the results here for completeness since these values will also be used during risk evaluation: "Minor" event probability is 71%, i.e., likely to occur and "negligible" events would almost certainly occur with 100% probability by definition (LOS A is the minimum level and therefore always present).

7.5.4 Risk Evaluation

Finally, the above results can be used to determine the risk level by using the matrix of Fig. 7.2. In our numerical example, the first calculation returned a possible likelihood with moderate consequences, thus resulting in level 3. On the other side, we also had a rare likelihood for major events, from which, using Fig. 7.2, we obtain level 2. Minor and negligible events correspond to a risk level of 2 and 1, respectively. To be conservative, we take the highest risk level, i.e., level 3, which tells us that the density profile considered in Fig. 7.4 represent a high risk scenario. Again, we would like to remind that the values used here are only for reference and crowd managers should set appropriate values taking into consideration the specifics of their scenario and the crowd involved (more discussions on this aspects will also follow later).

7.6 Limitations and Best Practices in Risk Assessment

Although we have already stressed out that the example presented above in addition to its related quantities and values are only meant for reference, we want to add a few words on limitations, alternatives, and future developments in regard to the presented risk assessment method.

7.6.1 Risk Assessment in Case of Sporadic Information

The density profile presented earlier in Fig. 7.4 represents a rather ideal situation in which data are collected continuously at very short intervals. However, in most of the cases, sensing data are provided with some delay and in a much more discrete manner. In these instances, the probability can be calculated from the values provided for each interval, as shown in the example of Fig. 7.5.

To make the example easier, we may assume that reliable sensors are used and estimated density is provided every minute, with the reference time t_{ref} being the same for the previous case (i.e., 10 min). Under these conditions, the calculation for the probability of an event of moderate consequences is as follows:

$$P(\rho \geq \rho_2) = \frac{t_4 + t_5 + t_6 + t_7 + t_8}{t_{\text{ref}}} = \frac{5 \text{ min}}{10 \text{ min}} = 0.5 \qquad (7.4)$$

Other consequences can be calculated in a similar manner as already presented before for Fig. 7.4. In the case of the density estimation from Fig. 7.5, we also have

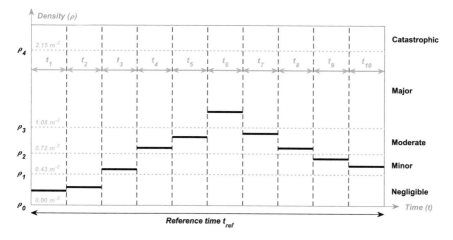

Fig. 7.5 Example on how to determine level of risk from a sensing system providing density at regular intervals

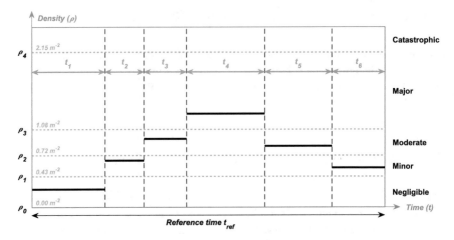

Fig. 7.6 Example on how to determine level of risk for systems in which interval is not constant

a risk level 3, corresponding to high risk (more in detail the results are: major event rare, moderate possible, minor likely, and negligible almost certain).

However, it is also possible that the sensing system cannot provide data on precisely scheduled intervals, like for the example shown in Fig. 7.6. This can occur for a variety of reasons, for example, in systems based on cameras where computational time could depend on a number of conditions or because of unexpected network problems (especially if data are transmitted using a mobile network that is shared by the visitors). Although it would be preferable to avoid such a condition and it is preferable to use many relatively short intervals rather than few long intervals, the risk level can still be calculated. For example, taking the previous reference time of 10 min, the probability of an event of moderate consequences will be:

$$P(\rho \geq \rho_2) = \frac{t_3 + t_4 + t_5}{t_{\text{ref}}} = \frac{1.20\,\text{min} + 2.20\,\text{min} + 1.90\,\text{min}}{10\,\text{min}} = 0.53 \quad (7.5)$$

Calculation of the risk level will follow as described above, leading also for this case to a level 3, i.e., a high risk.

7.6.2 Risk Assessment Using Multiple Quantities

In the examples above, we assumed for the sake of simplicity that risk assessment is based solely on crowd density. However, as often stated, speed and flow should be also considered in the same way of density, if possible. In other words, the analysis presented so far should be performed by considering all density, speed, and flow, while also adding additional quantities if available or needed. The same methodology will be applied for all quantities, thus resulting in a risk level for each. The worst outcome among the quantities considered will become the risk level in that section. For example, at a marathon start, density and speed may both lead to a risk level of 1, but flow may result in a higher risk level of 2, thus making the event at medium risk.

In regard to what explained above, we would like to remind that the risk of crowd incidents is high at major intersections and in passageways in which crowds can move freely in both directions, and this, although density may not be necessarily high. Historically, density has been the only factor in risk assessment for the sake of simplicity and because a better indicator is lacking at the moment, but the increasing precision of sensing technology will allow greater use of indicators other than density in the future. For example, the congestion index [8] briefly introduced in Chap. 4 has shown being a possible candidate to evaluate the condition of crowds with more fidelity compared to density alone and it may be particularly effective at evaluating scenarios like intersections and bottlenecks. In addition, the combination of congestion index and density may be an even better indicator for risk than density alone (both "crowdedness" and "smoothness" get mixed in this combination). However, more research is still needed to validate alternative approaches and find out their limitations, so care is always needed for newly presented quantities.

To complement the discussion above, it should be mentioned that, although, to some extent, some technologies are already existing and employed, in the future, it is likely that more subtle indicators acting as early warning alerts, such as the "mood" of a crowd, will increasingly be available through technologies such as image processing (or computer vision). Taking these sorts of psychological indicators into consideration will allow for more precise risk assessments to be carried out.

7.6.3   Choice of Numerical Values

In addition to what explained earlier, we should remind readers again, that values chosen here are not universal for any kind of location or event. In particular, the density related to a specific consequence as defined in Table 7.1 was based on the LOS for flat surfaces. If, for example, an area with a remarkable slope is considered, different values must be used since the potential to fall and result in a crowd accident is higher. If stairs are considered, even more conservative values are needed as the same density will result in much worst consequences should an accident occur.

7.6.4   Best Practices and Future Trends

In the previous example only one area close to the exit was used. However, ideally, the area targeted for crowd management, or, in other words, the whole surface where people are allowed to move should be divided up into, for example, 5 m square sections, and then chronological data from sensors and/or simulation would be calculated for each section. Using the results gained for a reference time of, say, 10 min, the likelihoods corresponding to the five consequence scenarios will be computed for that period of time and for each section. In the next step, the matrix of Fig. 7.2 will be used to define the risk level corresponding to each likelihood-consequence combination, with the item with the highest risk level defining the risk level in each section. This would allow to create a chessboard-like map of risks covering the whole facility in detail, which could be readily read and understood. The maximum level among all sections can determine the overall risk level, which we may also define as the level of alert. Ideally, this process is repeated every time new data are obtained from the sensors.

7.6.5 Taking Special Conditions into Account

To complete the discussion on limitations and ways to address shortcomings, it should be also noted that regions/sections with high density are clearly dangerous, but high density areas should be considered with an even higher risk when they are spread across different, smaller locations. This is because the presence of multiple small spots (usually only a few meters square) of high-density crowds tends to exacerbate the risk across the whole area. Also, it should be noted that multiple smaller risks may combine and accumulate, resulting in a knock-on effect that develops into a more serious situation. This cannot be predicted using historical data, which makes near-future prediction vital. This is also where human judgment comes into account when analyzing the results of risk assessment; experienced personnel will be able to "feel" risky situations by qualitatively interpreting the results, but it is important that they have access to reliable data (especially in case of large infrastructure where it is impossible or very difficult to visually monitor every location simply looking through the cameras). As an example for what discussed here, small issues such as equipment failure or a lack of communication prior to the event may accumulate into a larger risk over time as we have seen in Chap. 3. This means that is important to simulate the crowd across a variety of scenarios and for the organizer and crowd manager to have the logical ability to trace the effects of various causal relationships.

In this context, we should remind that not only the risk level, but also the difficulty in reducing it should be considered in the frame of the risk assessment. Response to any problems that may arise while dealing with the crowd is different with some issues being easy and other difficult to control. If controlling a problem is difficult, it is important to prevent it from occurring wherever possible. Although in some cases, the difficulty in solving a problem may be accounted by increasing its consequence, there are also many situations where this sort of issue cannot be assessed using the approach presented earlier based on the likelihood-consequence matrix. In these cases, the risk level will need to be determined directly.

7.6.6 Risk Assessment Diversification

Finally, it should be reminded that any successful safety protocol relies on diversity, redundancy and independence among the methods/systems used [9]. While redundancy and independence is actually related to the safety system itself (e.g., a backup system is always required should the main fail and a power generator is needed to become independent on electric supply in case of blackout), diversity also applies to the risk assessment method discussed here. For this reason, we would like to point out that the method for risk level calculation described in this chapter is only a single approach for using changes in density data to assess future risks, and crowd management that considers alternative methods to compute risks is needed in reality. In this sense, for example, having a protocol to evaluate the qualitative feedback from the staff on site could help making an alternative risk assessment.

7.6.7 Risk Assessment Accounting for Secondary Elements

To conclude the discussion in regard to risk assessment, we would like to move beyond the crowd and also consider secondary elements that should also be taken into consideration when performing the final evaluation. Here, we will focus on a method to combine primary crowd intrinsic risk with secondary elements, but a more detailed discussion on factors affecting crowd events will follow in the next chapter.

There are risk factors that are not directly associated to the crowd itself and are somehow secondary (but not negligible) in respect to the specific area/location considered. For example, weather, road closures, traffic conditions, train cancellations, and other elements can all have a great impact on the flow of people in any given area. Although the nature of such risks is very different, we would like to point out that the same methodology presented can be employed and may be implemented within the best-practice risk assessment system discussed above.

For instance, the risk level for a thunderstorm affecting an open-air festival is more closely related to weather forecast information than crowd condition observed as the storm approaches. So, if weather forecast predicts a thunderstorm with lightnings and hail with 80% probability in a short time, then we can assess its likelihood as "likely" and the consequence as "major," thus leading to a risk level of 4 and requiring immediate action. Similarly, if the threat of a terror attack is concerned, events having a political or religions meaning are more likely to become a target and the likelihood of an accident will be higher than for an academic conference, although consequences may be similar.

In addition to the previous example on weather, Table 7.3 also provides a more complete example where risk assessment is performed considering several secondary elements. As the example of Table 7.3 shows, sometimes it is not easy to consider each element separately and correlation among them often occur. For instance, hot weather itself already represents a health concern but has also an effect on intoxication as alcohol tends to dehydrate the body thus posing an even higher health risk on hot

Table 7.3 Risk level calculation example for an imaginary event in which several elements are taken into consideration. In this case, the risk level of the event is 3 (high risk) with health concerns representing the most critical issue. In this case, weather and transportation conditions could be estimated and predicted automatically through third services (weather forecast, traffic information), while violence, health, and intoxication would be treated as "static" elements

Element	Weather	Transportation	Crowd condition
Risk	Natural disasters	Service interruption, road closure, congestion, etc.	High density etc.
Condition	Forecast predicting clouds with occasional light rain, quite high temperatures	Train service often delayed or suspended but access by road usually available; most people will arrive by car	Undelimited area; crowd density is predicted to be low in general and medium at peaks
Likelihood	Unlikely	Likely	Rare
Consequence	Moderate	Minor	Minor
Risk level	2 (medium)	2 (medium)	1 (low)
Element	Violence	Health	Intoxication
Risk	Fights between participants, attacks, aggressions, etc.	Sickness, loss of consciousness, etc.	Unpredictable behaviors, health concerns, etc.
Condition	Episodes of violence have been rarely reported for similar events	Relatively large proportion of elderlies, heatstroke possible due to hot weather	Alcoholic beverage not sold on site, carry-in allowed but possibly limited to few people
Likelihood	Unlikely	Possible	Rare
Consequence	Moderate	Major	Minor
Risk level	2 (medium)	3 (high)	1 (low)

weather. In addition, high crowd densities are likely to be more dangerous under high temperatures. On the other side, a compact crowd may help heating up the body at very low temperatures but isolated individuals are at risk. Also, slippery surfaces become an important problem at low temperatures (several accidents occurred in these conditions). In short, both low and high temperatures represent risk factors for crowds. Similarly, a thunderstorm will directly affect the crowd but can also disrupt transportation and create health concerns (people may get wet if outdoor, which is particularly worrying at low temperatures). More on the risk elements that need to be considered, the effect they may have on an event and their correlation will be discussed in the following chapter.

When secondary elements are implemented it may not be possible to automatically update all of them. For instance, real-time weather conditions are easy to obtain and forecast services are often provided by reliable sources. Traffic conditions are also usually available for important connections, with congestion prediction possible and sometimes available through public or private services. However, violence or health conditions cannot be monitored easily or can only be provided as a form of verbal feedback from staff on site.

It is however possible to combine variable secondary elements with "static" ones that may be only available as a result of the evaluations performed during off-site risk assessment during planning. In this case, a risk level will be associated to each element, with "static" ones taking a value associated beforehand and considered as not changing during the event. When secondary information (both dynamic and static) is combined with data gained through sensors analyzing the intrinsic state of the crowd, the maximum risk level among all secondary elements and the crowd state will be used to define the level of alert (similarly to the example of Table 7.3).

7.7   From Risk Assessment to Crowd Control

Most of what outlined above only concerned risk assessment. However, obviously, once a risk has been identified and evaluated, crowd control is needed to minimize it. In this context, it is important that crowd control strategies or methods put into place are proportional to the assessed risk level in order to efficiently reduce it. As a general rule, higher risk levels require higher levels of control. This fundamental rule also combines to what already discussed in Chap. 6: Crowd control has to be designed in a progressive way in which "soft" solutions (such as simple, static information provision) are employed for low risks at the earlier stages and "hard" solutions (barricades or flow control for example) are gradually introduced if risk cannot be reduced. However, this also means that when risks get higher, multiple methods of crowd control, such as a mixture of information provision and guidance, have to be used in combination in order to be effective. While static information provision does not require human resources, higher levels of crowd control increasingly require numerous and specialized personnel. It is therefore important that human resources is planned in detail and people are able to take multiple and different roles if needed. For example, people working at information desks should be prepared to set up simple partitions to divide flow of people, set up queuing arrangements or extinguish small fires if necessary. Of course, for large-scale disasters police and/or firefighters will be called to assist and will take over in dealing with very dangerous situations, but, as already stated, risk management relies on preventive measures, so keeping people away from a small fire and extinguish it before it gets bigger can definitely prevent catastrophic outcomes. If properly designed, this sort of crowd control can eventually reduce risk by one or more levels.

At the planning stage for off-site crowd management, numerous scenarios should be created during preliminary evaluations, a large number of crowd simulations performed and the type of crowd control needed for each scenario considered accordingly. It is important to discuss various what-if and worst-case scenarios with stakeholders, in order to thoroughly identify and share the points at which risk could potentially occur. In particular, it should be clear for everyone which stakeholder will be responsible for a specific crowd control measure and which tasks can be partially shared by multiple stakeholders. As discussed above, extinguishing a fire is clearly a responsibility of firefighters in the same way as keeping under control a violent crowd is a role proper of the police, but it is important that other stakeholders (organizers or facility security for instance) can help when risk is still low: by extinguishing a small fire or start dividing fans from opposite teams if tension is perceived (but not yet seen in form of violence).

In some sense, it may be also useful to evaluate the risk that a crowd control strategy could fail due to human error, to evaluate which strategy is more likely to require alternative approaches or a larger amount of human resources. There are several factors that are known to contribute in increasing the likelihood that a person or a team may fail in carrying a task. Among the most relevant ones we may consider: time available, task complexity, stress, procedural guidance, training and experience, environment and human–machine interface (if applies) [10]. Although those factors can and should be used to identify which control strategy is more demanding for personnel (and thus more likely to fail), the same can be also be used to make the same strategy less demanding (and thus more likely to succeed). In short, if a strategy is likely to fail or would require too much human resources, both methods to improve it and alternatives should be investigated.

References

1. International Organization for Standardization: ISO 31000: Risk Management (2018)
2. Mitsubishi Electric Corporation: Mitsubishi Electric Develops World's First Real-Time Crowd-Congestion Estimation System. http://www.mitsubishielectric.com/news/2016/pdf/0818-b.pdf (2016). (online; accessed 17 March 2017)
3. Molyneaux, N., Scarinci, R., Bierlaire, M.: Design and analysis of control strategies for pedestrian flows. Transportation, 1–41 (2020). https://doi.org/10.1007/s11116-020-10111-1
4. Lopez-Carmona, M.A., Garcia, A.P.: Cellevac: An adaptive guidance system for crowd evacuation through behavioral optimization. Safety Sci. **139**, 105215 (2021). https://doi.org/10.1016/j.ssci.2021.105215
5. Thaeler, J.J., Patel, A.P.: Crowd Prediction and Attendance Forecasting (2014). US Patent 8,768,867
6. Anthony (Tony) Cox Jr, L.: What's wrong with risk matrices? Risk Anal.: Int. J. **28**(2), 497–512 (2008). https://doi.org/10.1111/j.1539-6924.2008.01030.x
7. Murakami, H., Feliciani, C., Shimura, K., Nishinari, K.: A system for efficient egress scheduling during mass events and small-scale experimental demonstration. Royal Soc. Open Sci. **7**(12), 201465 (2020). https://doi.org/10.1098/rsos.201465
8. Zanlungo, F., Feliciani, C., Yucel, Z., Nishinari, K., Kanda, T.: A pure number to assess "congestion" in pedestrian crowds
9. Littlewood, B., Strigini, L.: Redundancy and diversity in security. In: European Symposium on Research in Computer Security, pp. 423–438. Springer (2004). https://doi.org/10.1007/978-3-540-30108-0_26
10. Blackman, H.S., Gertman, D.I., Boring, R.L.: Human error quantification using performance shaping factors in the spar-h method. In: Proceedings of the Human Factors and Ergonomics Society Annual Meeting, vol. 52. SAGE Publications Sage CA, Los Angeles, CA, pp. 1733–1737 (2008). https://doi.org/10.1177/154193120805202109

Chapter 8
Planning of Mass Gatherings and Large Events

Abstract Planning an event or preparing for the opening of a new facility is not an easy task and requires months or years of preparation and a continuous discussion between all stakeholders. While crowd sensing and simulation is a technical work, requiring theoretical knowledge and know-how expertise, planning largely rely on experience and accumulated feedback from previous or similar events. Although it is impossible to list all elements that require attention while planning, there are some problematics on which crowd managers are often confronted. In particular two aspects are important during planning: (1) understanding the conditions under which an event is held and (2) setting up operating modes specific for those conditions. After addressing both aspects, a risk assessment is needed for both normal and abnormal operation and, if risk is judged too high, the analysis on conditions and operating modes is repeated until an acceptable risk level is reached. This chapter discusses relatively general aspects related to planning, while addressing more in details conditions and operating modes requiring particular attention.

8.1 Introduction

In the previous chapters, we examined all the methods and tools available to crowd managers. It is now time to discuss how these tools and methods can be used during off-site crowd management. But let us first provide a more comprehensive definition for off-site crowd management: this comprehends the set of decisions and actions performed in the preparatory stage before the start of the event, and is commonly referred to as "planning". In broad terms, it should be thought of as an activity that is performed between each event. In other words, it is an important part of the feedback process that involves analyzing the experience and data gained from past events, and reflecting on how they can be incorporated into better planning for the next event.

In this chapter, we will look at a summary of how to implement planning and consider the points that should be part of the actual planning process. Like for all activities involved in crowd management, also planning should be a comprehensive process, involving all stakeholders and considering a macroscopic perspective, and, as such, it should incorporate all of the points that we have looked at so far.

In presenting the problematics encountered during the planning phase we tried to consider the most common events and scenarios, but, obviously, every case is different and need to be considered in detail taking into account all peculiarities of the location, the crowd and other factors. Also, we should point out that although this chapter focus specifically on event planning, the preparatory phase leading to the opening of a new shopping mall, for example, is not much different and in that sense the presentation that follow may also help for such kind of scenarios.

8.2   Objectives of This Chapter

Being the concluding chapter of this book (the next final chapter only provides a succinct review on the most important points of crowd management), the reader should be able to get a more complete image on crowd management and understand how the mostly theoretical topics discussed so far relates when planning for an event. This chapter should provide starting points from which each reader can build her/his own plan and prepare for an event. In that sense, one of the aims of this chapter is to help readers eventually identify weak points and make use of the methods presented in the previous chapters to address them. In addition, this chapter aims at clarifying temporal and organizational elements related to event planning, helping readers to set up a timeline and create committees to achieve organizational goals with sufficient margin of time and eventually leading to a successful event.

8.3   Planning Approach

The first thing we should consider is when to start the planning process. In ultra-large-scale events such as the Olympic and Paralympic Games, the process is started more than four years before the next event begins. For annual events that are held on a regular basis, such as firework festivals, the process of reflection and the consideration of necessary changes often begin as soon as the previous event finishes. In the case of one-off events at which thousands of people are expected to gather, preparation should begin a year in advance (six months at the latest), but preparations should be started as soon as is feasible, especially if it looks like it will take time to manage the expectations of stakeholders. Even when doing something such as re-opening regular service at a large department store, crowd flow lines need to be checked during the floor plan creation stage in order to identify risks. Consideration should also be given at this point to areas in which stagnation is likely to occur, in order to reduce waiting times and implement higher levels of service.

The most important part of the planning process is conducting thorough risk assessments in advance, in order to eliminate the possibility that potential risk will turn into real threats and to keep risk levels under control. Typically, the planning process proceeds as shown in Fig. 8.1.

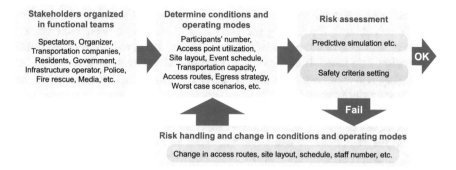

Fig. 8.1 The planning flow

The first part of this process is creating a list of all concerned stakeholders. Stakeholders will vary from event to event but, as mentioned in Chap. 1, they will most likely include visitors, facility personnel, transportation companies, local residents, the government (at various levels), event organizers, site security, emergency services, and the media. The next step is to select representatives of the stakeholders to form dedicated teams. Rather than having a single team that represents all stakeholders at once, these teams should be divided according to their function and purpose, such as ensuring smooth transportation or implementing security. Each team should be composed of representatives from every stakeholder that has relevant information for each subject.

In most of the cases, there should be a transportation team that is involved with the movement of people, an operations team that runs the venue, a security team, and a service team. This means that, for example, the transport team should include stakeholders that include event organizers, public transportation operators, the venue management company, and representatives from the security team. Additionally, each time should have a designated leader who can periodically meet with the leaders of the other teams to discuss the planning in detail, and share information with other stakeholders so that they can proceed with their own reviews. For reference, in the case of the 2020 Tokyo Olympics and Paralympic Games, stakeholders were divided into a total of 52 separate teams (referred to as "functional areas"), and the ones that were closely related to crowd management are as follows.

- Venue management (safe and efficient operations, crisis management)
- Event service (defining pedestrian routes, managing crowd flow)
- Security (event security, access control, emergency crisis management)
- Signage (creating and managing signs for venues and surrounding areas)
- Transportation (providing smooth mobility services, managing traffic)
- City operations (coordination with municipal governments, maintaining normal operations of host cities or communities).

The next stage of the process is to determine the given conditions that will form the basis of crowd management, such as number of expected visitors, and use this information to determine parameters for operations, such as the design of visitor flow lines. In this context, the term "given conditions" includes the event's content and schedule, venue layout, number of visitors, closest transportation links, and other information. The schedule of the event is usually decided by the organizer, but care must be taken to avoid rushed or unreasonable timings and, of course, safety should be given top priority at all times.

The (given) conditions can be determined in a number of ways that we will not detail here, but should include not only reflecting on lessons learned from similar events in the past, but also using questionnaires to profile potential visitors or to predict, among others, what are the expectations from visitors or which image local residents have on the event and how they plan to change their routine when the event will be held. When it comes to set conditions related to transportation and local traffic, but also to grasp the profile of local users, the use of mobile phone location data to estimate the movement of people on a regional basis and get a first-hand image on their attributes have become common in recent years.

Setting up the conditions of an event strongly relates on the image that the organizer has of that event and therefore, rather than being set by the crowd management team, most of the details will be considered as part of the natural path along the event planning process, unless there are particularly unexpected circumstances.

Next, taking the given conditions as static properties defining the boundaries within an event that must be managed, the so-called operating modes are created, which should dynamically ensure (through crowd and environment control) that those boundaries are never exceeded. Operating modes include visitor flow lines, control methods for admission and exit, guidance and crowd control, both inside and outside the venue. Guidance implementation should consider visitor attributes such as age and cultural background, and people with disabilities should be accounted for when drawing up plans for access methods. It should also be noted that the flow of people can vary a great deal depending on whether the venue is indoors or outdoors, and the timing of the event. If, for example, the event is due to take place during evening rush hour, it will be necessary to coordinate with local residents and commuters. All of these many variables will need to be taken into consideration when planning the operation of the event.

Furthermore, given that these conditions and their implementation may change during the planning process and alter the level of associated risk, it is advisable to estimate the conditions as accurately as possible and then provisionally set the operating modes before proceeding with the risk assessment. At any rate, allowing a certain amount of leeway is necessary when considering the conditions. It is important to consider multiple possibilities for flow lines, station share ratios, entrance/exit positioning, and so on, as this will make it possible to maintain flexibility throughout the planning process.

It is especially important to consider a range of what-if scenarios when considering operating modes, such as emergency planning for fire or earthquake evacuations, or problems with the operation of the transportation system. There are many potential factors at play, of course, but all teams must consider some abnormal operations and make sure that everyone is mindful of worst-case scenarios.

This makes it possible to conduct risk assessments at the same time as defining the conditions and their implementation as operating modes. At this scope, using available data and conditions to create scenarios to be simulated through crowd simulations can be a solid approach in order to see if there are any problems with proposed operating modes. However, given that it is not always possible to perform detailed crowd simulations due to time, budget, or technical constraints, the alternative methods that are described below can be used to make estimations. Furthermore, as an alternative to simulations, social experiments or small-scale experiments with human participants can be performed in advance at the venue for the scope of risk assessments. For example, the time taken to check visitors' luggage can be better estimated by performing tests on-site rather than by simulation.

If the risk assessment concludes that there is no risk at all, then the planning process is complete. However, a one-time assessment cannot normally be expected to produce such an optimistic result. In the event that this does happen, it may be because the margins specified in the conditions and operating modes are too large, and the assessment should be performed again under tighter and more stringent conditions.

If certain areas are particularly high-risk, risk reduction countermeasures must be implemented in each area in order to ensure that the established risk criteria are met. It may be necessary, therefore, to reconsider the placement of visitor flow lines and/or the positions of entrances and exits. In some instances, it may also be necessary to restrict the number of visitors by limiting ticket sales. This loop, of performing risk assessments again after any changes are made to conditions or operating modes, should be repeated many times, until all stakeholders are satisfied that all problems have been mitigated. We will take a closer look at the planning process itself in the following sections.

8.4 Setting Conditions and Operating Modes

After all the relevant teams of stakeholder have been created, the first task is to determine the conditions under which the event will be held. For sporting events, these will include various related data, such as the competition schedule, number of visitors, passenger share for stations that are used (i.e., the proportion of visitors using a specific station when several stations give access to the venue), background traffic volumes, and layouts of other venues. Depending on the nature of the data available, multiple teams will need to cooperate to share the information necessary to make the needed decisions (see Table 8.1). Depending on the constraints of the event, flow lines configuration may become a condition (such if there is a single road linking the only access point to the venue, providing little alternatives to the use of access routes), but, most of the time, only "static" data are to be used as conditions and aspects such as flow lines should be later determined based on those fixed conditions (for instance, dividing both in- and outflow along the single route may be considered as part of the operating modes).

Table 8.1 Examples of stakeholders that are associated with various conditions and operating modes

Condition/ operating mode	Relevant information and decision-making	Related stakeholders
Conditions		
Guest number	Audience: managed by the number of tickets, maximum seats at the venue, station(s) capacity; visitors: non-ticket holders estimates based on similar events	Visitors, facilities, transportation, media, etc.
Guest attributes	Mobile information data, registration in dedicated online service, image recognition by camera, etc.	
Traffic generated from commuting people	Survey of the number of employees working at nearby companies, or the number of people who pass through station ticket gates on weekdays	Local residents, transportation, operations, media, etc.
Resident-generated traffic	Determined using municipal demographic data, etc.	
Entrances/exits	Refer to flow lines and queuing spaces inside and outside the venue	Facilities, sponsors, security, etc.
Toilets	Consider additional temporary toilets (number/position) and refer to event schedule	
Operating modes		
External flow lines	Determined based on the passenger share of each nearby station, the width of the sidewalk, the presence of traffic lights, etc.	Visitors, facilities, transportation, security, sponsors, media, etc.
Internal flow lines	Eliminate counterflows and intersections, consider impact of bottlenecks	
Access control	Entry: determine priority, prepare group gates; exit: simultaneous exit, staged exit	Organizer, transportation, security, etc.

8.4.1 *Conditions*

Condition 1: Schedule

The event schedule is a prerequisite for crowd management, and is usually set by the organizer or sponsors based on factors such as the performers involved or broadcast time. In practice, however, the schedule is sometimes set without taking the requirements of crowd management into consideration. It is therefore essential to be prepared to operate under conditions that are unfavorable. Furthermore, if more than one event is scheduled per day at the venue, this will require audience changes (empty the venue to later accommodate the next audience) that will cause confusion if the flow lines in the venue are not properly laid out. Holding several events with continuous changes in audience gets more difficult when a venue is a long way from transportation links. For example, if shuttle buses must be provided as part of the crowd flow lines, setting up a proper service in line with events' schedule and train timetable is not an easy task and require close collaboration between multiple stakeholders. The situation becomes even more complicated if there are other events being held nearby at the same time of the main event that is being planned. It would be best to avoid these sorts of issues if possible, but there will always be cases when complications are unavoidable for various reasons, so it is important to be able to include this condition in the final review and proceed as necessary. Then, once the risk assessment has been performed, if this kind of complication poses a high risk that cannot be avoided, consider prioritizing safety and changing the schedule of the event(s). With this in mind, it is important to set stakeholders' expectations in advance and make them aware that safety should always have highest priority.

Condition 2: Visitors' number

The number of expected visitors is a particularly important condition and needs to be estimated with a high degree of accuracy. This should be determined not only by looking at the capacity of the venue, but at past events and the relative appeal of this event in particular. For venues that do not have seats, capacity can be estimated by available area, and a limit set at, for example, 0.5 people per square meter, in order to make a simple estimation of the maximum capacity. Although it is possible to manage the number of visitors by restricting the issuance of tickets, there may be those who come to buy tickets at the venue or come for the spectacle even without a ticket, which can be difficult to factor into estimates. This is why there have been recent trials of using mobile phone location data to estimate the number of visitors by looking at the number of people moving between regions. If there is any uncertainty about attendance levels, it is important to always err on the side of higher potential risk, and set the number of attendees as slightly higher than expected.

Condition 3: Visitors' attributes

Crowd management needs to be based on an understanding not only of the number of visitors but also the attributes of those who will be attending an event. In particular, factors such as age, gender, cultural identity, grouping patterns (the presence of families or social groups, etc.), disabilities, whether those attending are likely to have luggage, and how well guests know the area (if they have visited before or not), are all known to have a sizable influence on crowd flows.

It is possible to have a rough understanding of the age and gender of fans at, for example, a concert for a singer, but this is more difficult to predict at sporting events. Additionally, since there is a high probability that groups will stay together once they arrive, it may be necessary to take measures such as setting up dedicated routes or gates for them in advance if large groups are expected. If people from foreign countries are likely to attend the event, multilingual signs and information provision should be considered (by possibly also adding a system of symbols universally understood). Accessibility should be ensured for people with disabilities, and dedicated barrier-free routes should be considered. In recent years there has also been an increase in the number of people carrying large luggage such as suitcases and, just as is the case for people with strollers, this can have a major impact on flow because of the large area they take up.

Visitors' familiarity with the area around the venue will also have a major impact on crowd flows. If a large number of attendees are likely to be unfamiliar with the location, many signs and guides will be needed at road junctions, since visitors who are unfamiliar with the venue will increase congestion when they search for their seats or for the toilets. On the other hand, those who are familiar with the venue may not follow the flow lines set out in planning, and may decide to take the shortest possible route to their destination. This causes disturbances in the movement of people around them, which is undesirable from the perspective of crowd management. It is therefore necessary to put additional countermeasures in place, such as increased security in high-risk areas.

Condition 4: Volume of background traffic

Those inside the venue are not the only people with a connection to the event. Nearby companies and those who work for them are also stakeholders, and should be included as targets of crowd management. The flow of these people is referred to as "background traffic" and, when they occupy the same paths that are used for visitor traffic flow, estimating their flow is an important condition. The combination of local users and visitors is also challenging in relation to the points discussed above as local users are likely to stick to habits, while first-time visitors will follow signs and use navigation services. In this sense, it is also a responsibility of management to ensure that people around the event are not disturbed by congestion. This can be worked out to a certain extent, based on demographic data, daily surveys, and surveying local companies. It is also important to note that background traffic volume is different on weekdays, weekends, and holidays. It is necessary to accommodate this through operational measures, such as reserving part of any active flow lines for background traffic volume.

Condition 5: Venue-related data

Data about the venue, such as the width of internal and external passageways, the positioning of stairs, information about bottlenecks and other obstacles, and the space that is available for static crowd, are all essential conditions. Furthermore, routes for stakeholders and VIPs will need to be prioritized, as well as the logistics for loading and unloading at the venue, which means that these also need to be considered as conditions. On this scope, it is important to provide several type of maps each easily understandable by each stakeholder and organization involved. Companies involved in the logistics need to know parking space for trucks, internal storage space and the size of freight gates. Guidance personnel will need a completely different type of map, where access routes, flow lines, toilets or medical assistance location are clearly recognizable. The complete and often complex map providing any sort of information should be used only within the company managing the facility by personnel familiar with its details.

Additionally, gates and security checks are usually present at the entrances of venues at which events are held. Entrance gates need to be evaluated in detail, in terms of their effect on crowd density, risk and service level. Information such as the number and location of gates, their processing capacities, and their opening times, are therefore required conditions, and additional gates should be added if deemed necessary after evaluation.

8.4.2 Operating Modes

Once all the conditions have been set in the manner outline above, the next step is to begin evaluating the operating modes based on the available data. The important thing at this stage is deciding on visitor flow lines and the operating modes to be implemented for guests entering and leaving the venue.

Operating mode 1: Visitor flow lines

Some or all of the flow lines may be set as a condition when there are constraints in place on operations. However, typically, designing routes for safe movement from the station to the event, and lines within the venue itself, is fundamentally a core part of the operational review process. Deciding where to place security guards along the flow lines is also a necessary part of their design. Their placement should be decided through cooperation between the organizer, facility manager, and the transportation, operations and security teams. Information on road closures or construction, and construction plans for nearby commercial facilities and other structures is an extremely important part of this process, which means that it is necessary to gather the relevant data and use it as the basis of the discussion between stakeholders.

It if fundamental that routes are set so that the flow lines for entry and exit do not intersect, so as to avoid confusion (and congestion) between the paths. Security guards and signs need to be placed at points of intersection, branching, and accumulation. Routes to be used by fire and rescue service, stakeholder and VIP access should be prioritized in the decision-making process and set at an early stage, and flow lines for general visitors should be set around them.

If there are multiple public transport stations near the event venue, the number of visitors that will be arriving from each station and their relative share will need to be predicted in advance. This information is often set as a condition, but it may also be decided on when planning operations. Knowing this information allows traffic flow lines to be set with the number of passengers at each station and the width of the nearby sidewalks in mind. It is helpful if there is data available from similar events in the past, but if this information does not exist then the values should be considered as a range of possible numbers.

Visitors will stay on sidewalks if they are close to the venue, but they may need to cross the road at intersections with signals. If this is the case, they will be stopped at the red light for a period of time, and it is important to be careful about the accumulation that can occur. In order to prevent a large number of people from accumulating in a small space, consideration must always be given to the available waiting areas when setting flow lines. If there is little space available, it may be necessary to restrict traffic, stop cars, or fully pedestrianize an area. However, this will have a great impact on logistics and the movement of local residents, which means it is important to carefully consider the issue with stakeholders before implementing traffic restrictions.

If the venue is a long way from the nearest station and many people use their cars to go there, parking at the venue may reach capacity, which means that it is usually necessary for the organizer to operate a shuttle bus service (or found some extra parking space). When a shuttle bus service is implemented, it is important to set the bus operation system so that it matches the event schedule and venue capacity. It is also important to keep in mind the route between the bus stops, station, and venue, and the space that is available for accumulation while people wait for buses.

It is also necessary to check to see whether other events are planned in the vicinity of the venue. If other events will be happening, it is important to design flow lines for each event so that they do not intersect, and those involved in organizing the other events should be included in the stakeholder discussion.

Next, consider flow lines in the venue. Venues have many bottlenecks, such as narrow sidewalks, obstacles, and stairs, and it is important to design routes that avoid them as much as possible. Safety should always be given top priority, even if this means planning a deliberate detour. The location and number of toilets and restaurants are also important to consider when planning internal flow lines. It is necessary to ensure that accumulation area for those queuing for facilities are kept separate from flow lines, because the lines that form may disturb the flow of other crowds. When merchandise is being sold at the venue, the location and number of vendors should be carefully considered. Long lines may occur here, which means that it is important to not only design flow lines around queues, but also to decide the number of vendors that are needed to meet visitors' needs and ensure that they do not have to wait for an excessive amount of time. Furthermore, wheelchair users will need routes that do not have steps and that allow smooth mobility, both inside and outside the venue.

As a general rule, the movement of people inside and outside the venue should not be considered independently of one another. It is best practice to set routes optimally as a coherent whole, so that the flow line from the station to the seat in the venue and vice versa intersect as little as possible.

Operating mode 2: Entrances and exits

The next step is to decide how the entrances and exits to the venue will operate, as these form the contact point between the exterior and interior of the venue. Ticketing and security checks are usually performed at venue entrances, which means there is a high possibility of large groups of people accumulating around them, depending on the time of the day. It is possible to use the data gained while examining conditions regarding the number of gates, their processing capacity, and the distribution of visitor arrival to make an approximate estimate of the number of people that will be accumulating at the gates. Queuing theory and crowd simulation can also be used to gain some idea of the number of people and how long they will be waiting, and this information can be checked against whether there is enough available space to accommodate the people who will be waiting in line. It is also necessary to consider how the queues will be arranged at the entrances, in terms of how they will be lined up, and whether there should be priority or group lanes available.

Furthermore, consideration should be given to what happens to people who are not permitted entry at the gate, such as when, for example, a visitor has an error on their ticket, or it is invalid. In these instances, if the gates need to be passed as again after their tickets are checked, the waiting time for the queue behind them will keep growing. It is therefore desirable to guide these visitors to a separate area for responding to unusual circumstances, in order to obstruct the main flow of guests as little as possible.

Operating mode 3: Internal venue operations

If the capacity of the exits or the nearby station(s) is limited, leaving the venue simultaneously will expose visitors to danger. In these instances, it is possible to divide the audience into blocks and have them exit in order for safety reasons. This can be done at events where the audience is seated, where their exit can be staggered according to, for example, the blocks in which they are seated. If timing is accurately chosen, crowd density can be reduced without having a large influence on total egress time [1]. However, in those sports where the result is known (or quite clear) before the end of the game, some spectators will leave before the end of the game. In these cases, it is relatively uncommon for everyone to leave at the same time but, at the end of a concert by a singer, it is likely that all the spectators will leave simultaneously. For sporting events it should be also reminded that people movements may depend on the result of the match and that this may change in unpredictable ways, so a flexible a approach is required. Operating modes can be set by paying attention to this kind of event attribute. In regard to what said earlier, security should be in high alert at the end of a game as people leaving may suddenly try to re-enter if the result suddenly change.

Controlling entrance to the venue is generally difficult, but it is possible to make predictions about the distribution of arrivals by looking at the timetables of nearby stations and judging from past experience. It should also be noted that if there are a lot of unreserved seats, many people will begin to line up for the event early. Anticipating this kind of entrance and exit distribution is an important part of crowd simulation.

Furthermore, if it looks likely that there will be an increase in the number of visitors, it is necessary to decide on various operational responses, such as preparing additional seats or standing areas and providing protection from the heat or rain when the event is held outdoors. Apart from this, other crowd behavior policies should be well-defined and clearly communicated to visitors. Rules about alcohol sales, re-entry, left luggage, and smoking areas are examples of the important points that will need to be discussed.

Additionally, it is important to take extra care when the venue is used for multiple purposes. For example, when a venue is used for multiple events in one day, the flow of people may change a great deal depending on the nature of each event. If bulky materials are to be loaded and unloaded due to changes in event fixings, truck flow lines will also need to be secured. Attention should be paid not only to fixed operations, but to time-sensitive changes in operating schedules.

It is also necessary to prepare the infrastructure that is needed to provide information to visitors, through such methods as bulletins, internet pages, and public broadcasts.

The nature of the operating modes described above may be partly determined by cost and time, as well as administrative restrictions such as noise regulations. The number of security guards that can be deployed and the available communication methods are also often determined by budget. Taking such operational constraints into account allows for better facility design and flow line planning.

8.5 Risk Assessment for Normal Operation

The next stage is to perform risk assessment for normal operation. On this purpose density needs to be estimated in various places and at different moments considering multiple possible scenarios. At this point we should note that, in contrast to the on-site approach discussed in the previous chapter, where density was accurately known; in the off-site risk assessment presented here only (rough) estimates for crowd densities are possible. It is however important to set up scenarios that are as realistic as possible, while being slightly conservative, to ensure a reliable risk assessment.

Simulators may become useful on this purpose, but, when not available, alternative methods are needed. One approach would be to use historical data from previous, similar events, but, such data may not always be available. For recurring events it is usually easy to get access to such data, and it is therefore essential that a feedback is kept after each event (possibly both in form of numerical and qualitative information). It is not rare that data on previous or similar events is available but poorly maintained, making it difficult to perform a reliable risk assessment. For new events or when a new location is used, it is important to look for similar locations or events elsewhere. It is usually always possible to find comparable cases and simulation results from a number of realistic scenarios can be combined with data collected from various sources to get a more complete and accurate image. For new locations/events, diversifying the source of information can help getting a better idea on what is possibly easy to predict and what is largely influenced by the specific conditions occurring on-site. On this scope, any piece of information can be useful in identifying dangerous areas in advance.

In addition to the complex simulators, a simple, alternative method only relying on predicted in- and outflow of visitors may be also used to get a rough estimate of crowd density. By estimating the number of people going into and leaving a facility it is possible to obtain the number of occupants at any given time, as presented in Fig. 8.2. On this purpose, the event schedule can also play an important role in creating an approximate and yet reliable estimate on how many people will move in and out at specific times. This sort of calculation can be easily done by using a simple spreadsheet software. Finally, by dividing the area's total space by the number of people, a rough estimate of density can be obtained, which allows to determine the risk level. In other words, it can be used to check the balance of flows at bottlenecks to find where imbalances between entry and exit are likely to cause lines of waiting people, such as entrances, stairs, security check, toilets, kiosks, parking lots, pedestrian crossings, and station platform. This also allows time to be factored into risk assessments for potentially dangerous areas. As the numeric example of Fig. 8.2 shows (and discussed earlier), people tend to arrive gradually before an event starts but usually leave almost simultaneously around the closing time (obviously, this also depends on the nature of the event).

Once density has been estimated, the risk level has to be determined. Since crowd conditions are very difficult to be predicted in advance an approach like the one described in Chap. 7 for on-site risk assessment is not possible. For this reason, off-site risk assessment for normal operation is often simply done by using the Level of Service (LOS) described in Chap. 2 to work out maximum crowd densities for each location. Put simply, this method of risk assessment estimates fluctuations in density over the course of a day at a certain place, and considers the risk acceptable if the maximum density value corresponds, for example, to LOS level D or below. It

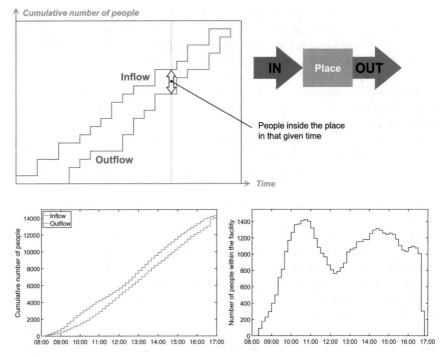

Fig. 8.2 Method to estimate total number of occupants by using entrance and exit rates. The numerical example is quite typical for crowd events taking place during the day (like a trade exhibition or an amusement park). In this example visitors are allowed into the facility from 10:00 to 17:00

should be noted that the acceptable LOS value will vary depending on the country and the circumstances of each event, which means the setting will need to be set on a case-by-case basis after reaching agreement with stakeholders. Additionally, there are cases where only high-risk areas, such as bottlenecks at entrances, exits, intersections, and stairs, will need to be reviewed in detail, instead of assessing the entire venue. Again, it is also necessary to look at prior experience from previous events, as past data can help to identify areas where risk is high.

It is also essential to not forget that crowd density can be said to be the most important variable when making assessments of crowd safety, but as we have already noted, the criteria used to judge this are typically different depending on the location of the crowd, as shown in Table 8.2.

People who are walking on a sidewalk need a certain amount of space to move their legs, and crowd densities at LOS level A, in which completely free walking is possible, are below $0.31\,\mathrm{m}^{-2}$. If the density exceeds $2.15\,\mathrm{m}^{-2}$ shown in level F, walking may be difficult, and the flow may grind to a halt. Areas in which the flow has stopped completely make accidents more likely, and care is needed here.

Table 8.2 LOS level by density (units are m^{-2}) [2]

LOS	Sidewalk	Stairways	Waiting lines
A	< 0.31	< 0.54	< 0.83
B	0.31–0.43	0.54–0.72	0.83–1.08
C	0.43–0.72	0.72–1.08	1.08–1.54
D	0.72–1.08	1.08–1.54	1.54–3.70
E	1.08–2.15	1.54–2.69	3.70–5.26
F	≥ 2.15	≥ 2.69	≥ 5.26

On stairs, the range of movement is limited to the next stair that is available, so densities are somewhat higher than would be typical of a sidewalk where free movement is possible. However, stairs also have a higher risk than sidewalks of causing accidents such as falls, and it is absolutely necessary for people to avoid stopping walking when stairs are too crowded. Furthermore, if the spaces at the top or bottom of the stairs are crowded, there is a risk that the congestion will immediately spread to the stairs and stop the flow of people who are walking on them. As this is also an extremely dangerous situation, stairs need to be carefully checked during the planning stage to ensure that the flow in front, behind and on the stairs themselves is sufficient to avoid congestion.

People do not move when they are waiting in line, so densities for those who are waiting are highest, but some caution is also required here. Densities are not uniform throughout lines of people, and tend to be higher at the front. This will lead to crowd compression, and happens because people tend to naturally pack forward when waiting for something. It is therefore effective to bend lines of people back on themselves a number of times to release the pressure that arises from people packing forward.

Risk levels should be checked against Table 8.2, and places that are level E or higher should be considered unacceptable to guarantee a good service and potentially dangerous thus in need for countermeasures. In other words, levels C and D or below are acceptable.

When even getting a rough estimation of the density is difficult, it is possible, by recalling the definition of risk defined in the previous chapter, to calculate the probabilities for cases that have occurred at similar events in the past. In other words, likelihood may be computed by working out how many times an accident occurred under conditions similar to the scheduled event and which consequences could cause. For example, religious events tend to have a long history. If we assume that for an yearly event the medical personnel has reported 30 cases of people falling from the stairs over the last 60 years, all resulting in light or negligible injuries (like someone losing footing in a sparse crowd), we may conclude this accident is possible (50% probability) and consequences minor (only light injuries). To continue the example, if, however, this year has a particular importance in the frame of the religious tradition and five times more pilgrims than usual are expected, we may conclude serious injuries or even fatalities could occur (density will be higher) and therefore consequences are major to catastrophic. Using the risk-level matrix of Chap. 7 as an example, this combination of likelihood and consequence will relate to an extreme risk.

8.5.1 Important Points to Check

In light of what discussed above, the important points that should be checked during normal operation can be summarized as follows.

Check 1: Intersections

Intersections here are intended as all the conditions in which people's flows mix, thus taking a broader meaning to what employed in Chap. 3. This task includes checking all flow lines that can be expected in normal conditions and includes not only main visitor traffic lines but also toilets, refreshment areas, entrance and exit locations, and making sure that the situation in the intersecting point is continuously monitored over time. It is also important to check the intersection of flow lines and places where queues are likely to form. If flow lines intersect multiple times, or if there are counterflows, these should be rectified. Specifically, make sure that entrance and exit flow lines are separated and the route used for both is different. Even if this involves a detour, if there are shops and restaurants on the route, then local businesses will take advantage, which may be a win-win solution in terms of safety and economic benefits.

Check 2: Evenness of distribution

Even in high-capacity venues, people tend to congregate in a limited number of popular spots at certain times, which leads to high density. If the schedule allows it, layouts and programs should be arranged so that two or more events are held at different places concurrently, to ensure that people are well-dispersed throughout the venue. Crowds should always be evenly distributed in the venue, and it is important to consider operations from a perspective of global/macroscopic optimization.

Check 3: Management boundaries

Generally speaking, the interior and exterior of the venue are divided into various parts and responsibility for the management of each part falls to a separate management entity. For example, the venue is operated by a company managing the facilities, the restaurants are operated by catering companies, entrance security is provided by a security company, and the local station is run by a railway company. It is often the case that problems arise at the management boundaries between these companies. If traffic in area A is flowing smoothly but area B, which is adjacent to it, becomes crowded, the inflow to area B should of course be stopped immediately. However, if real-time communication does not happen, those in charge of area A will assume that everything is normal and flow of people will continue from area A, while B will be in a condition of elevated risk. It is important to take this kind of situation into account and check management boundaries when planning. Furthermore, it is good to clarify the chain of command (or command hierarchy) for when it looks like something might happen, and to properly clarify who is in charge of the boundary itself.

To get more in detail, Table 8.3 lists some more specific and practical suggestions to be used in facility management for places where accumulation or congestion can be expected.

8.6   Risk Assessment for Abnormal Operations

Up until this point, we have been looking at planning for normal operating conditions, but it is of course necessary to also review whether safety can be properly maintained in the event of abnormalities. Given that this type of planning largely depends on the situation in question, we will look at multiple what-if scenarios and consider various recovery methods for situations that may occur.

For many of these scenarios, an important point to consider is whether or not it is possible to evacuate in multiple and possibly independent locations of the venue. There is a need to escape from many abnormal situations, such as an outbreak of fire or crime. If there is only one evacuation route when these situations occur, the crowd will flood toward the exit and the ensuing density can be dangerous, and if the evacuation route becomes blocked by fire, it will not be possible for people to escape at all. Multi-directional evacuation can be said to form the core of emergency response. Accordingly, it is important to set multiple routes for evacuation, and to clearly define the command system and methods of communication that will be used in an emergency.

It is important to have mechanisms in place that can be quickly put into use based, to some extent, on the judgment of those who are at the scene. If emergency responders have to report to central headquarters and wait for a decision to be made, the response may be delayed, and the situation may become more serious. It is therefore necessary to grant a certain amount of authority to people who are likely to respond, to thoroughly educate them about appropriate responses, and to properly codify countermeasures in a response manual. That said, responsibility should not lie solely with those in the field. It is also important to record abnormal situations in as much detail as possible, and to clarify how the situation changes over time, so the cause of the problem can be investigated, and lessons learned for future countermeasures.

Table 8.3 Potential risks and relative countermeasures for critical locations

Feature	Typical location	Risk	Countermeasures
Vertical movement	1. Stairs, steps, slopes 2. Escalators 3. Elevators	1. Speed is halved on stairs, access points gets crowded; risk of falls 2. Crowded landing platform, dropped luggage 3. Crowd intersection at doors	1. Wide stairs and spaces above and below, separated flows for up and down traffic 2. Make sure wide landing space is available at exit, supervise on both sides 3. Dynamically manage elevator stopping floors by eventually skip some and promote stair use
Queuing / waiting	1. Service counters, cashiers, ticket gates 2. Toilets, bus stops, etc. 3. Tourist attractions, information boards	1. Accumulation when capacity exceeded 2. Queues grow and intersect with other flow lines 3. Stopping to photograph or look hinders other pedestrians	1. Set appropriate capacity, reduce/simplify staff tasks, examine installation locations 2. Specify queue starting points and queuing lane 3. Ensure pedestrian flow lines are kept clear
Passing through bottlenecks	Doorways (entrances and exits)	Accumulation occurs when capacity exceeded; accident risk during evacuations	Extend width, ensure obstacles do not block flow
Avoiding obstacles	1. Pillars, signs in paths 2. Deformations (puddles, slippery surfaces, etc.)	1. Impedance causes accumulation 2. Falls or detours disturb flow	1. Remove obstacles or make them visible from a distance if removal not possible 2. Eliminate deformations, smooth surfaces and ensure proper drainage
Direction change	1. Corners 2. Branching paths	1. High congestion on inner flow line 2. Accumulation when direction is unclear	1. Install mirrors, ensure flow lines are kept separate 2. Provide easy to understand guidance
Intersections of people	1. Corridors 2. Station platforms 3. Junctions	1. Collisions from counterflow, deadlock 2. Queuing crowds cause collisions 3. When flow increases crossing becomes difficult, collisions are likely	1. Divide corridor into two directions 2. Separate flow lines, install proper signage and mark queuing positions 3. Widen paths, install easy-to-see signs, set priority direction
Intersections with vehicles	1. Pedestrian crossings 2. Parking lot entrances	1. Stepping into road at signal 2. Interaction with cars	1. Ensure sufficient space for people waiting at the curb 2. Set guidance staff to switch from vehicular to pedestrian traffic upon necessity

It is extremely important to factor in the following examples when considering the possibility of abnormal situations arising. It is also important to note that these abnormalities can occur in combination with each other and should not be considered only as entirely independent events.

8.6.1 Risk Factors

Risk 1: Abnormal weather

It is vital to take measures against summer heat and winter cold when conducting outdoor events. It is also important to make provisions for rain. As an example, a sudden heavy downpour may cause a crowd to rush indoors, causing falls in the process. Furthermore, hurricanes or typhoons may paralyze public transportation, and flooding rivers may cause damage. As it is difficult to make long-term forecasts of sudden changes in weather, judgment should be made immediately beforehand. It is therefore necessary to properly define the criteria for canceling the event before abnormal events occur, and that management agrees that safety must take priority over business. In particular, conditions and timing for canceling an event should be clear among all stakeholders, since last-minute decisions could lead to confusion among intended visitors and people may have already started traveling to the venues despite the absence of staff there.

Risk 2: Sudden illness

Both visitors and event staff may suddenly fall ill due to a range of causes, whether this is loss of consciousness, illness, food poisoning, or pre-existing conditions. In any case, proper routes for emergency vehicles should always be secure, so that ambulances can get close to the scene. It is also important to establish a first aid station and clearly inform visitors of its location and how it may be contacted. Needless to say, medical personnel should be proportional to the number of visitors and other conditions such as weather or crowd's properties.

Risk 3: Transportation delays or suspensions

Transportation may be suspended due to injury (not rare in railway operation), equipment failure or weather (like in case of snow), which could cause significant deviation in the movement of the crowd from the planned flow line. If, for example, several stations serve a venue, it is therefore necessary to create alternative flow lines and manage them dynamically, in case one of the train lines is suspended. Furthermore, real-time communication between venue management and the station staff is essential, as is ensuring that systems are in place to provide visitors with up-to-date information. Finally, it is important that visitors trust information from organizers as the most reliable source. Although the best practice is to include transportation information providers among the stakeholder, applications available to search for train connections may take some time to report service interruptions. In that case, visitors should be aware of the situation and follow security guidance instead of their phone suggestions. If reliable information is provided before and during the event, it is more likely visitors will trust organizers also in case of disruptions.

Risk 4: Fighting/violence

Many sports events are contested between bitter rivals and, in these cases, there is a possibility that the crowds of fans will become agitated and clash with each other. Trouble between visitors is also more likely to occur where alcohol is available. Accordingly, sale of alcoholic beverage should be forbidden in events judged for high risk. The basic rule for events potentially leading to riots is to keep visitors segregated, but it is also good to have in place better monitoring and security than would otherwise be present. Also, it may be appropriate to have at least part of the security randomly distributed among the crowd of visitors. When security is distributed across the crowd the feedback to organizers is more accurate and actions can be quicker. However, it is important that visitors do not perceive this presence as restrictive and therefore a long-standing dialogue with representative of problematic fanclubs is necessary.

Risk 5: Power outages

There are many systems in place at venues that will become non-functional in the event of a power outage. Modern technology is especially vulnerable to problems with the power supply, and critical systems should have backup power generation in place in case of an outage. Power outages have many causes but are sometimes caused by rats eating through electric cabling, which makes daily infrastructure inspections extremely important. Also, blackout and fire are often correlated (a short circuit may cause fire and fire may cause a blackout). It is therefore essential to ensure that if one problem happens it will not escalate adding the second issue. Finally, it is extremely important that in case of power outage exit get open although this may allow people to get in in that case. It is not uncommon that doors get automatically closed in case of blackout, making it more difficult for firefighters to enter and people to leave, if necessary.

Risk 6: Traffic accidents

Accidents between vehicles will usually mean that the section of road where the accident happened is closed off for a period of time. In these instances, the sidewalk may also not be usable, and the flow line may suddenly change as a result. Further-more, accidents at railroad crossings will have a knock-on effect on the operation of trains and cause chaos at nearby stations. The location of traffic accidents cannot be predicted in advance, which makes it unrealistic to try to create backup flow lines in advance. Accordingly, roads that will cause the most trouble if they are cut off should be identified, and plans for how to divert traffic in an emergency should be drawn up. Long-term road closures can also lead to major logistics issues, including making it difficult to transport food and water, event performers and sporting equipment. Alternative routes should therefore be drawn up for all important transportation.

Risk 7: Event trouble

Events do not always proceed according to schedule. For example, if traffic is dis-rupted, athletes, staff, and many spectators may arrive late, causing problems with the running of the event. It is therefore necessary to consider clear standards for delay or cancellation of the event before issues arise. Necessary infrastructure or the IT system may also be compromised during an event, and it is important to review both during normal operations and implement backups as needed. Also, schedules need to be flexible to a certain degree and alternative schedules have to be prepared as backup in case of sudden circumstances.

Risk 8: Outbreak of fire

In the event of a fire, the fire department must be contacted immediately, and the crowd must be evacuated along the routes that were previously drawn up. For the purposes of this scenario, consider the various places where fire is most likely to break out, and ensure that evacuation along multiple routes is possible. It goes without saying that the venue should be checked for combustible materials and any hazardous items should be removed. Fire and smoke prevention countermeasures are also needed, and restaurants that use fire in food preparation should perform evacuation drills in advance. Furthermore, fire doors must be checked to ensure they are unlocked, obstacles should be removed from evacuation routes and guide lights should be checked to make sure they are in proper working order, before any issues arise.

Risk 9: Earthquakes or major natural disasters

Following each country's and local regulations, the venue's building should be prop-erly checked for earthquake resilience, and a manual should be prepared that details the kind of evacuations that should take place depending on the magnitude of the earthquake. Real-time information should also be monitored for information on any fires or other natural disasters that occur in the aftermath, and methods for guiding and controlling crowds should be drawn up by stakeholders so that optimal evacuation behavior is possible. Although some countries are relatively safe in regard to earthquakes, natural disasters are not to be underestimated. Strong winds may blow up roofs of permanent structures and knowing weaknesses of a facility in regard to natural disasters is essential to prepare for worst-case scenarios.

Risk 10: Outbreak of infectious diseases

At a basic level, the spread of infectious diseases should be controlled at ports and airports, but it is important to share information that helps to stop the spread of deadly diseases that are already at risk of developing into more serious outbreaks. Isolation is the important principle when dealing with cases of suspected symptoms, and it is therefore necessary to implement a medical system that is able to cut off a suspected patient's contact with others before any issues arise. It is also important to avoid anxiety or fear that would be caused by excessive media coverage. Usually, infectious diseases do not affect management on-site since they do not spread in a short time, but their likelihood should be taken into account when planning as it may lead to cancellation or a reduction in the number of visitors. Also, stakeholders should have valid consultants to judge whether a cancellation is necessary.

Risk 11: Crimes such as terrorism

Events with large numbers of people can easily become soft targets. Because of this, police share information about terrorists with foreign countries and have surveillance systems in place that can be used at the time of large-scale events. In the event of an emergency, the government, police, and counter-terrorist police should be provided with all necessary information, and all stakeholders should follow the police's instructions.

8.7 From Planning to On-Site Operation

We have looked at the whole picture of the planning process above, but once risk assessments have been completed and operating modes have been agreed upon, the specific details must be properly shared with the people who are on the scene. It is therefore necessary to fully brief them with the results of the planning process once it has been completed and before the event has begun. If this is not done correctly, there is a danger that, even if various risks have been considered in planning, the correct countermeasures will not be deployed in the field. It is particularly important to explain why the crowd's flow lines have been set in the way they are, and detailing the many ideas for risk aversion that lie behind the reasoning involved. Doing so will help improve understanding of the increased risk that may occur if on-site staff guides arbitrarily change the flow line or fail to regulate visitors who do not keep to the intended paths.

However, overly rigid and strict enforcement of the rules in a dynamic situation may also pose a risk. Given that this is the case, it may be necessary for a person with experience in the field to be on-site to judge and decide. That said, as mentioned earlier, sole responsibility should not rest with those who are on-site, and the person in charge with an overview of the whole picture should be in constant communication.

Furthermore, the flow lines that have been created in the planning stage before the event should be shared with as many people as possible. This can be done by creating and distributing pamphlets and/or smartphone applications that contain venue maps, and by publicizing them through the internet and other media.

To further reduce the risk inherent in dangerous places by as much as possible, demand management for visitors is essential. This should take place from the early stages of the planning, right up until the day of the event, and can involve asking companies in the local area to telecommute on the day in an effort to reduce background traffic volume, announcing the date and times when congestion is to be expected in the media, and other activities designed to encourage restraint of movement.

Through all activities performed at the planning stage it should be possible to avoid that risks become a real threat and prepare for on-site crowd management.

References

1. Murakami, H., Feliciani, C., Shimura, K., Nishinari, K.: A system for efficient egress scheduling during mass events and small-scale experimental demonstration. Roy. Soc. Open Sci. **7**(12), 201465 (2020). https://doi.org/10.1098/rsos.201465
2. Fruin, J.J.: Pedestrian planning and design. Tech. rep, Metropolitan Association of Urban Designers and Environmental Planners (1971)

Chapter 9
Conclusion: The Seven Knows

Crowd management must always give the highest priorities to protecting people's lives. This is the foundation on which everything in the philosophy of preventive safety is built. The management system described in this work can be summarized in the list of "the seven knows" provided in this chapter.

> ## > Know the other

This means knowing the crowd that is to be controlled. As crowd's behavior changes greatly depending on its attributes, it is important that you build up an understanding of the people in the crowd in advance by sharing information properly with the stakeholders.

> ## > Know the past

The main purpose of crowd management is to prevent crowd incidents. However, no matter how careful the management systems that are put in place, there will unfortunately always be incidents. Learning from past cases of failure and understanding the causes that led to historical incidents helps to prevent them from occurring again in the future.

C. Feliciani et al., *Introduction to Crowd Management*,
https://doi.org/10.1007/978-3-030-90012-0_9

> Know the present

Knowledge of the current state of the crowd should form the basis for all decisions in on-site management. It is important to understand crowd behavior in real time by deploying a range of different methods for sensing and through the feedback from staff on-site.

> Know the future

It is important to try to predict the future based on the current situation and to identify risks in advance. With this in mind, it is necessary to use the data obtained through real-time sensing to anticipate future actions through simulation, and to evaluate risk countermeasures.

> Know the danger

Anticipating various dangers for the crowd and performing assessments to determine risk level is an important function of management. When risks are predicted, it is important that they are fully understood in a quantitative manner, and that this understanding is used to determine risk priority.

> Know the control methods

Crowd control must be used to reduce anticipated future risk. This is achieved through various methods, and choosing the appropriate response depends on the situation and the level of risk involved. It is important to know the control methods available and to prepare accordingly.

> Know the self

The "self" referred to here is the team that manages crowds together, and information sharing and collaboration between stakeholders is essential for successful management. Proper clarification of responsibilities is needed in order to unify the decision-making process.

Appendix A
Historical List of Crowd Incidents

This appendix provides a list of crowd accidents that occurred over a period of 120 years between 1900 and 2019 (see Table A.1). Although we tried our best to make this list as complete as possible, we are perfectly aware that there are possibly many accidents which we were not able to find, especially those small accidents only reported by local newspapers on languages not known by the authors or the ones occurring before internet became a predominant tool for information retrieval (and thus are possibly only reported on paper in local archives). Nonetheless, we believe the list is complete enough to provide a systematic overview on the common characteristics of crowd accidents, the type of location where they mostly occurred and the chain of events that caused them.

Given the length of the list and the extensive literature on which we relied to collect information we decided to avoid listing all references (for each accident we relied on one or more sources, thus making the number of references totaling several hundreds of items). An additional reason leading to the decision to not list references is given by the fact that many internet pages on which we relied may not be accessible in the future, thus making references potentially unreachable as this book will become old. However, as we found out while confirming the validity of each accident's report and checking for details, in most of the cases, an internet search in which date, country, facility and keywords such as "stampede", "crush", "disaster" or "tragedy" would be enough to get access to reports or newspaper articles providing details.

Our investigation started by considering lists of crowd accidents provided by several sources. Scientific articles [1–19], books [20–26], tables provided by people well-known in the crowd research community [27] and trusted internet services [28–30] were used to collect a first draft of this archive. Later, each accident was verified individually to check whether original information was correct and gain more insight into causes and circumstances.

However, not all accidents found during the investigation were included in this appendix. Inclusion criteria (i.e., conditions under which an accident was included/excluded in the list) are given as follows:

- **Number of fatalities**: Accident is included if one or more fatalities are reported. We did not differentiate whether fatalities occurred almost instantaneously or people passed away after some time in hospitals.
- **Number of people injured**: We also included accidents without fatalities if ten or more people got injured. We did not distinguish between injuries requiring medical assistance on-site and the ones requiring treatment in the hospital.
- **Crowd implication**: We excluded the cases in which smoke intoxication played the most important role in causing fatalities or when casualties were directly caused by fights closely related to hooliganism or widespread violence (in particular if injuries were all caused by weapons). We nonetheless included accidents caused by people fleeing a starting riot, because, while such a sudden change in crowd behavior may be difficult to predict, improper crowd management often has an important role especially when escaping routes are not available.
- **Structural failure**: We excluded the relatively rare cases in which some structural elements apparently failed due to constructional negligence (e.g., construction company failed to follow constructional guidelines) or in locations external from the managed facility (like a wall collapsing relatively far from a stadium after riots started). We nonetheless included the cases in which a structure failed due to overcrowding as this is related to crowd management. However, determining whether structural failures had been related to improper crowd management or not was not always trivial and sometimes not even possible.
- **Reliable sources of information**: We only considered reports from reliable sources, these being well-established newspapers or press agencies (Reuters, Associated Press, BBC, New York Times, etc.), official reports, scientific articles, etc. We also included those accidents for which several sources of somewhat reliable information apparently not linked to each other's were available, but only in case they all provided same or very similar evidences.

- **Availability of the report in an understandable language**: Thanks to the support from colleagues we were able to consider English, Italian, Japanese, German, French, Spanish, and Chinese. In addition, for a few cases, we made use of machine translation, but obviously considered with special regard those (translated) reports.
- **Minimum number of information available:** In some cases, an accident is reported without giving figures on casualties and with little or no information on the circumstances. Those cases have been excluded.

In addition, we would like to point out that in several cases there were inconsistencies between the reports, often in relation to the chain of events, but also in reporting the number of fatalities and people injured. If reports were contrasting on one specific aspect we either decided to include all versions or excluded that aspect in the summary provided here. Generally, all sources tend to agree on the spatial configuration of accidents, but the cause for the change in behavior or the reason leading to a worsening of the situation often differ among sources and/or several contrasting opinions are given.

In relation to the above, we would also like to remind that numbers provided (for fatalities and people injured, but also and particularly for attendance) are to be considered as an estimate presenting the magnitude rather than a precise indication. Injuries reported during crowd accidents may lead to hospitalization with victims passing away after days, weeks, or longer periods (in some cases even years [31]), thus making it sometimes difficult to accurately assess even the number of deaths. Nonetheless, the overall number of fatalities and people injured can be seen as an indicator showing the magnitude of the disaster (even if figures are approximate an accident with one casualty could be said as being "less tragic" than one having hundreds of deaths).

Finally, concerning the information contained in the summary of each accident, we tried to focus on aspects related to crowd motion. More in particular, our aim was to show the failures from which crowd managers can learn something from the past. As it can be noticed from this historical list some accidents are fairly similar, showing that some mistakes are repeated over time and sometimes lessons from the past are unfortunately not enough to avoid a recurrence.

Table A.1 Historical database for crowd accidents throughout the world from 1900 to 2019

Date	Country	Number of fatalities
September 19, 1902	USA	Fatalities: 115

Around 3,000 attendees at a sermon misheard the word "fight" as "fire" and tried to evacuate the building simultaneously in the ensuing chaos. Many people were killed when they fell over in the staircase outside the exit. Most of the fatalities were women.

January 11, 1908	UK	Fatalities: 16

A movie screening for children was held at a public hall. The supervising staff directed children to the lower floor when the upper floor became overcrowded. The crowd that attempted to go down the stairs were not able to, due to overcrowding on the lower floor. 16 children died and 17 were slightly injured.

December 24, 1913	USA	Fatalities: 73

Someone at a miners' Christmas party held on the second floor of an assembly hall shouted "fire", and attendees rushed to escape down the stairs. The crowd was squeezed against the inward-opening doors at the bottom of the stairs. Of the 73 people who died, 59 of them were children.

February 4, 1914	UK	Fatalities: 0

A brick wall collapsed under the swaying weight of the crowd in a game played in front of a record home crowd of 43,000 people. 75 people were injured, some of them critically. Reasons for the collapse are unclear, but some pointed out the absence of an adequate number of police, while others blamed materials used for construction.

December 31, 1929	UK	Fatalities: 71

The projector began to emit smoke during a packed movie screening. Around 1,000 children tried to evacuate at once. Children piled up down the stairs, in front of the emergency exit, which was padlocked shut.

January 8, 1934	Japan	Fatalities: 77

A crowd of around 10,000 people, far in excess of the station's capacity, gathered to see off new recruits to the army. Before the train carrying the recruits was able to depart, pushing broke out on the stairs to the station overpass, causing members of the crowd to fall over. 77 people were killed and 74 injured.

February 17, 1934	UK	Fatalities: 1

In the day representing the record attendance at Hillsborough stadium (72,841 people) a men was pressed against a gate when trying to get into the already closed stadium (some suggest the locked gate collapsed due to crowd pressure).

April 1, 1939	UK	Fatalities: 2

Hundreds of people climbed the roof of an already capacity filled stadium despite the police asking them to refrain doing so. The roof collapsed over the spectators killing two and injuring another 15.

October 23, 1942	Italy	Fatalities: 354

(continued)

Table A.1 (continued)

The day before a large air raid had dropped tons of bombs, so, at the day of the accident, when the raid alarm rang, people rushed into a tunnel shelter and some fell from the stairs while people outside kept trying to get in.		
March 3, 1943	UK	Fatalities: 173
A woman carrying a child fell over on the stairs while a large crowd tried to enter the station to use it as an air raid shelter during an air raid, resulting in many people getting killed.		
March 9, 1946	UK	Fatalities: 33
A fence in the stands at a crowded soccer game collapsed, and many in the crowd fell over and were killed. It is estimated that 85,000 attended the match.		
April 9, 1952	Venezuela	Fatalities: 53
Almost 6,000 people gained for a religious event and tried to leave simultaneously when someone yelled "fire". Many people tried to leave from a gate, unaware that is was closed. It is believed "fire" was said by some people having criminal intentions.		
March 9, 1953	USSR	Fatalities: 109
Several hundreds of people got killed in the crowd during Stalin's public funeral as citizens tried to pay their respects to Stalin's casket. Exact number is unknown with some believing being over thousand.		
January 2, 1954	Japan	Fatalities: 16
When a rope restricting pedestrian access to the bridge was lifted, the crowd surged forward into the newly available space. An old woman stumbled and fell, causing a chain reaction of people falling over each other.		
February 3, 1954	India	Fatalities: 500–800
A surge in the crowd at an important Hindu religious event (Kumbh Mela) and a destination for pilgrimages, caused a fence to collapse and a crowd accident. It is believed 5 million pilgrims gained for the 40-days festival in which bathing plays a fundamental role.		
March 30, 1955	Chile	Fatalities: 7
Ticket sales for a highly expected game was set to take place at the stadium on the day of the match. Thousands of people started to pack days before the sale started and when gates suddenly opened people rushed in, eventually leading to a crowd collective motion. More than 150 people were injured.		
January 1, 1956	Japan	Fatalities: 124
Crowds attempting to leave an important religious ceremony via the third gate of the shrine ran into a crowd trying to gain entrance to the ceremony, resulting in a stairway accident. 77 people were seriously injured.		
December 14, 1957	UK	Fatalities: 1
Crowd surged forward after a goal was scored eventually leading to the collapse of a wall whose bricks fell over children seating beneath. One boy was killed. Wall construction was judged as sound, but the absence of dedicated barriers contributed to pressure built-up.		
September 16, 1961	UK	Fatalities: 2

(continued)

Table A.1 (continued)

A last minute-draw, when people already started leaving, resulted in a surge in an already crowded stairway as people tried to get back to join celebrations.

| January 27, 1962 | UK | Fatalities: 0 |

Several people were injured after a barrier collapsed during a game attended by an estimated 42,000 people. Reports suggest 15 people were treated for their injuries at a local hospital.

| May 24, 1964 | Peru | Fatalities: 328 |

An unpopular call by a referee resulted in a pitch invasion, and police fired tear gas in response. Scared spectators fled the stadium via the stairs leading outside. The exits were closed, and the resulting crowd density caused people to get killed.

| December 7, 1966 | Netherlands | Fatalities: 0 |

During a game played in thick fog, fans at the back of the terrace pressed forward for a better view, resulting in an accident in which 200 people were injured and 31 taken to the hospital.

| March 15, 1967 | UK | Fatalities: 0 |

Fans tried to enter an already started game after turnstiles were shut. A barrier collapsed due to growing crowd pressure injuring 32.

| September 17, 1967 | Turkey | Fatalities: 43 |

A riot broke out between fans of opposite teams and the fleeing of people from violence resulted in an accident in front of the stand exit.

| April 30, 1968 | UK | Fatalities: 0 |

A barrier collapsed as a crowd of thousands tried to enter an already packed stadium. Gates had been closed a few minutes before the start. It is believed 50,000 people tried to enter the stadium having a capacity for 30,000. 49 people were injured.

| June 23, 1968 | Argentina | Fatalities: 71 |

Extreme behavior by some spectators scared the rest of the crowd, which tried to evacuate via the stairs leading outside. The exits were locked, and the resulting crowd density led to an accident. Approximately 150 people were injured.

| January 2, 1971 | UK | Fatalities: 66 |

Spectators attempting to leave the stadium at the end of a soccer game all tried to access the narrow stairs at once. A single person falling over caused a large number of other people to fall in a chain reaction. It is believed more than 80,000 fans attended the game.

| March 4, 1971 | Brazil | Fatalities: 2 |

On the re-inauguration of the expanded stadium rumors about a possible collapse of the stadium resulted in a tumult as people rushed to the pitch. Several thousands were hurt in the stadium filled with over 100,000 spectators (some even reporting as much as 150,000).

| February 17, 1974 | Egypt | Fatalities: 48 |

Venue for the match had been changed to a stadium with a capacity lower then the one where the game was initially planned. Worried they will not be able to get in fans rushed to the new venue and a wall collapsed under the pressure of the crowd. At least 48 lost their lives and 50 were injured.

(continued)

Table A.1 (continued)

March 10, 1975	USSR	Fatalities: 20

An accident occurred on stairs as people were leaving after a hockey match. Is believed fans rushed to get souvenirs, although other factors (such as lights getting off) apparently contributed to the accident (details are unclear). Attendance was reportedly below capacity. Actual number of fatalities is not clear.

December 11, 1976	Haiti	Fatalities: 0–3

A fire cracker lighted after a goal scared fans, who knocked down a soldier, who in turn accidentally killed two children with his gun. The confusion generated by the escalating situation resulted in several people getting killed in the moving crowd, although numbers are unclear. The soldier eventually committed suicide later on.

May 1, 1977	Turkey	Fatalities: 27

Some people started shooting during a political rally attended by 500,000. Intervening security forces entered the scene with sirens and explosives, further scaring the crowd already trying to flee. From autopsy results it is believed that 27 people died due to crush injuries (with others being killed by bullets).

June 9, 1979	Germany	Fatalities: 0

Fans celebrating created pressure on the ones standing on the lower side of the terrace, where a protection net broke resulting in 71 people getting injured.

September 16, 1979	Indonesia	Fatalities: 9

An estimated number of 200,000 fans attended a concert in a stadium designed for 30,000. As a result the stadium collapsed, killing nine. It is reported that over 90,000 tickets were printed. All fatalities involved children, with dozens more injured.

December 3, 1979	USA	Fatalities: 11

Believing that the concert had started earlier than expected, a large number of people with first-come-first-served tickets flooded the entrance to the venue. People pushing to get to the entrance caused a rise in crowd density, resulting in a serious accident. 26 people were injured.

January 12, 1980	UK	Fatalities: 2

To avoid a possible clash between fans, exit was staged with home supporters leaving first. Pressure built up among visiting supporters standing in front of the gates resulted in the collapse of a brick wall.

May 4, 1980	Zaire	Fatalities: 9

People struggled to enter the venue as gates opened in front of a huge crowd that gathered to see an important religious leader. Half a million people are said to had gathered to the event. 72 were injured, some of them critically.

July 9, 1980	Brazil	Fatalities: 3–7

Stadium gates' were forced open by a large crowd trying to enter the venue during the visit of an important religious leader. The crowds surged through the open gates where fatalities occurred. More than 30 people were injured.

August 14, 1980	Iraq	Fatalities: 59

People rushed to the exit after a confined electric fire developed in a cinema. Most of the victims were children. 45 people were injured.

August 16, 1980	India	Fatalities: 16

(continued)

Table A.1 (continued)

People escaped from an escalating violence among fans of opposing team in a stadium without divisions between both groups of supporters. Spectators perished at the exit gates trying to escape the riot. More than 100 were injured.		
February 8, 1981	Greece	Fatalities: 21
Fans rushed out of the stadium to celebrate after a game, but, as a result of some of the stadium exits being partially closed, the crowd density of leaving spectators increased, leading to an accident where 11 people died and more than 50 were injured.		
April 11, 1981	UK	Fatalities: 0
A goal caused a crowd surge leading many fans to move out of the terrace. 38 people had been injured. Radial fencing was used at the time of the accident.		
October 20, 1982	USSR	Fatalities: 66
Fans from the home team tried to go back to the stadium after a goal was scored 20 s before the end. Because of the low attendance only one exit was used and groups from both directions clashed on the partially frozen stairs. Dispute exist on the number of fatalities, some reporting up to 340 people.		
November 18, 1982	Colombia	Fatalities: 22
People started to flow out of the stadium as result seemed certain. A quick draw led some to come back but were blocked by others escaping from rowdy fans who started urinating from the upper deck. An accident occurred at the exit where a railing collapsed. More than 100 were injured.		
November 26, 1982	Algeria	Fatalities: 10
A packed roof collapsed after 20,000 people gathered in a stadium with a capacity for 15,000. 584 people were injured. Most of the deaths were children.		
February 14, 1984	UK	Fatalities: 0
24 people were injured as a crowd surge following a goal resulted in a wall collapse.		
May 26, 1985	Mexico	Fatalities: 8
People died inside a tunnel as they tried to enter an already full stadium before the start of a well anticipated game. Reports speculate that false tickets were sold and point out weaknesses of doors, which allowed people to force their entry.		
May 29, 1985	Belgium	Fatalities: 39
A riot broke out between home fans and visiting supporters before the start of a soccer game. The rest of the crowd tried to flee, and those at the front were squeezed against a fence, resulting in 39 deaths.		
April 14, 1986	India	Fatalities: 47
Around 20,000 pilgrims had been waiting for two hours in a police cordon to cross a bridge during the Kumbh Mela. After the crowd surged forward the police responded with a mild baton charge creating confusion in the crowd and resulting in 47 fatalities and several injuries.		
December 10, 1987	China	Fatalities: 17

(continued)

Table A.1 (continued)

A thick fog led to the suspension of ferry service, leaving people waiting at the terminal for several hours. When the service was finally resumed and a ferry arrived, the crowd hurried to board, causing an accident. 70 were injured. It is estimated 30,000 to 40,000 had been waiting.		
December 26, 1987	China	Fatalities: 28
Elementary school students leaving their classrooms for early morning assembly flooded a dark stairwell in which the lights had been switched off. A fall on the stairs resulted in the deaths of 28 people.		
March 13, 1988	Nepal	Fatalities: 93
A sudden hailstorm at a soccer game caused an accident in the exit tunnel leading from the terrace as the spectators tried to evacuate. The stadium doors had been locked, preventing the crowd from escaping.		
August 20, 1988	UK	Fatalities: 2
Around 50 people fell over about 13 m from the stage when the excited crowd at a rock concert surged forward. Two people died.		
April 15, 1989	UK	Fatalities: 96
A large number of spectators tried to enter the stands of a stadium at the start of a soccer match, despite the stands being surrounded on all sides by fences, which led to an increase in density. 96 people died as a result of being pressed into the pitch-side fencing.		
July 2, 1990	Saudi Arabia	Fatalities: 1426
An incident occurred as a large number of pilgrims moved down a tunnel 550 m long and 10 m wide. Some people fell from a bridge onto pilgrims exiting the tunnel causing people to accumulate within it. That day outside temperature was 44 °C.		
January 13, 1991	South Africa	Fatalities: 42
An unpopular decision by the referee led to fights breaking out between spectators at a soccer match. The remaining spectators scared out and were pushed against riot control fences as they attempted to escape, resulting in the deaths of 42 people.		
January 24, 1991	USA	Fatalities: 3
13,000 excited spectators surged toward the stage at a rock concert, leading to the deaths of three people.		
February 13, 1991	Mexico	Fatalities: 41
A large number of pilgrims surged into the atrium of a church in order to receive blessings from God, leading to a crowd incident. 55 were injured.		
September 24, 1991	China	Fatalities: 105
People moving against the flow of the crowd at a lantern festival in a park led to an incident on a bridge with poor lighting. Some of the 105 deaths were caused by people falling from the bridge itself.		
December 28, 1991	USA	Fatalities: 8
A large number of spectators trying to enter an already crowded gym to watch a basketball game led to an incident in a small stairwell at the entrance. More tickets had been sold than the gym had capacity. There were eight deaths and 29 injuries.		

(continued)

Table A.1 (continued)

February 18, 1992	India	Fatalities: 30

A crowd surge occurred during a religious event after the chief minister arrived for a holy dip. Reports are rather unclear and it appears that some deaths were related to a collapsed building but many also due to the density of the crowd. Two gates were used for about ten thousands pilgrims.

May 5, 1992	France	Fatalities: 18

A temporary terrace collapsed killing 18 and injuring 2,300. The temporary facility was built to increase stadium capacity by 50% for an important match. The structure collapsed before the match started.

July 19, 1992	Brazil	Fatalities: 3

A grid collapsed leading to people falling 8 m over people sitting beneath them. It is unclear what led people moving toward the grid, although it was found that structural failure was possibly caused by corrosion and lack in maintenance.

January 1, 1993	Hong Kong	Fatalities: 21

More than 15,000 drunk people gathered at the intersection of different red light districts for the New Year countdown. The high-density crowd that formed led to an incident. 21 people died and 67 were injured. The area in which they had gathered was on a steep slope.

October 30, 1993	United States	Fatalities: 0

Pressure accumulated on the crowd as fans were celebrating, eventually leading to the failure of the front rail throwing them to the field. 73 people were injured, six of them critically.

May 23, 1994	Saudi Arabia	Fatalities: 270

A crowd incident occurred among pilgrims attending the stoning of the devil ritual. Details on the accident remains mostly unclear.

November 23, 1994	India	Fatalities: 113

Security police baton-charged a crowd of about 40,000 people after order broke down at a demonstration. The incident occurred as the crowd tried to escape. At least 113 people died, primarily women and children. Fences and barbed wire barricades had been installed prior to the incident.

June 16, 1996	Zambia	Fatalities: 9

An accident occurred as people tried to flee the stadium and a wall collapsed. Reports are conflicting on what caused the sudden crowd motion, but the stadium was reported being well over capacity. At least nine people died.

July 14, 1996	India	Fatalities: 39

Devotees tumbled in a narrow staircase inside a temple complex killing 39 people and injuring 35. Some were wounded by bamboo and steel wires as they were thrown against a temporary barricade. Gates' opening was delayed, apparently to let in VIPs first.

July 14, 1996	India	Fatalities: 21

Devotees got killed as they were crossing an overcrowded bridge used on both directions to take a holy dip, resulting in 21 fatalities and 40 people injured. It is said that more than 2 million people had gathered for the event.

July 31, 1996	South Africa	Fatalities: 15

(continued)

Table A.1 (continued)

Private security guards closed gates and attempted to control the crowd using electric cattle prods to prevent those without tickets to board a train after a campaign to crack down fare beaters was started.		
October 16, 1996	Guatemala	Fatalities: 84
An accident occurred before the game started in a reportedly overfilled stadium (possibly due to counterfeit tickets) leading to the collapse of a fence separating different areas. 147 people were injured.		
January 1, 1997	UK	Fatalities: 0
A crowd of about 400,000 attended New Year celebrations. Railings collapsed at a concert leaving 300 people injured. Underfoot conditions were hazardous due to the presence of snow.		
April 5, 1997	Nigeria	Fatalities: 5
Only two of the five gates were mistakenly opened at the end of a 40,000 packed soccer game. Crowds moved to the exits unaware that some of them were locked. It is believed stadium was over capacity.		
April 9, 1998	Saudi Arabia	Fatalities: 118
Another incident among pilgrims attending the stoning of the devil ritual killed 118 people and injured 180. Details are unclear.		
April 18, 1998	Zimbabwe	Fatalities: 4
A collective rush happened during celebrations for the independence day as thousands of spectators scrambled for seats for events, which included a free soccer match between two popular teams.		
December 25, 1998	Peru	Fatalities: 9
A tear gas bomb was exploded inside a nightclub facility and nine people were killed as they tried to escape outside. The only door available was closed by security personnel believing a gang wanted to enter to steal or start a fight. Only 30 or 40 of the 250 people present managed to leave the nightclub.		
January 14, 1999	India	Fatalities: 53
A landslide occurred at a temple during a religious pilgrimage, causing 200,000 male pilgrims to get scared and flee, which in turn caused a crowd incident. Some died in the landslide, but most were killed from the crowd itself. Most of the pilgrims were not familiar with the location as they came from far away.		
May 30, 1999	Belarus	Fatalities: 53
A sudden thunderstorm during an outdoor concert caused many young attendees to attempt to take shelter in a nearby subway station. Some people slid and fell over on the wet sidewalk, causing a crowd incident.		
December 4, 1999	Austria	Fatalities: 6
As attendees left at the end of a snowboarding contest, many people slipped on the dark, steep slopes and fell into a barrier at the bottom of the hill. Dozens of people had been injured and were taken to the hospital, some in serious conditions.		
March 24, 2000	South Africa	Fatalities: 13

(continued)

Table A.1 (continued)

A tear gas canister was throw inside a nightclub in the afternoon when children were filling the facility. The emergency door was locked and the only way out was down a narrow staircase leading to the main entrance. Fatalities are said to have occurred on the staircase, where a wall also collapsed.

| April 16, 2000 | Portugal | Fatalities: 7 |

Two canisters of gas were set off in a popular nightclub at the same time when lights went out, leading to a blind escape. The nightclub recently passed safety regulations inspections.

| April 23, 2000 | Liberia | Fatalities: 3 |

A crowd surge occurred in an apparently overfilled stadium. One person died jumping from a fence to escape the dense crowd while others passed away for its consequences.

| May 26, 2000 | Pakistan | Fatalities: 8 |

An accident occurred in a circus as guards used batons to break up an unruly crowd. It is believed people without ticket tried to force their entry in a break between shows when spectators were leaving the circus. A special show was held that day close to where a religious congregation was also held.

| June 5, 2000 | Ethiopia | Fatalities: 14 |

An accident occurred in an amphitheater during a memorial ceremony attended by thousands as children began running to cover from a rainstorm. More than 50 were injured, all victims were children.

| June 30, 2000 | Denmark | Fatalities: 9 |

Excited spectators surged toward the stage during a concert, resulting in nine deaths and 26 injuries.

| July 9, 2000 | Zimbabwe | Fatalities: 12 |

An accident occurred as police responded with tear gas to fans throwing plastic bottles in a near-capacity crowd causing many people to urge toward the exits. Fans leaving the stadium found more gas outside.

| December 30, 2000 | Brazil | Fatalities: 0 |

A fence collapsed over crowd pressure after some people apparently tried to escape from fighting. More than 60 fans were injured. Other reports suggest injuries occurred as fans tried to jump over the protective barrier.

| January 26, 2001 | Australia | Fatalities: 1 |

A teenage got killed in a mosh pit during a music festival. Barriers were not employed to split the crowd and were introduced in later editions following the incident.

| March 2, 2001 | South Africa | Fatalities: 7 |

An accident occurred as commuters rushed down stairs toward a main-line passenger train. Dynamics is not clear although it is believed security locked the gates and an announcement on the sudden closure was made only 10 minutes before departure, leading passengers to rush.

| March 5, 2001 | Saudi Arabia | Fatalities: 35 |

An incident occurred among pilgrims attending the stoning of the devil ritual.

| March 18, 2001 | Indonesia | Fatalities: 4 |

(continued)

Table A.1 (continued)

Teenage girls got killed at the front of the stage during a performance of a boy band in a shopping mall. The band performed without a stage. The accident occurred as the band started signing autographs. A similar appearance was canceled after 20,000 stormed the venue.		
April 1, 2001	Pakistan	Fatalities: 44
Thousands of men crammed into a narrow street leading to the main door of a shrine. A collective rush occurred as the opening of the shrine was delayed by more than 3 h with about 100,000 people waiting. Becoming restless amid the delay some of them opted to seek entry through a secondary gate out-of-bound leading to a scramble in which 44 got killed and about hundred were injured.		
April 11, 2001	South Africa	Fatalities: 43
A crowd of fans who were trying to find tickets for a soccer match surged into an already over-capacity stadium when the match began to heat up, destroying the perimeter fence in the process. The sudden flow of people caused a crowd incident near the entrance gate.		
April 29, 2001	DRC	Fatalities: 14
Police fired tear gas to unruly fans who had invaded the pitch leading to an ensuing crowd accident. Fans were believed to had thrown objects at each other. The main exit was blocked leading to no way out.		
May 6, 2001	Iran	Fatalities: 15
A roof collapsed as spectators reportedly sat on top of a temporary scaffolding in a crammed stadium said to have been well above capacity. Hundreds have been injured.		
May 9, 2001	Ghana	Fatalities: 126
Extreme behavior from some of the fans at a soccer match led to the police responding with tear gas. Many spectators tried to evacuate simultaneously. A crowd incident occurred because there were too few exits and the exits that did exist had been locked.		
July 21, 2001	Japan	Fatalities: 11
An incident occurred just before the end of a firework display, as a crowd of spectators trying to leave ran into a crowd of people going in the opposite direction on a pedestrian bridge between the railway station and the venue. 247 sustained injuries. The exit stairs of the pedestrian bridge acted as a bottleneck, as they were half the width of the bridge itself.		
August 8, 2001	Bangladesh	Fatalities: 23
A worker in a garment factory sounded the alarm after seeing flames shooting from an electric circuit board. Workers converged to the stairs to find the single exit locked and the security guard absent.		
December 15, 2001	Brazil	Fatalities: 4
A crowd of about 60,000 people attended a gift distribution event. A wall collapsed and the resulting confusion killed four and left several injured. 10 members of the army were reportedly on-site to manage the large crowd, although 70 were planned to be on service.		
December 21, 2001	Bulgaria	Fatalities: 7
A crowd incident occurred as attendees tried to enter the venue for a Christmas party because the stairs that led into the venue had become frozen and were slippery. Six people between the ages of 11 and 15 died.		

(continued)

Table A.1 (continued)

September 23, 2002	China	Fatalities: 21

Students in a middle school attempted to leave evening classes in complete darkness. Not being able to see, students could not understand the situation and kept pushing. Eventually a guardrail collapsed killing 21 and injuring 47. It is said two teacher were on duty to manage 1,563 students and the school was designed for 800.

September 28, 2002	India	Fatalities: 16

During a commotion people tried to protect others from becoming involved. As a result of this event the crowd was pushed down the stairs toward the two platforms, increasing crowd density at the end. In the chaos some climbed on an arriving train and got electrified by the overhead high tension wire. A lot of people were arriving for a political rally.

January 5, 2003	China	Fatalities: 3

A power loss occurred in a middle school in the afternoon. As power could not be restored it was decided to cancel evening classes and let the students go home. Students in the classroom upstairs rushed down the stairways as students in the playground rushed upstairs to get their bags, eventually clashing on the stairs. 19 were injured.

February 11, 2003	Saudi Arabia	Fatalities: 14

An incident occurred among pilgrims attending the stoning of the devil ritual.

February 17, 2003	USA	Fatalities: 21

Security guards trying to break up a fight at a club used pepper spray, causing chaos among the 1,500 attendees as many believed that they were being attacked by terrorists and tried to flee toward the exit. The exit was at the bottom of a steep flight of stairs and the door to the street was narrow, and opened inward. 21 people died from suffocation.

May 3, 2003	Benin	Fatalities: 13

An accident occurred as stadium gates were opened for a concert by a popular artist. Gates opening was delayed by a previous event held in the same venue.

August 27, 2003	India	Fatalities: 39

The throwing of silver coins to a crowds of pilgrim leading to a religious event was believed to have caused a collective rush, which killed 39 and injured about 150. A different source said the collective motion was caused as pilgrims rushed for the holy dip after sadhus (holy men), already late in their bathing, had finished.

December 11, 2003	China	Fatalities: 5

An accident occurred on stairs after students were leaving a middle school in the darkness due to a power loss. 15 children were injured, four of them seriously.

February 1, 2004	Saudi Arabia	Fatalities: 251

An incident occurred among pilgrims attending the stoning of the devil ritual. Over 200 people were injured.

February 5, 2004	China	Fatalities: 37

A large number of people moving against the flow of the crowd caused an incident on a bridge between two venues that were separated by a river at a New Year lantern festival. 37 people died, many of them women and children. There were reports that the bridge was crowded with people watching fireworks at the time of the incident.

(continued)

Table A.1 (continued)

March 12, 2004	Syria	Fatalities: 5
An accident occurred as spectators escaped from rioting fans. More than 100 people were injured.		
April 12, 2004	India	Fatalities: 21
About 10,000 women with babies and small children attended a rally held in a park. The accident occurred as the end of the event was broadcast and it was announced people could collect gifts at the reception counter. This led to a large number of women hurrying toward the reception counter near the exit. 21 women and children died.		
May 3, 2004	Bangladesh	Fatalities: 6
The explosion of an electric transformer nearby initiated an evacuation in a six-story garment factory. Workers rushed on the stairwells killing six and injuring at least 30.		
September 1, 2004	Saudi Arabia	Fatalities: 3
A furniture store held an event at which the first 50 people to attend would each receive a gift certificate worth 500 Rial, and the next 200 attendees would each receive 100 Rial vouchers. More than 8,000 people gathered outside the store before it opened. Despite being scheduled to open at 10 a.m., the store opened at 9 a.m., and the crowd broke through the safety barriers.		
October 10, 2004	Togo	Fatalities: 4
At the end of a soccer game lights went off due to a power outage causing fan to run for the exits. Another eight people were injured, three critically. The stadium was recently built.		
November 13, 2004	India	Fatalities: 5
Passengers rushing to catch a leaving train struggled on stairs during one of the biggest holiday of the year. It is believed two women slipped on the stairs triggering the accident.		
November 20, 2004	Togo	Fatalities: 13
People got killed at the gates as they tried to surge into the president's palace when the gates were thrown open. That day a political march was organized, with the number of participants (hundreds of thousand) underestimated. Some reports suggest people were hoping for banknotes handout from the president.		
January 25, 2005	India	Fatalities: 291
A pilgrim at a religious festival attracting more than 300,000 people fell on the steep and narrow stairs to the temple, which had become slippery with palm juice used in the offerings, and caused a crowd incident. Subsequently, an electric wire short-circuited at a nearby store, causing a fire that spread to cooking gas cylinders, which then exploded.		
February 26, 2005	Burkina Faso	Fatalities: 2
An accident occurred on the more shaded area as stadium gates for a film festival were opened in a scorching day. That day also featured a concert by a well-known singer. Between 10 and 20 people were injured.		
March 25, 2005	Iran	Fatalities: 5
An accident occurred after the game when 100,000 spectators moved to the exits. About 40 others were hurt, five of them in critical condition. No reason was given for the rush to the doors.		
April 6, 2005	Bangladesh	Fatalities: 7

(continued)

Table A.1 (continued)

An accident occurred during a bathing religious festival. It is believed some people slipped while walking on the path connecting two holy pools where pilgrims were dipping. Dozens were injured.

August 16, 2005	USA	Fatalities: 0

An estimated 5,500 people turned out at a shop in a rush to purchase largely discounted laptops. 17 people were injured as the gates opened.

August 31, 2005	Iraq	Fatalities: 953

One person in a crowd of about a million pilgrims on their way to a temple shouted that another pilgrim was carrying explosives. Fearful of suicide bombers, the crowd surged toward a closed bridge. Despite the gates at both ends of the bridge being locked, the crowd forced their way in but were unable to escape from the far end, causing deadly overcrowding. Many people also fell off the bridge and drowned.

September 8, 2005	Sri Lanka	Fatalities: 1

A bomb hoax resulted in a sudden evacuation aboard a plane that was about to take off. 62 passengers were wounded in the accident. Emergency exits were opened to let passenger evacuate the plane. 424 passengers and 19 crew members were on board.

October 6, 2005	Bangladesh	Fatalities: 8

Several accidents of various extent took place several times over two days as thousands of people gathered at the residence of an industrialist to collect gifts. Details remains unclear, although it is believed another 50 were injured.

October 24, 2005	China	Fatalities: 0

As the bell rang students in the playground rushed upstairs at the same time when other students attempted to reach the playground from upstairs. 10 students were injured as both groups clashed at the stairs.

October 25, 2005	China	Fatalities: 12

As students were about to leave after evening classes a blackout occurred and someone shouted "ghosts", getting everyone rushing to the staircase where the accident occurred. Another 27 have been injured, some seriously.

October 30, 2005	Saudi Arabia	Fatalities: 7

An accident occurred as a man was distributing cash in a car park. As voices started to circulate more and more people rushed causing a collective motion killing seven and injuring 40.

November 6, 2005	India	Fatalities: 6

People began to gather very early for a food relief supply campaign organized in a school. As soon as the gates were opened people stormed in leading to the accident. Dozens were injured.

December 18, 2005	India	Fatalities: 42

At 3 a.m. a crowd of about 4,500 people began to gather at a distribution center offering relief supplies (open was scheduled for 9 a.m.). Shortly afterward it began to rain heavily and rumors spread that distribution of supplies would be limited to 1,000 families. At around 4 a.m., the crowd broke through a police cordon and surged into the entrance of the building. People at the front of the crowd slipped and fell on the sloping ground of the entrance-way. There were enough supplies for 45,000 families.

January 12, 2006	Saudi Arabia	Fatalities: 345

(continued)

Table A.1 (continued)

An abandoned luggage caused an incident among pilgrims attending the stoning of the devil ritual. Pilgrims got killed as they stumbled over the luggage left at the entrance of a bridge and were overrun by the crowd behind.		
February 4, 2006	Brazil	Fatalities: 3
The excited crowd rushed the stage at a concert, killing three and injuring 42.		
February 4, 2006	Philippines	Fatalities: 73
Around 30,000 people gathered outside a stadium for a public event. Games with cash and luxury goods as prizes were scheduled to start at 6 a.m., with tickets only available on the day at the venue. Once the festival began, the organizers announced that only the first 300 people could participate in the prize games. This lead to a huge crowd surge. The security hurried to close the gates, but the crowd behind did not stop, and the gate collapsed, causing the accident.		
April 9, 2006	Pakistan	Fatalities: 30
An accident occurred on stairs during a 10,000 packed religious event attended by women. Reports are unclear, but they agree that a women stopped on stairs to assist a child, leading some to stumble and ultimately leading to a collective motion toward the only narrow exit located below the stairs. Over 100 people suffered injuries.		
August 20, 2006	Hungary	Fatalities: 0
1.5 million people gathered around the capital city for a firework display. A severe storm hit the city leading people to rush for a shelter. Three people were killed and dozens injured, although it is not clear whether injuries were caused by the weather, the crowd itself or other factors. Some reports suggest the storm was predicted (or predictable).		
September 12, 2006	Yemen	Fatalities: 51
A crowd incident occurred as participants left a stadium that was used as a venue for a presidential election rally. It is believed people in the overcrowded stadium rushed toward the stage to get a glimpse of the president, leading to the collapse of an iron fence. More than 200 were injured.		
November 4, 2006	India	Fatalities: 4
An accident occurred as doors of a temple were opened and thousands of devotees tried to enter. Around 50,000 pilgrims were waiting for hours to enter the shrine. All dead were over 70 years old.		
November 18, 2006	China	Fatalities: 6
After an evening class, middle school students swarmed into the staircase of a three-story building killing six and injuring 39. It is unclear what triggered the collective motion, with a witness suggesting someone was seen squatting to tie shoelaces on the stairs as hundreds rushed downstairs.		
December 17, 2006	Pakistan	Fatalities: 27
During a wedding, high intensity lights sparked a blaze and people were killed while escaping from the fire, also leading to the collapse of a wall under crowd pressure. It is unclear whether fire or crowd had the major role in the fatalities, but the collapse of the wall suggests crowd density was rather high.		
April 30, 2007	Tunisia	Fatalities: 6
A major surge occurred during an open air concert as enthusiastic spectators saw stars appearing on stage. Several people fell down eventually resulting in the fatalities.		

(continued)

Table A.1 (continued)

June 2, 2007	Zambia	Fatalities: 12
Spectators leaving a soccer game rushed for the free shuttle buses, causing a crowd incident. Another 40 people were injured.		
September 7, 2007	Zambia	Fatalities: 4
A brick wall collapsed as victims were trying to reach a free mosquito net handout in a community hall. Some people tried to reach the location by climbing the walls causing the collapse. Six more people were injured.		
October 3, 2007	India	Fatalities: 14
As three overcrowded trains carrying thousands of pilgrims to a religious event arrived at a station, a platform change was announced. A crowd incident occurred as the passengers tried to make their transfers. 14 women died and more than 40 were injured.		
October 5, 2007	North Korea	Fatalities: 6
A crowd incident occurred as 150,000 spectators were leaving a stadium after watching a public execution. Another 34 were injured. Details remain unclear.		
October 13, 2007	India	Fatalities: 12
An incident took place on a bridge leading to a hilltop temple during a religions event used on both directions. It is reported that thousands of people crowded a narrow path leading to the temple. Some pilgrims are thought to have been pushed off the bridge while others fell over.		
November 11, 2007	China	Fatalities: 3
A supermarket offered a 20% discount on cooking oil. As the store opened, a large number of customers who had been waiting outside were admitted at the same time, causing a crowd incident. Three people were killed and more than 30 injured.		
January 3, 2008	India	Fatalities: 6
An accident occurred as thousands of pilgrims attempted to garland a statue in a temple, killing six and injuring another 15. More than 100,000 pilgrims gathered at the hill-top temple, which had only one gate used for both entry and exit.		
February 9, 2008	Indonesia	Fatalities: 10
A deadly accident occurred after a concert as people tried to get in at the same time when hundreds attempted to get out through the only gate. Unconfirmed reports suggest the venue was filled over its capacity of 700.		
March 27, 2008	India	Fatalities: 9
A high-density crowd of 100,000 pilgrims gathered at a temple for a religious event. Crowd pressure caused a fence to collapse and many of the pilgrims fell over, causing a crowd incident.		
June 1, 2008	Liberia	Fatalities: 10
An accident occurred as gates were closed, leaving thousands of people wanting to enter the full stadium outside. It is believed that many fake tickets were in circulation, leading the stadium to get filled as people were still trying to enter. All the casualties occurred in front of a single gate.		
June 20, 2008	Mexico	Fatalities: 12

(continued)

Table A.1 (continued)

Police raided a nightclub filled with 500 young people for drugs and underage drinking, causing the guests to flee. The only emergency exit was locked, and a crowd incident occurred, killing 12 people.		
July 4, 2008	India	Fatalities: 6
An accident occurred in front of a temple's gate as the deity was taken out. A crowd surge occurred that caused those accompanying the deity to fell down. 12 were injured. It is said one million people congregated for the 9-days festival.		
August 3, 2008	India	Fatalities: 146
A rain shelter collapsed at a temple where 3,000 followers had gathered for a religious event. Someone who saw the collapse shouted that there had been a landslide, and those in the crowd who heard this rushed toward the perimeter fencing that had been installed by the police, causing a crowd incident in which the fence collapsed and 146 people died. It was raining at the time.		
September 14, 2008	DRC	Fatalities: 13
Riots started between fans after a player conducted a "witchcraft" to weaken the opposite team. Crowd escaping the riot resulted in an accident, killing 13 and injuring others.		
September 30, 2008	India	Fatalities: 224
An accident happened at the moment the door of a temple was opened resulting in the destruction of the barricades. A slope leading to the temple resulted in many people to loose footing. Rumors have blamed a bomb blast nearby and possibly also a collapsing wall could have caused the collective reaction. More than 425 people were injured.		
October 2, 2008	Tanzania	Fatalities: 19
Children were killed by a possible combination of lack of oxygen and crowd pressure in an overfilled disco hall. Occupancy was reported being twice the recommended number.		
November 28, 2008	USA	Fatalities: 1
A crowd of over 2,000 people gathered at a store on the day before a bargain sale. As the opening time of the store approached, the crowd smashed the glass doors at the store's entrance. Five minutes before the store was scheduled to open, a store employee got killed under the collective crowd motion. The store was due to open at 5 a.m. and the crowd had begun to gather at about 9 p.m. on the previous day, filling the available space by 3:30 a.m.		
December 16, 2008	China	Fatalities: 0
After a singing competition ended, 3,000 students headed upstairs to put their stools in classroom and later return to the cafeteria on the first floor. Students from both directions clashed on the stairs at the first floor injuring 25.		
March 29, 2009	Ivory Coast	Fatalities: 19
A crowd of fans without tickets had gathered outside the stadium, and rushed the entrance just before the start of the match. The entrance collapsed due to the sudden crowd pressure, causing an incident. Over 100 people were injured.		
May 23, 2009	Morocco	Fatalities: 11
An incident occurred as spectators attempted to leave in a hurry a 70,000 packed free concert leading to the collapse of a wire fence. The event was moved to a larger venue to meet a growing demand. Delays in the concert schedule may have contributed to the sudden move and some blamed police decision to close some gate.		

(continued)

Table A.1 (continued)

September 9, 2009	India	Fatalities: 5

A rumor started among a group of students who had got wet in the rain on their way to school that rain leakage had caused a short circuit and they were at risk of electrocution. In the ensuing chaos, a counterflow occurred on the stairs as students tried to flee, causing a crowd incident. There were five deaths and 33 injuries.

November 15, 2009	UK	Fatalities: 0

Fans rushed the stage at an event by a popular artist, causing a crowd incident when fencing collapsed. More than 60 people were injured.

November 25, 2009	China	Fatalities: 0

Students trying to move upstairs clashed with others moving downstairs between the second and third floor. Five were seriously injured and dozens more required medical assistance.

December 7, 2009	China	Fatalities: 8

52 classes ended simultaneously meaning that between 2,000 and 2,500 students left their classrooms at the same time. The crowd became concentrated on the single staircase close to the student dormitories, causing a crowd incident. It was raining heavily outside. Eight people were killed and 26 were injured.

December 20, 2009	India	Fatalities: 8

A disaster occurred as gates of a temple were opened during a ceremony, which could accommodate 50,000 people despite the estimated 100,000 present. It is believed somebody slipped triggering the disaster.

January 14, 2010	India	Fatalities: 7

An accident occurred at a jetty as people surged to board a boat during a religious festival. It is believed only a bamboo barricade stood between the crowd and the jetty, which easily crumbled. Dozens were injured.

February 25, 2010	Mali	Fatalities: 26

An accident occurred at the entrance of a mosque as people had to squeeze through a narrow road because the main road was closed for construction. Another 55 people had been injured.

March 4, 2010	India	Fatalities: 63

A rumor claiming someone had been electrocuted by faulty electric wiring spread among a crowd of 10,000 people that had gathered at a temple distributing free food and clothes. The crowd all tried to flee at once, rushing through a gate that was still under construction, and the gate collapsed. Subsequent crowds tried to get through, leading to a crowd incident. Many of the victims got killed under the collapsed gate.

March 8, 2010	India	Fatalities: 1

Around 30,000 to 40,000 aspirants showed up in a recruitment center to apply for a police job. In total 100,000 forms were given out although 3,600 positions were available. The accident occurred as the gates were opened. 11 people were hurt.

April 15, 2010	South Africa	Fatalities: 1

A person died while queueing for World Cup tickets as thousands of people waited overnight. A seizure while in the line was identified as the apparent cause of death. Ticket sale system had been recently changed from internet to ticketing offices to allow a wider access to the public.

(continued)

Table A.1 (continued)

April 30, 2010	India	Fatalities: 5
Conflicting reports exist to explain a sudden surge that occurred during a religious function. Some believe a women mistook a thick rope for a snake and started screaming, others believe the surge was caused by a sprinkling of holy water. A structural collapse was also blamed by some. A squall hit the venue during the function.		
May 4, 2010	Netherlands	Fatalities: 0
A men started screaming during a memorial service causing fear among the thousands of visitors. It was later confirmed the man had a long history of drug-related offenses and was in a "confused state". At least 30 people were injured.		
May 16, 2010	India	Fatalities: 2
A last minute platform change triggered a collective motion during summer rush with many people carrying luggages. 15 people were injured.		
June 6, 2010	South Africa	Fatalities: 0
14 people sustained minor injuries as they tried to enter a stadium for a game whose tickets were sold and handed out outside the stadium. A first rush occurred when gates were opened. Gates were closed and a second rush occurred as they were re-opened to be finally closed.		
July 24, 2010	Germany	Fatalities: 21
An accident occurred when a crowd of people trying to get to a concert venue encountered a crowd that was trying to leave on a connecting road with a shared entrance and exit. More than 500 people were injured. The access road to get to the venue had a gentle uphill slope.		
October 16, 2010	India	Fatalities: 10
An argument over sacrificing goats during a religious festival triggered a simultaneous motion of the 40,000 people who had gathered at the temple. It is believed a commotion occurred as people tried to get their goats sacrificed first. Another 11 people were injured.		
October 23, 2010	Kenya	Fatalities: 7
An accident occurred as fans were trying to force their way into a stadium when a gate collapsed. It is believed the group did not have the tickets and did not want to pay, although other reports point out that gates were already closed despite the stadium being not filled. At the time it was raining heavily.		
November 22, 2010	Cambodia	Fatalities: 347
4 million people attended a festival held on an island. The island and the mainland both became overcrowded. A crowd of about 7,000 people became trapped on the bridge to the island by the crowds on both sides and were unable to move for several hours. Rumors spread through the crowd that the bridge would collapse and that they were at risk of electrocution, causing widespread chaos. 347 people were killed and 755 injured.		
November 29, 2010	China	Fatalities: 0
Students pushed to squeeze through a narrow staircase eventually resulting in an accident, which injured at least 41. Some report that the steps of the staircase were 1.5-m wide. The building housed 1,800 students.		
January 14, 2011	India	Fatalities: 106

(continued)

Table A.1 (continued)

According to several sources, an out-of-control jeep collided with pilgrims coming back home in an unlighted steep narrow forest stretch. The event triggered pilgrims to flee, ultimately leading to 106 deaths and injuring more than 450. However, details remains mostly unclear.		
January 15, 2011	Hungary	Fatalities: 3
An accident without an apparent trigger occurred in an overcrowded nightclub killing three and injuring 14. It is reported that about 2,500 were in the nightclub, designed for 307, while 4,000 tickets had been printed. A witness said he could not touch the ground for five to ten minutes due to extreme crowd density.		
February 12, 2011	Nigeria	Fatalities: 11
People were leaving a packed stadium after a presidential rally. A police officer apparently shot in the air in an attempt to control the crowd, but resulting in a surge. Main gate was said to be locked forcing people to use narrow passageways. Some report that people were trying to leave while others attempted to get in at the same time.		
February 21, 2011	Mali	Fatalities: 36
An accident occurred as people were leaving a stadium where a religious ceremony had been held. The crowd surged against a metal barrier, killing 36 and injuring 64, most of them women. Some reports suggest the stadium was filled over capacity.		
May 27, 2011	Nigeria	Fatalities: 25
About 5,000 supporters of a political leader gathered for a valedictory party. Party leadership asked supporters to queue and started distributing gifts. After hours in line, when it started to get dark, believing the presents may be insufficient, people started jumping the queue resulting in an accident killing 25.		
July 9, 2011	Republic of the Congo	Fatalities: 7
An accident whose details are rather unclear happened at the entrance of a stadium where a music festival was held. It is said a large crowd gathered, with people outside outnumbering people inside.		
October 19, 2011	UK	Fatalities: 2
An apparent announcement about couches leaving had people rush toward the exit in a nightclub (coach travel was included in ticket cost). Some reports suggest a fire alarm was also triggered, worsening the situation. It is unclear whether capacity was exceeded or not.		
November 8, 2011	India	Fatalities: 20
An accident occurred as people were trying to enter a sacred place during a religious festival for which around 200,000 gathered. It is believed the accident occurred as pilgrims were climbing stairs to cross a bridge leading to the venue. Crowd management was said to be handled by volunteers. 50 pilgrims were injured.		
November 22, 2011	Indonesia	Fatalities: 2
Thousands of fans gathered outside a sold-out stadium in the hope to get tickets on the spot. When a gate was momentarily opened fans rushed to get in leaving two people dead. In the days preceding the match disorders occurred as the tickets sold out.		

(continued)

Table A.1 (continued)

January 9, 2012	Pakistan	Fatalities: 3
After a concert in a private college, private security guards used batons to push back a group of fans who rushed toward a singer to get his autograph. This led to a second rush toward the exits where the accident occurred. The main gate was closed although details on the reasons are unclear. Venue was said to be over capacity.		
January 10, 2012	South Africa	Fatalities: 1
A woman was killed in a dense crowd as thousands of students attempted to seek precious remaining slots from a university. The accident occurred as the gates were opened. Three people were critically injured. Most of the people were poor students who were not able to apply online and had to apply on-site.		
January 14, 2012	India	Fatalities: 12
Pilgrims attempted to pass through the closed gate of an area hosting the fire oven on which the faithful walk. An accident occurred killing 12 and injuring four. Police attempt to force back the crowd was blamed by some, while police suspect some may have succumbed due to the severe cold.		
February 1, 2012	Egypt	Fatalities: 74
Violent home supporters stormed into the field leading the opposite team and their fans to run into their side to shelter from the attack. An accident occurred during the escape as stadium gate was closed. Many fatalities were caused by knife injuries or direct violence, but apparently also improper crowd management had an impact. More than 500 were injured.		
February 19, 2012	India	Fatalities: 6
A collective rush apparently occurred after brakes of a four-wheeler failed at a fair venue. Tens of thousands of devotees had gathered for the fair concluding a religious event.		
March 18, 2012	Egypt	Fatalities: 3
During the funeral of a religious leader attended by ten thousands of people, three participants got killed and another 137 were injured. The accident happened at the cathedral square. A non-lethal incident was also reported as gates were opened, before church officials scrambled to close the doors again.		
September 23, 2012	India	Fatalities: 3
It is believed that time constraints to perform an "auspicious sight" led to an accident in which three people died. A dozens sustained serious injuries. Some claims the accident occurred as devotees were passing through the exit and police was absent. Police claims the deaths were caused by hearth attack after climbing the stairs.		
September 24, 2012	India	Fatalities: 12
An accident occurred inside the hall of a religious institution possibly after an elderly women slipped and fell, leading others to fall over in overcrowded conditions with no space to move. Crowd control was performed by temple volunteer inside the institution with police staying outside. 30 were injured.		
September 25, 2012	India	Fatalities: 1
An accident occurred late at night after devotees had been waiting in line for the whole night. Some indicate a person fainted leading to the accident, others blame the use of force by the police. The hot weather and high humidity possibly had a contribution, with some also reporting only one out of five exits were used.		

(continued)

Table A.1 (continued)

November 1, 2012	Spain	Fatalities: 5

An accident occurred in an exit corridor of an arena during a large music party. Venue was found to be over capacity (which was not clearly defined since music events had been never hold in the sport facility) and not long before the accident a cargo gate (not intended for pedestrian access) was opened letting many people in. Crowd control was missing or nearly missing within the premises.

November 19, 2012	India	Fatalities: 17

A power outage in the darkness sparked a rush among devotees close to a river to get to the main road resulting in an accident where at least 17 people died. Some claims electricity was cut after a report of a naked electricity wire. It is reported that police control room received the information of the accident more than 1.5 h later from a journalist.

January 1, 2013	Ivory Coast	Fatalities: 60

An accident occurred as people were going back home after a firework display. The incident occurred as people exited the stadium and according to some witnesses two large crowds moving in opposite directions collided causing the tragedy. It is believed around 50,000 were on the streets. 200 were injured.

January 1, 2013	Angola	Fatalities: 16

Several people have been killed while trying to enter an overcrowded stadium for a church vigil. The accident occurred at the gates as many more than the 70,000 expected people turned up. According to reports all gates were used and the tragedy occurred as people were moving in through a partially slippery surface.

February 10, 2013	India	Fatalities: 42

An accident took place at the railway station where millions of pilgrims were converging to take a holy dip for the Kumbh Mela religious festival. Reports are conflicting on the cause, some suggesting a railing collapsed others blaming police use of force to control the crowd.

February 27, 2013	China	Fatalities: 4

Students from a primary school attempted to leave the dorm to take morning class but the gate was not open as usual, blocking the flow and causing the accident. When the gate was opened it was already bent by the pressure of the crowd.

May 19, 2013	Ghana	Fatalities: 4

An accident occurred as worshipers attempted to get holy water distributed for free for a special occasion. The number of people attending was underestimated with police and army unable to control the crowd attempting to enter the church.

July 14, 2013	Indonesia	Fatalities: 18

People escaping a riot between spectators during a boxing match scrambled out of the stadium killing 18 and injuring more than 40. The facility accommodating 1,500 the day of the match had two exits.

October 13, 2013	India	Fatalities: 115

Many pilgrims were killed on a 7-m wide and 400-m long bridge when a 25,000 estimated crowd was over it. Rumors saying the bridge was about to collapse resulted in a collective rush as some people drowned after jumping from the bridge. Sources are however conflicting on what caused the collective rush.

(continued)

Table A.1 (continued)

October 16, 2013	Nigeria	Fatalities: 20

An accident occurred when a political leader was giving out gifts and money to his supporters. Similar accidents already occurred in the same place under similar circumstances.

November 2, 2013	Nigeria	Fatalities: 28

An accident occurred during a vigil in a church. It is believed more than 50,000 people (some suggesting 100,000) gathered for the event while the church could accommodate only 5,000. It is unclear what caused the accident, some relating it to a commotion, others to people shouting "fire."

January 5, 2014	China	Fatalities: 14

An accident occurred outside a mosque as a crowd rushed to take offerings of a traditional food. Possibly organizers were not sufficiently prepared for the high number that showed up as the event was held on a Sunday.

January 15, 2014	India	Fatalities: 3

An accident occurred in a fair as people were watching a dance in a theater. The accident was possibly caused by a clash between two groups or rumors of fire. Lighting was reportedly insufficient at the venue.

January 18, 2014	India	Fatalities: 18

Supporters assembled in front of the residence of a spiritual leader to mourn his death. An accident occurred as gates were opened and people burst in. 18 people died and 56 were injured.

March 15, 2014	Nigeria	Fatalities: 10

As part of a recruitment program 100,000 applicants tried to enter a stadium with a capacity of 60,000 where tests were scheduled. Gates remained closed by security men and an accident occurred as anxious job-seekers tried to jump fences to enter the venue. The resulting chaotic situation killed 10 and injured more than 40. Nationwide 6.5 million people had paid an application fee to apply for 4,000 positions.

March 15, 2014	Nigeria	Fatalities: 4

An estimated 28,000 job-seekers tried to enter the stadium with a capacity of no more than 15,000. They had all already paid an application fee to take part to the tests scheduled on the venue. The crowd started to run for safety after soldiers started shooting in the air in an attempt to control the crowd. Three of the victims were pregnant women, more than 20 were injured.

March 15, 2014	Nigeria	Fatalities: 3

A school was used to perform tests for a nationwide job application. The venue was successfully filled with 11,000 candidates by 7 a.m. However, a two kilometers long line formed in front of the venue. Fearing the situation would escalate personnel resorted to tear gas, causing seven people to collapse and resulting in the death of three. Space around the venue was limited due to the large number of vehicles parked there by applicants.

March 15, 2014	Nigeria	Fatalities: 5

About 25,000 applicants were invited for a job interview in a stadium accommodating 16,000. Several job-seekers arrived early in the morning but were not allowed into the main bowl and some gates were locked. As one gate was opened people stormed in leading people at the front to collapse. Some also report that rifles were fired in the air in an attempt to control the crowd.

(continued)

Table A.1 (continued)

April 25, 2014	DRC	Fatalities: 23

Power generators were cut out during a tribute concert to a recently deceased singer, plunging the stadium into darkness. An accident occurred as people tried to leave the venue, killing more than 20.

May 11, 2014	DRC	Fatalities: 15

During an important soccer match fans began throwing stones to the pitch to which police responded with teargas, eventually leading to the crowd fleeing toward one exit where the accident occurred. Another 10 people were injured. It is believed the stadium was packed beyond capacity.

July 30, 2014	Guinea	Fatalities: 34

Hundreds of people leaving a concert on a beach troubled while rushing through the single exit. The accident happened at the end of the show, which was attended by up to 10,000 people. Dozens were injured.

August 25, 2014	India	Fatalities: 10

Thousands (reportedly 50,0000) of devotees gathered to celebrate a religious event. During the procession a live electric wire shocked a woman and set off chaos, triggering an accident in which people broke through rope barriers. 10 pilgrims were killed and another 12 were injured.

October 3, 2014	India	Fatalities: 32

Tens of thousands of people gathered to watch a religious event on a lawn ground surrounded by buildings. An accident occurred as people were rushing to leave after the event, some blaming a rumor of a live high tension wire falling on the ground. Around 15 people were injured.

October 10, 2014	Pakistan	Fatalities: 8

An accident occurred at a political rally as people rushed together toward the main gate as a speech ended. Circumstances remain unclear, with some blaming that only two of the five gates were opened and other reporting lights were switched off. Over 100 people were injured.

November 21, 2014	Zimbabwe	Fatalities: 11

An estimated crowd of 30,000 leaving a stadium from a single exit after a religious service caused an accident killing 11 and injuring 40. Since only one exit was open, some tried to break off parts of the wall to leave, prompting the police to fire teargas thus causing a rush in the crowd.

December 31, 2014	China	Fatalities: 36

A crowd of 300,000 gathered to assist to New Year celebrations. An accident occurred on a stairway leading to a viewing platform as people were moving on both directions. Reasons for the rush on both directions are unclear, some blaming rumors of a show cancellation, other reporting cash coupons were thrown on the crowd.

February 8, 2015	Egypt	Fatalities: 25

Police used tear gas to attempt dispersing crowds of about 6,000 ticket-less fans who were making their way into the stadium for a soccer game. After three years of restrictions on games' attendance, 5,000 tickets were up for public sale, with another 5,000 distributed through the club. Fans were known for their history of battling the police.

(continued)

Table A.1 (continued)

February 17, 2015	Haiti	Fatalities: 18
An accident occurred during the carnival parade as a man on-board of a float hit an overhead power line creating a spark, which triggered a sudden rush within the surrounding crowd. The man survived the shock but 18 from the bystanders were killed and another 78 injured.		
March 27, 2015	Bangladesh	Fatalities: 10
An accident occurred on the riverbanks as pilgrims were moving through narrow passages to take holy dips. The annual festival usually attracts one million people, but on this edition the number was much higher since it came on a public holiday. Some report that rumors emerged about a collapsing bridge, although the main cause is not clear.		
April 16, 2015	Chile	Fatalities: 5
Metal fences collapsed killing several fans during a concert in an underground club. It is believed a group of people tried to enter the venue by force despite the premises were already at full capacity, although others blame the use of force by guards with whom a clash took place.		
July 9, 2015	Bangladesh	Fatalities: 23
An accident occurred after a large crowd gathered for clothes that were being donated. More than 1,500 people had assembled outside the clothing factory and a collective rush occurred as people tried to force their way through a small gate. More than 50 people were injured.		
July 14, 2015	India	Fatalities: 27
An accident occurred at the riverbank where devotees were taking a holy dip. The accident occurred at a narrow entrance to the banks as people leaving the river clashed with people trying to bath in a particularly auspicious time. The festival is held once every 144 years and 40 million pilgrims were expected over 12 days. 15,000 policemen and 171 cameras were used to monitor the situation.		
August 10, 2015	India	Fatalities: 11
An accident occurred around 5 a.m. as some of the 150,000 pilgrims who gathered for a religious festival surged toward the entrance of the temple after doors were opened. People sleeping in the kilometers-long queue were overran as others pushed toward the entrance. Around 50 were injured.		
September 24, 2015	Saudi Arabia	Fatalities: 2236
An accident occurred at a T-intersection between two streets leading to a bridge during the annual Hajj pilgrimage. Exact dynamics of the incident is unclear and also the number of victims is disputed. That year temperatures were extremely high and political tensions existed between countries from which most of pilgrims arrived.		
October 14, 2015	Poland	Fatalities: 3
An accident occurred during a party organized in a university. Due to a lack of control at the entrance, organizers were not able to keep the number of attendees under control, reaching a total of 1,500. The tragedy occurred at the connection between two buildings as people tried to move in opposite directions under high crowd density.		
October 21, 2015	Cameroon	Fatalities: 1
An accident occurred during a religious event held in a stadium at 1 a.m. A report claims that when people were leaving the venue from the single exit others started to get in, while another version claims the accident was caused by a robbery attempt.		

(continued)

Table A.1 (continued)

October 25, 2015	Afghanistan	Fatalities: 12

Students of a high school got killed as they rushed to escape the school building after chaos broke out following a strong earthquake. More than 30 were injured. The school was not damaged by the quake.

November 15, 2015	Malta	Fatalities: 0

A glass banister collapsed under crowd pressure as people were trying to leave all at once down a staircase after someone sprayed a gas inside a nightclub. 74 people were injured.

February 2, 2016	India	Fatalities: 4

Four people drowned following a collective rush in a temple pond. Causes remain unclear but officials sources admitted they failed to estimate the actual number of pilgrims and were not able to keep the crowd under control as rituals started in the early morning. The accident came as the deity was taken toward the pond.

October 2, 2016	Ethiopia	Fatalities: 52

An accident occurred after police used tear gas during a protest at a religious festival. Rubber bullets and baton charge were also used. It is believed some threw stones to the police. An estimated two million people gathered for the event in a period during which several protests started in the country.

October 9, 2016	India	Fatalities: 2

An accident occurred on stairs as people were moving out during a political rally through the only gate (although some reports suggest two were employed). It is reported that the accident occurred under intense heat. According to some sources 100,000 people attended the rally.

October 15, 2016	India	Fatalities: 24

An accident occurred as people heading to a religious event tried to cross a bridge at once. 4,000 people were expected but 50,000 showed up. The surging crowds killed one man and rumors that the bridge could collapse fueled more chaos.

October 16, 2016	Angola	Fatalities: 8

An accident occurred as people were leaving a stadium where a music festival was being held. It is reported 15,000 tickets were sold for a venue with a capacity of 8,000. Some reports claim doors had been locked and police was looking for criminals inside the venue. Another 40 were injured.

December 10, 2016	Nigeria	Fatalities: 3

A crowd of worshipers struggled to pass through the doorway of a synagogue to attend the healing service of a famous prophet. In the process three people collapsed and died. The accident occurred at 4:30 a.m. when thousands of people already filled the venue.

January 15, 2017	India	Fatalities: 6

A collective rush broke out while people were waiting to board a boat from an island where a religious event was being held. Other sources attributed the fatalities to hearth attack. A large crowd was waiting for a boat as many urged to come back as they would have had to wait 8 hours for the high tide to dip again. At least 1.5 million people took their holy dip over two days.

February 10, 2017	Angola	Fatalities: 17

An accident occurred as hundreds of supporters stormed the stadium gates. The crowd pushed against barriers after failing to gain entry to the venue before the match. It is believed the stadium would have not be sufficient to accommodate the crowd. At least 60 were injured.

(continued)

Table A.1 (continued)

March 6, 2017	Zambia	Fatalities: 8
Competition over food aid resulted in an accident as thousands of people in need struggled to claim food handouts. It is reported 35,000 people jostled to enter the stadium where the distribution was organized. 28 others were injured.		
March 11, 2017	Argentina	Fatalities: 2
Two people were were killed when spectators rushed to the stage during an open air concert. The show was attended by 350,000 people, although the event was planned to handle half of that number. Dozens were injured.		
March 22, 2017	China	Fatalities: 2
An accident occurred in a primary school when students gathered in the bathroom in a short period of time. The incident happened during a 10 minutes break while preparing for monthly examinations. Some reports suggest the wall of the bathroom collapsed. More than 20 were injured.		
May 28, 2017	Honduras	Fatalities: 4
Hundreds of fans (allegedly in possess of a ticket) tried to break past stadium's barricades during an important match. Some reports claim the stadium was oversold, possibly due to fake tickets being sold. Police fired tear gas and used water cannons in an attempt to control the crowd. Another 25 were injured.		
June 3, 2017	Italy	Fatalities: 3
An accident occurred during a public viewing in a square attended by thousands as some people shot pepper spray in an attempt to steal valuables. This caused a rush in the crowd, which eventually led to the collapse of a railing leading to an underground garage. More than 1,600 people were injured, many because of the broken bottles on the ground.		
July 6, 2017	Malawi	Fatalities: 8
An accident occurred at a free soccer game in a stadium. Gates' opening time was delayed by about three hours and when the gates finally opened the accumulated crowd rushed in the stadium, killing eight and injuring around 40, mostly children. Some report the gates were force opened and police fired tear gas.		
July 15, 2017	Senegal	Fatalities: 8
Around the end of an important match, a wall collapsed under crowd pressure after fans tried to escape from violent supporters throwing projectiles between them. Police fired tear gas at clashing supporters in an attempt to disperse them causing what could have exacerbated the situation. More than 40 were injured.		
July 29, 2017	South Africa	Fatalities: 2
An accident occurred as fans attempted to pour through a gate for a well-anticipated derby. The situation went under control when all gates were opened. It is believed the sale of fake tickets at entry gates contributed to the accident. The stadium had a capacity for 87,000 spectators and was sold out.		
September 15, 2017	Bangladesh	Fatalities: 3
An accident occurred in a refugee camp hosting tens of thousands as clothing were thrown from relief trucks. It is reported the distribution was not authorized by the agencies managing the refugee camp and similar accidents already happened as private distributions were improvised on the camp.		

(continued)

Table A.1 (continued)

September 29, 2017	India	Fatalities: 23
An accident occurred on the stairs of a tiny overbridge connecting platforms of a train station as four trains arrived simultaneously during rush hour. At the time it was raining and possibly someone slipped on the already packed stairs, which were used also as shelter from the heavy rain. Another 30 were injured.		
September 30, 2017	France	Fatalities: 0
A barrier collapsed after fans surged forward to celebrate a goal in a stadium. The accident occurred as the stadium was being refurbished. More than 20 were injured and some were taken to the hospital. A report found that proper calculations were not performed when designing the barrier and the company managing the stadium did not perform proper maintenance.		
November 4, 2017	India	Fatalities: 3
An accident occurred at a narrow lane that was used by pilgrims to reach and leave a river where they were taking a holy dip during a religious event. All victims were elderly women. The event was attended by thousands of devotees. Another 10 were injured.		
November 19, 2017	Morocco	Fatalities: 15
An accident occurred during annual food aid distribution at a local market. It is reported a crowd of 800 (larger than usual) was attracted in the town with 8,000 inhabitants. Another 40 were injured. Details on the accident remain unclear, although some report that barriers collapsed.		
November 24, 2017	UK	Fatalities: 0
A fight between two people in a subway platform led to false reports of gunshots on a day when shoppers were filling the streets of a popular shopping area attracted by special discounts. As people tried to seek shelter some fell and 16 were injured, some requiring hospital treatment.		
December 18, 2017	Bangladesh	Fatalities: 10
An accident occurred at the end of the funeral service of a political leader when ritual food was arranged in a venue. The accident occurred as gates of the community center were opened and people rushed despite the announcements that enough food was available to everyone. It is reported around 8,000 people took part to the event.		
January 10, 2018	India	Fatalities: 1
An accident occurred during an army recruitment drive after the gate of the ground was opened at 3 a.m. Applicants were asked to wait in line but when the gate opened people began jostling to enter the venue. An estimated 4,000 aspirants had been waiting in cold weather. Another four were injured.		
May 12, 2018	Sierra Leone	Fatalities: 1
An accident occurred at a presidential inauguration held in a stadium. Thousands of people had been waiting in queue from the morning, but president's supporters tried to force their way through a gate for cars of invited guests. This sparked police response, which resulted in the accident. 90 were injured.		
May 14, 2018	Bangladesh	Fatalities: 10
Over 20,000 people had assembled for gift distribution (food and money) in front of a mosque. When the gate was opened at 9 a.m. some fell and got overrun. Many have been waiting the whole night. It is reported the ground could hold 3,500 people at most and security was very limited. Another 50 were injured.		

(continued)

Table A.1 (continued)

May 27, 2018	India	Fatalities: 0
A large number of students were in a train station to appear for an examination when a rumor of an earthquake triggered a collective motion, which injured 58. The accident occurred at night as many students were sleeping in the station.		
June 16, 2018	Venezuela	Fatalities: 19
Following a fight during a student's party attended by 500, some individuals threw a tear gas canister. Participants attempted to evacuate the venue, but the only narrow exit was located at the bottom of a staircase and was closed, leading to an increase in crowd density killing 19. Reasons for the door being closed remain unclear.		
August 8, 2018	India	Fatalities: 5
A crowd surge at a hall entrance occurred as public was allowed to pay homage to the remains of a deceased political leader. Police were letting in people in batches but a rush occurred and they were not able to control the crowd, resorting to force to push it back. More than 20 were injured.		
September 9, 2018	Madagascar	Fatalities: 1
Supporters started to form kilometers-long queues from the early morning for an important match scheduled at 2:30 p.m. The accident occurred as some supporters wanted to get in despite the gate being closed because the stadium was full. At least 37 people were injured.		
September 16, 2018	Angola	Fatalities: 5
Soccer fans were killed as they flooded out a stadium after a game. The accident happened as supporters found the gates shut after the match. When the police finally opened the gates, people rushed out with some falling down and ultimately killing five and injuring another seven.		
December 8, 2018	Italy	Fatalities: 6
Some individuals sprayed an "irritant substance" inside a nightclub prompting the occupants to flee the venue. However, only one emergency exit was open and a metal railing on the way out collapsed, causing people to fall off the walkway. About 1,400 were in the venue with a capacity of about 470 (it is believed some few hundreds sneaked into the venue). 200 people were injured.		
December 28, 2018	South Africa	Fatalities: 3
People from a religious community assembled at the show ground of a church to attend a service by a famous preacher. When heavy downpour started, people push each other in a scramble to find shelter. The accident left three dead and another nine injured.		
January 28, 2019	Malaysia	Fatalities: 2
More than 1,000 people showed up at an indoor market for free food coupons given out to elderly people, but only 200 were available for the buffet meal. Two people (78 and 85 years old) passed away as they were waiting in the pushy crowd. Only four people at a time were allowed to get into the office and register for the coupons.		
February 12, 2019	Nigeria	Fatalities: 15
An accident occurred during an afternoon rally as thousands of supporters tried to follow the president's convoy out of the stadium through a partially locked gate. People were seen rushing and pushing to each other to leave the stadium. Around 15 people died and dozens were injured (sources vary on the exact number).		

(continued)

Table A.1 (continued)

March 17, 2019	UK	Fatalities: 3

An accident took place in a nightclub when the gate was opened to get a crowd of more than 600 in the venue accommodating a maximum of 500. Shortly afterward a forward rush occurred and the whole queue collapsed, killing three people and injuring four. It is said 100 people collapsed to the ground after the surge occurred.

June 26, 2019	Madagascar	Fatalities: 16

An accident occurred at a stadium during the independence day. After the military parade finished, gates were open to let people in for a free concert by a famous singer. However, gates were suddenly shut afterward. Believing entry was possible the crowds kept moving toward the closed gates, killing 16 and injuring about 80.

August 22, 2019	Algeria	Fatalities: 5

An estimated 30,000 people gathered at a stadium for the concert of a famous singer. The accident occurred as fans thronged through the entrance. The concert was scheduled for 7 p.m., but people started gathering from mid-afternoon. It is said there were only four entrances allowing people to enter one at a time and the stadium could accommodate only 15,000.

September 10, 2019	Iraq	Fatalities: 31

Pilgrims gathered for a traditional run of 2–3 km through the built environment. During the run, attended by hundreds of thousands, an accident happened, probably because a walkway collapsed or somebody stumbled, leading others to fell over him. 31 people were killed and more than 100 were injured.

November 9, 2019	Venezuela	Fatalities: 4

People climbing over entry barriers during a free concert organized in a park and attended by around 8,000 people caused the barriers to give way ultimately leading to a collective rush killing four and injuring more than 30. It is said that queue had formed from the early morning with the concert scheduled for 10 a.m.

December 1, 2019	Brazil	Fatalities: 9

Armed criminals escaping from the police entered a street party as they continued firing. The 5,000 people who had gathered for the party fled in search for a shelter, as police closed the street and threw pepper spray canisters. The rush for shelter resulted in nine people getting killed and injuring around 20.

References

1. Bista, D.B.: Nepal in 1988: many losses, some gains. Asian Survey **29**(2), 223–228 (1989). https://doi.org/10.2307/2644583
2. Elliott, D., Smith, D.: Football stadia disasters in the united kingdom: learning from tragedy? Ind. Environ. Crisis Q. **7**(3), 205–229 (1993). https://doi.org/10.1177/108602669300700304
3. Nicholson, C.E., Roebuck, B.: The investigation of the hillsborough disaster by the health and safety executive. Safety Science **18**(4), 249–259 (1995). https://doi.org/10.1016/0925-7535(94)00034-Z
4. Vaze, B.: Gowari deaths: crucial issues neglected. Econ. Polit. Weekly, 1959–1959 (1995)

5. Bowley, D.M., Rein, P., Scholtz, H.J., Boffard, K.D.: The ellis park stadium tragedy. Eur. J. Trauma **30**(1), 51–55 (2004). https://doi.org/10.1007/s00068-004-1230-2
6. Wise, K.: Attribution versus compassion: the city of chicago's response to the e2 crisis. Publ. Relat. Rev. **30**(3), 347–356 (2004). https://doi.org/10.1016/j.pubrev.2004.05.006
7. Lee, R.S., Hughes, R.L.: Exploring trampling and crushing in a crowd. J. Transp. Eng. **131**(8), 575–582 (2005). https://doi.org/10.1061/(ASCE)0733-947X(2005)131:8(575)
8. Ahmed, Q.A., Arabi, Y.M., Memish, Z.A.: Health risks at the hajj. Lancet **367**(9515), 1008–1015 (2006). https://doi.org/10.1016/S0140-6736(06)68429-8
9. Johansson, A., Helbing, D., Al-Abideen, H.Z., Al-Bosta, S.: From crowd dynamics to crowd safety: a video-based analysis. Adv. Complex Syst. **11**(04), 497–527 (2008). https://doi.org/10.1142/S0219525908001854
10. Zhen, W., Mao, L., Yuan, Z.: Analysis of trample disaster and a case study-mihong bridge fatality in china in 2004. Safety Sci. **46**(8), 1255–1270 (2008). https://doi.org/10.1016/j.ssci.2007.08.002
11. Vendelo, M.T., Rerup, C.: Weak cues and attentional triangulation: The pearl jam concert accident at roskilde festival. In: Academy of Management Annual Meeting, Chicago, IL, pp. 1–38 (2009)
12. Akhter, S., Salahuddin, A., Iqbal, M., Malek, A., Jahan, N.: Health and occupational safety for female workforce of garment industries in Bangladesh. J. Mech. Eng. **41**(1), 65–70 (2010). https://doi.org/10.3329/jme.v41i1.5364
13. Rogsch, C., Schreckenberg, M., Tribble, E., Klingsch, W., Kretz, T.: Was it panic? an overview about mass-emergencies and their origins all over the world for recent years. In: Pedestrian and evacuation dynamics 2008, pp. 743–755. Springer (2010). https://doi.org/10.1007/978-3-642-04504-2_72
14. Helbing, D., Mukerji, P.: Crowd disasters as systemic failures: analysis of the love parade disaster. EPJ Data Sci. **1**(1), 7 (2012). https://doi.org/10.1140/epjds7
15. Memish, Z.A., Stephens, G.M., Steffen, R., Ahmed, Q.A.: Emergence of medicine for mass gatherings: lessons from the hajj. Lancet Infect. Diseases **12**(1), 56–65 (2012). https://doi.org/10.1016/S1473-3099(11)70337-1
16. Hsu, E.B., Burkle, F.M.: Cambodian bon om touk stampede highlights preventable tragedy. Prehospital Disaster Med. **27**(5), 481–482 (2012). https://doi.org/10.1017/S1049023X12001057
17. Illiyas, F.T., Mani, S.K., Pradeepkumar, A., Mohan, K.: Human stampedes during religious festivals: a comparative review of mass gathering emergencies in India. Int. J. Disas. Risk Red. **5**, 10–18 (2013). https://doi.org/10.1016/j.ijdrr.2013.09.003
18. Wagner, U., Fälker, A., Wenzel, V.: Fatal incidents by crowd crush during mass events.(un) preventable phenomenon? Der Anaesthesist **62**(1), 39–46 (2013). URL https://doi.org/10.1007/s00101-012-2124-z. (in German)
19. Kok, V.J., Lim, M.K., Chan, C.S.: Crowd behavior analysis: a review where physics meets biology. Neurocomputing **177**, 342–362 (2016). https://doi.org/10.1016/j.neucom.2015.11.021
20. Thompson, P., Tolloczko, J., Clarke, N.: Stadia Arenas and Grandstands: Design. CRC Press, Construction and Operation (1998)
21. Reilly, T.: Science and Soccer. Routledge (2003)
22. Darby, P., Johnes, M., Mellor, G.: Soccer and Disaster. Psychology Press (2005)
23. Gad-el Hak, M.: Large-Scale Disasters: Prediction, Control, and Mitigation. Cambridge University Press (2008)
24. Nauright, J., Parrish, C.: Sports Around the World: History, Culture, and Practice. Abc-Clio (2012)
25. Still, G.K.: Introduction to Crowd Science. CRC Press (2014)
26. Elwood-Stokes, C.: Football Disasters: The Moments we will Never Forget. Independently Published (2019)
27. Still, G.K.: Crowd disasters (2019). https://www.gkstill.com/ExpertWitness/CrowdDisasters.html
28. Wikipedia: List of human stampedes and crushes (2021). https://en.wikipedia.org/wiki/List_of_human_stampedes_and_crushes. (online; Accessed 24 August 2021)

29. Wikipedia: List of human stampedes in hindu temples (2021). https://en.wikipedia.org/wiki/List_of_human_stampedes_in_Hindu_temples. (online; Accessed 24 August 2021)
30. Wikipedia: List of soccer stampede disasters (2021). https://en.wikipedia.org/wiki/List_of_soccer_stampede_disasters. (online; Accessed 24 August 2021)
31. Wikipedia: 2017 turin stampede (2021). https://en.wikipedia.org/wiki/2017_Turin_stampede. (online; Accessed 24 August 2021)

Glossary

Crush Controversial term often used to describe crowd accidents in which people get pressed against a structure (e.g., a wall or a gate) or get compressed from the crowd. It is unclear whether this is caused by a crowd domino/crowd avalanche or whether it can happen without people actually falling to some extent (i.e., by having people pressed to death against a wall). Regardless on the mechanism, it is nonetheless known that suffocation is the most common final cause of death in crowd accidents, possibly explaining the widespread use of "crush" to describe the accidents. Due to its controversial definition, in this book it is not used.

Cellular Automata (CA) A computational method conceived by mathematicians Stanislaw Ulam and John von Neumann in which space is divided into a computational grid and system dynamics is computed over successive time steps. CA is used in a variety of fields and is particularly suited to simulate crowd behavior. The dynamics of the system (i.e., crowds) in CA simulations can be seen as a chess game in which the rules are defined by each model.

Congestion Index Measure to quantify the "smoothness" of crowd motion. The congestion index is 0 when people move in a perfectly aligned manner and get close to 1 when movements get more disorganized and random. As the name suggests, it can be used to estimate the level of congestion in pedestrian crowds.

Crowd Avalanche Accident occurring at high crowd densities where the close physical contact between people allows forces to travel through the crowd. This condition leads to instabilities within the crowd where a turbulent-like motion is observed, ultimately leading to locally very high-density areas while also allowing the creation of a empty spots. Some person may fall in this open spot leading to an avalanche-like motion in which people pack over the ones on the ground, causing death by internal injuries or suffocation.

Crowd Domino Accident possible at even relatively low crowd densities (roughly 3–$5\,\mathrm{m}^{-2}$) and caused by people at the back of a crowd accidentally falling into those in front of them. This could result into a knocking cascade in which each successive person falls in a linear manner like in domino rows.

Crowd Management Proactive security activities that bring safety and comfort to individuals by facilitating efficient movement of crowds.

Crowd Manager A person whose role is to ensure that crowd management is performed in order to guarantee safety and comfort of the crowd by acting as coordinator between the various stakeholders.

Crowd Control The set of actions intended to change the way in which crowds move and behave. Crowd control may involve "soft" measures such as information provision and guidance or more "hard" methods such as barricades to ensure its effectiveness.

Crowd Sensing All activities involved in detecting the state of a crowd of people. Depending on the technology and method used, it may range from simply counting people in a given area or obtain more complex information related to their physical or psychological state.

Fundamental Diagram The name given to the density–speed or density–flow relationship in transportation systems. The fundamental diagram has been originally introduced to describe changes in speed occurring due to varying levels of vehicular density, but is also used for other transportation systems (from planes to trains, while also including biological processes), with pedestrian traffic being one of those. The density–flow fundamental diagram is particularly important as it allows to define a threshold for congestion (and thus define capacity more systematically).

Hajj Annual Islamic pilgrimage to Mecca (Saudi Arabia) usually attended by millions of people. The pilgrimage includes several rites to be performed over a number of days.

Level of Service (LOS) Concept introduced by John J. Fruin to indicate the quality of pedestrian areas. The LOS is defined on a scale from A to F and is intended to be used in the design, to set specific goals in regard to pedestrian spaces, or in the evaluation phase, to judge whether an intervention is needed. In the LOS, "A" represents the safest and most comfortable environment and "F" represents a condition, which should be reached only in exceptional situations.

Kumbh Mela A large religious festival in Hinduism in which ritual dip in the waters takes a central role. The festival is celebrated in a cycle of approximately 12 years in various river-bank pilgrimage sites. Several dozens of millions of people are said to attend the festival in the most crowded days.

Social Force (model) A common model used in crowd simulators. The concept behind the social force model is that people are repelled from each others' and are attracted toward their destination. Although the original formulation was proposed by Dirk Helbing in 1995 a number of improvements have been proposed over the years.

Trampling Literally meaning the act of "step heavily on something or someone" it is however sometimes used as a general term to indicate crowd accidents (especially the ones involving injuries or fatalities). Often (but not always) media refer to "trampling" for accidents that occur on stairs or when boundaries limiting the crowd are lifted (e.g., barrier collapse, opening of a gate). Its use in scientific literature is also often debated, with researchers focusing on crowd behavior sometimes associating it to a mechanism close to crowd domino and medical practitioners defining "trampling accident" based on the type of internal injuries. Due to its controversial definition, in this book it is not used.

Stampede   General term used to describe crowd accidents. Although the literal meaning only refers to a "sudden, impulsive and spontaneous mass movement", it has been often used to describe crowd accidents, especially the ones with fatalities. Mistakenly it is also often associated with mass panic being the trigger of that "sudden mass movement". To avoid misunderstandings given by the widespread incorrect use of "stampede" (especially in media), in this book we avoided its use and, if necessary, "stampede" will be employed as a general term to indicate any sort of sudden collective motion, regardless on the presence of injuries, to align closer to its original definition.

Stoning of the Devil   A rite part of the annual Hajj pilgrimage during which Muslim pilgrims throw pebbles at three walls.

Index

A

Abnormal weather, 255
Access gates, 207
Action (evacuation process), 35
Akashi Pedestrian Bridge Accident, 67
Audio messages (dynamic), 195

B

Background traffic, 244
Barricades, 204
Barriers, 204
Behavioral detection, 112
Behavioral (discrete-choice) models, 144
Behavioral levels (crowd simulation), 125
Bluetooth sensing, 96
Bottleneck effect, 208

C

Causality of crowd incidents, 56
Cellular automata, 132
Characteristics of crowds, 18
Chemosensors, 104
Choosing a commercial software, 150
Color in signs, 186
Commercial simulation software, 148
Communication with the crowd, 198
Computer vision, 79
Condition (planning), 243
Constricted areas, 62
Continuum models, 145
Crimes, 258
Crowd accidents classification, 56
Crowd avalanche, 54
Crowd behavior in emergencies, 32

Crowd behavior under normal conditions, 23
Crowd classification, 16
Crowd definition, 16
Crowd domino, 53
Crowd incident mechanisms, 52
Crowd manager, 9
Crowd size estimation by total mass, 101
Crowd theories, 27

D

Data-driven prediction (model-free approach), 145
Dead ends, 60
Definitions and fundamental principles (crowd management), 3
Deindividuation theory, 28
Density (crowd), 38
Density estimation (computer vision), 85
Design, construction, and implementation of wayfinding systems, 179
Detection and tracking (computer vision), 80
Detection of complex crowd patterns, 111
Disabled pedestrians, 189
Distance sensors, 89
Doorways, 60
Dynamic information provision, 189
Dynamic routing, 211

E

Earthquakes, 257
Elaborated Social Identity Model (ESIM), 29
Elements of wayfinding, 183
Emergent norm theory, 28

Emerging phenomena in crowds, 23
Emotional state and mood detection, 113
Enclosed spaces, 62
Entrances and exits, 60
Entrances and exits operation, 247
Evacuation process, 34
Evaluation of simulated motion, 152
Evenness of distribution, 252
Event schedule, 243
Event trouble, 257
External environmental factors, 58

F
Feature/object detection, 111
Fighting/violence, 256
Fire outbreak, 257
Flow control, 208
Flow lines, 245
Flow pattern, 63
Flow (pedestrian, crowd), 40
Fundamental diagram, 43
Future and emerging trends in sensing technology, 111

G
Gate/transit counting, 100
Global Positioning System (GPS), 93
Group mind theory, 27
Guidance staff, 211

I
Improving simulation results, 154
Inertial sensors, 103
Infectious diseases, 258
Influencing individual behaviors in crowds, 32
Information desk, 200
Information management (crowd control), 173
Instrumented detection, 96
Internal (crowd) factors, 63
Internal venue operations, 247
Internet pages, 194
Interpretation (evacuation process), 35
Intersections, 252
ISO31000, 218

L
LADAR, 89
Lan Kwai Fong Accident, 66

Level of Service (LOS), 46
LiDAR, 89
Localization technologies, 93

M
Macroscopic simulation models, 121
Management boundaries, 252
Manual counting, 101
Maps use in wayfinding, 187
Microscopic simulation models, 124
Multi-scale approach (crowd simulation), 125

N
Natural disasters, 257
Network models (details), 139
Network models (introduction), 123
Nudge approach in crowd control, 212

O
On-site operation, 258
Operating modes, 245
Optical flow (computer vision), 84
Outsourcing (crowd simulation), 148

P
Panic, 34
Physical methods for crowd control, 202
Place scripts, 31
Planning approach, 238
Planning of wayfinding, 177
Post-implementation evaluation of wayfinding systems, 182
Power outages, 256
Preparation (evacuation process), 35
Pressure sensors, 104
Purpose of assembly, 68

Q
Qualitative crowd characteristics, 15
Quantitative crowd characteristics, 36
Queuing systems, 205

R
Result visualization (crowd simulation), 156
RFID chip, 96
Risk analysis, 225
Risk assessment, 222

Risk assessment for abnormal operations, 253
Risk assessment for normal operation, 248
Risk definition, 218
Risk evaluation, 228
Risk identification, 224
Risk management framework, 220
Role of crowd management (in preventing accidents), 71

S

Self-categorization theory, 29
Self-organization in crowds, 23
Self-regulation approach, 213
Sensing accuracy, 110
Sensing method selection and comparison, 105
Sensor fusion, 112
Sign layout, 186
Sign material, 188
Sign media, 188
Signs in wayfinding, 183
Simulation code development, 148
Simulation scenario setup, 127
Simulator comparison, 146
Simulator selection, 146
Social force model, 136
Social identity model of crowd behavior, 29
Social identity theory, 29
Social media, 201
Soft crowd control, 173
Space representation in crowd simulators, 121
Speed (walking or crowd speed), 36
Spoken communication, 199
Stages of crowd control, 167
Stairways, 61
Stakeholders and information on crowd, 6

State-of-the-art modelling approaches, 125
Static information provision, 175
Sudden illness, 255
Symbols use in wayfinding, 187

T

Terrorism, 258
Thermocamera, 102
Ticket control, 207
Time constraints and competition, 69
Traditional media, 201
Traffic accidents, 256
Transportation delay, 255
Transportation suspension, 255
Types of crowds, 17
Types of crowd simulators, 121
Typography, 186

V

Velocity-based models, 143
Venue-related data, 245
Visitors' attributes, 244
Visitors' number, 243
Visual messages (dynamic), 193

W

Waiting lines, 205
Walking/mobile information staff, 200
Wayfinding design process, 176
Wayfinding (introduction), 175
Wayfinding issues, 189
WiFi sensing, 96

Y

Yahiko Shrine Accident, 66

Printed in the United States
by Baker & Taylor Publisher Services